Teaching Pilates for Postural Faults, Illness and Injury

For Elsevier:

Publisher: Heidi Harrison
Associate Editor: Siobhan Campbell
Commissioning Editor: Rita Demetriou-Swanwick
Development Editor: Veronika Watkins
Project Manager: Emma Riley
Designer: George Ajayi
Illustration Manager: Merlyn Harvey
Illustrator: Graeme Chambers

Teaching Pilates for Postural Faults, Illness and Injury

A practical guide

Jane Paterson

Exercise illustrations by Marie Robinson
Photographs by Antonia Reeve

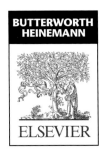

BUTTERWORTH
HEINEMANN

ELSEVIER

EDINBURGH LONDON NEW YORK OXFORD PHILADELPHIA ST LOUIS SYDNEY TORONTO 2009

Butterworth-Heinemann is an imprint of Elsevier
The Boulevard, Langford Lane, Kidlington, Oxford OX5 1GB, UK
30 Corporate Drive, Suite 400, Burlington, MA 01803, USA

First edition 2009
  Reprinted 2009, 2010, 2011 (three times)

Notice
No responsibility is assumed by the publisher for any injury and/or damage to persons
or property as a matter of products liability, negligence or otherwise, or from any use
or operation of any methods, products, instructions or ideas contained in the material
herein. Because of rapid advances in the medical sciences, in particular, independent
verification of diagnoses and drug dosages should be made

British Library Cataloguing in Publication Data
A catalogue record for this book is available from the British Library

Library of Congress Cataloging-in-Publication Data
A catalog record for this book is available from the Library of Congress

ISBN: 978-0-7506-5647-4

For information on all Butterworth-Heinemann publications
visit our website at www.elsevierdirect.com

Printed and bound in China

11 12 13 14   10 9 8 7 6

Contents

Acknowledgements

I owe a great debt to the following people who have been involved at different stages of this project. First Pat Millard for her time and friendship over the 5 years she has spent with me at our respective homes in Oxford and Edinburgh. She has devoted many hours to sitting at the word processor refining the text and associated tables over and over again, and I feel that without her unerring patience and stamina I would not have seen this project through.

Next, I gratefully remember my students, student teachers and colleagues not only in Oxford, but also in London, Birmingham and Edinburgh. They provided inspiration and supported me as I developed and documented my specific approach to teaching the exercises. This in turn led to my producing my Open College Network Foundation Training Programme for Teachers of Pilates that has been successfully delivered in several centres, including the Alan Herdman's studio in London. Then I must thank Andy Adamson for the considerable time he spent with me ensuring that my text accurately followed the details of the exercises, and my great friend Eileen Fry, whose experience, knowledge and skills were a key to finalizing the chapter on contemporary teaching methods. Artist Marie Robinson produced all the original, simple, but realistic drawings and Antonia Reeve all the lovely photographs, whilst Katerina Swinton, and Indigo and Ron Reeve kindly acted as such willing and excellent models, together with Chris Blagdon, who also made his studio available for the photographic sessions.

I had continued and loyal support from many others in particular Sylvie Essame and Susie Roberts, whilst my husband Gordon provided constant advice and input and contributed to the chapter on medical conditions.

Lastly, I must acknowledge the patience shown by all at Elsevier in waiting so long for me to complete this manual.

Thanks also to Stuart Porter for his advice.

DEDICATION

To my parents Bill and Marie Richards for gifts of love, curiosity and a desire for learning, Alan Herdman with whom I first embarked on Pilates in this country and my family: Gordon, Angus, Jennie, Olivia and Ione who never allowed me to forget that 'Plus est en vous – there is more in you than you know'

Preface

This text is the outcome of an idea I conceived many years ago when I first became involved in training aspiring professional dancers. I hope it will prove to be a useful educational tool for dance, physical fitness and sports teachers, as well as medical practitioners and allied health professionals involved in rehabilitation through exercise.

For as long as I can remember, I have loved music, movement and dance. I began studying ballet as a child in Australia and went on to train as a classical dancer and subsequently performed and taught professionally for several years. However, a back injury during a particularly extreme training session forced me to change direction and I decided to limit my professional dance work to teaching whilst I underwent training in general nursing. This proved to be very important over the years as it gave me a basic understanding of human anatomy and common medical conditions, and helped to develop my keen interest in injury prevention and health promotion through lifestyle, correct posture and exercise techniques.

There followed an ongoing desire to understand how the extraordinary talents and abilities seen in elite ballet dancers and sports persons depends not only on self-sacrifice and drive, but also on inherent qualities of physique, posture and effective movement patterns. I also needed to understand how there would always be a risk of injuries specifically associated with extreme exercise regimens, irrespective of an individual's natural talent and ability.

When I was training in Australia it was generally assumed that strenuous, rather than gentle or thought-ful, physical exercise would be most effective in the promotion of physical and mental wellbeing, but the pain and exhaustion experienced as exercise tolerance approached its limit indicated not only muscle fatigue, but also adverse changes in mental concentration, posture, balance and technique.

However, I was fortunate enough to study with an extraordinary Australian teacher who was many years ahead of her time. Although lacking formal medical training she understood the importance of good posture and correct spine function and the harm that might occur during strenuous but poorly executed exercise sessions. She also expected students to learn how to take responsibility for their own progress and we were all quickly taught self-assessment tools so as to understand our personal difficulties with technique and exercise performance.

This proved invaluable for me then, and subsequently has enabled me to enhance my technical and performance skills, so as to maintain my body shape and posture not only in normal everyday life, but also throughout four successive pregnancies. I now realize that what I had been taught as a young student in Australia proved an invaluable introduction to the underlying principles on which Joseph Pilates and other movement specialists based their exercises.

Such principles remain as integral basis for all efficient movement and this manual, therefore, aims to show how postural faults can be identified and effectively addressed through detailed attention to exercise techniques.

History of Joseph Pilates

I must be right. Never an aspirin. Never injured a day in my life.
The whole country, the whole world, should be doing my exercises.
They'd be happier.

Joseph Hubertus Pilates,
in 1965, aged 86

Joseph's original principles and exercises comprised the following.

Principles:
- Breathing
- Concentration
- Control
- Centring
- Precision
- Flow.

EXERCISES:

The Hundred, Roll-Up, Roll-Over, Leg Circles, Rolling Back, Single Leg Stretch, Double Leg Stretch, Spine Stretch, Open Leg Rocker, Corkscrew, See-Saw, Swan Dive, Single Leg Kick, Double Leg Kick, Neck Pull, Scissors, Bicycle, Shoulder Bridge, Spine Twist, Jackknife, Side Kick, Teaser, Hip twist with outstretched legs, Swimming, Leg Pull Front Support, Leg Pull Back Support, Side Kick Kneeling, Side Bend, Boomerang, Seal, Crab, Rocking, Control balance, Push-Up.

As a teenager, increasingly frustrated by the debilitating consequences of his rheumatic fever, rickets and chronic asthma, Joseph Pilates began to explore alternative methods of overcoming his disabilities. Through extensive physical study of Zen meditation, yoga and the rigorous exercise regimens of the ancient Greeks and Romans, Pilates' health and strength improved to such an extent that by the age of 14 he was an accomplished gymnast, boxer and skier.

Born in Germany to Greek parents, it is thought that as a young man Pilates may have joined a group of Chinese acrobats and in 1912, at the age of 32, moved to England where he became a professional boxer and self-defence teacher, counting members of the British police force among his trainees. However, his involvement with the police did nothing to protect him as shortly after the outbreak of World War I, Pilates, along with other United Kingdom residing German Nationals, was interned as an 'enemy alien' in a camp at Lancaster for a year of enforced inactivity. It was during this period that Pilates began to refine his beliefs in health and physical fitness and, with his fellow inmates as guinea-pigs, started devising a series of exercise combining physical fitness with mental acuity and control of breathing to build core physical strength and flexibility.

Transported to the Isle of Man to work as a hospital orderly for the latter part of the war, Pilates witnessed at first hand some of the human consequences of the conflict in the many disabled and bedridden victims attempting to recuperate from battle injuries, wartime diseases and enemy internment. From his own earlier experiences as a young man, Pilates realized the importance of strengthening muscles to aid recovery from these injuries and so he began gently and systematically moving patients' arms and legs using his own body to bear their weight. The hospital medical staff noticed improvements in recovery times in those patients with whom Pilates was working and encouraged him to continue developing his ideas, for which he had now begun to incorporate the use of springs taken from one of the old-fashioned hospital beds. He believed that springs could provide progressive resistance similar to human intrinsic muscular activity and simultaneously bear the weight to enable muscles to heal.

After the war, Pilates returned to Germany where he continued to develop his exercises and equipment working with the Hamburg police. He was also building relationships with the dance community, striking a lasting professional and personal friendship with the pioneering Slovakian dancer, choreographer and dance theorist, Rudolph von Laban. However, by the mid-1920s his work was attracting unwelcome attention from the German Army that insisted he train their troops. Therefore, in 1923, with increasing pressure from the militia but with no desire for his techniques to aid their cause, Pilates emigrated to America to start a new life in New York. It was during the long sea crossing of the Atlantic that he met his future wife, Clara, who was to become his patient as he taught her his techniques to help her overcome her chronic arthritis. Clara later became his business partner when they set up his first studio in 1924 on Eighth Avenue in the heart of the dance neighbourhood. Word of this new studio spread swiftly through the dance community and, with the endorsement of such legends as Martha Graham, Tanya Holm and George Balanchine, the studio and its Pilates techniques soon became renowned, not only for aiding rehabilitation of their dancers' injured muscles, backs, knees and other joints, but also as complementary exercise techniques to promote strengthening and balancing.

Whilst initially the exercise sequences were performed on mats, it was during this golden period that Pilates developed his fully mechanical machine, the 'Universal Reformer', now more commonly known as the 'Plie Machine', a sliding horizontal bed that could incorporate up to four springs and thus be adapted to meet the requirements of specific exercises as well as match the individual's strength. Over the ensuing years, Pilates developed other pieces of equipment, all designed like the Reformer to stabilize the torso during exercise and help his clients increase their range of movement, correct misalignments and weight distribution, control muscles and monitor their energy expenditure.

In the 1940s Pilates became increasingly aware of his own mortality and, keen to leave a legacy, began to train three of his students as teachers. These 'Master Teachers' – Eve Gentry, Ron Fletcher and Romana Krysanowska – were the first of a now worldwide network of Pilates teachers and, following Joseph's death in 1967, Krysanowska supported Clara at the New York studio by becoming its Director during the 1970s. Meanwhile, other 'Master Teachers' – Bruce King, Kathleen Stanford-Grant and Carola Trier – trained in the 1950s, then Mary Bowen in the 1960s. It was Carola Trier's own student, Robert Fitzgerald, who, in the late 1960s alongside Trier, trained Alan Herdman, who first brought the Pilates Method to the United Kingdom.

Herdman, formerly a chemical engineer, had gone to train at the London School of Contemporary Dance and was working as a teacher and dancer when he was encouraged by the artistic director of the London Contemporary Dance Theatre to go over to New York to study the Pilates Method. Whilst there he worked intensively with Trier and Fitzgerald and, on his return to the United Kingdom in 1971, Herdman set up Britain's first Pilates studio, the Body Control Studio at the London School of Contemporary Dance. As with Joseph Pilates' original New York studio, his first clients were actors, dancers, singers and athletes, but as word of the method's success spread, doctors and physiotherapists began referring patients struggling with chronic injuries to the Body Control Studio as a rehabilitating measure. Following the success of his first venture, Herdman trained the first United Kingdom Pilates teachers and, as his training schemes grew, new studios were opened in London, as well as throughout the rest of the country and in Europe and Australia.

After Clara Pilates' death in 1977, Romana Krysanowska continued as Director of the New York studio and during the 1980s the Pilates Method experienced something of a comeback during a period of renewed interest in the technique throughout the United States, the United Kingdom and Europe. As a result of this, in 1991 the Institute for the Pilates Method, Santa Fe, was formed for the purpose of protecting Joseph Pilates' original technique from distortions and to offer a formalized training scheme for the technique. Originally formed with Michelle Larson as Director and Joan Breibart as President, and joined by the original six Master Teachers as the Advisory Board of Directors, in 1995 the Institute was legally required to change its name as in the United States only Joseph Pilates' original studio and the teachers it trains were to be permitted to use the name 'Pilates'. Renamed The Physical Mind Institute, this body still exists, as do the spirit and techniques created and nurtured by Joseph Pilates, whether carrying his name or not.

The legacy of Joseph Pilates and his striving for physical perfection through an implicit understanding of the human body and how it works and moves survives to this day, helping countless dancers, actors, athletes and laymen to rehabilitate after injury and so recover their full physical potential.

Reference

Pilates JH 1988 Your health. Revised edition, Robbins J (ed). Presentation Dynamics, Incline Village, NV. First published, 1934

Note to the reader

This text is for dance and movement teachers who need to be able to recognise and address common postural faults as well as for physiotherapists and allied medical professionals using pilates exercises within treatment or rehabilitation programmes.

The anatomy covered should not be regarded as a definitive text; it has been included as an "aide-memoire" when teaching. Further reading for anatomy students is given in the appendix.

Anatomical body charts

(Reproduced with permission from Thibodeau GA, Patton KT 2007 Anatomy and physiology, 6th edn. Mosby, St Louis)

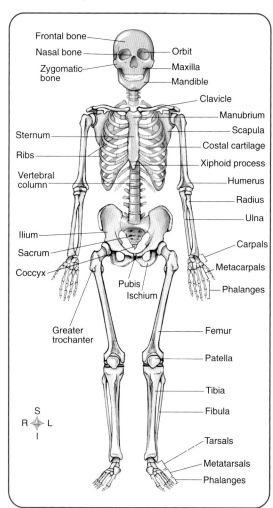

Skeleton – anterior view

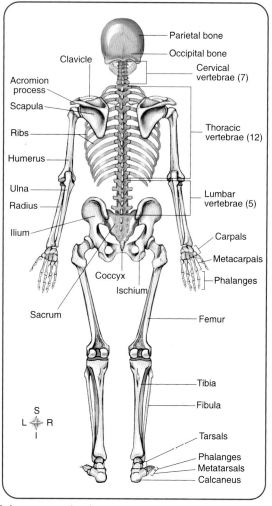

Skeleton – posterior view

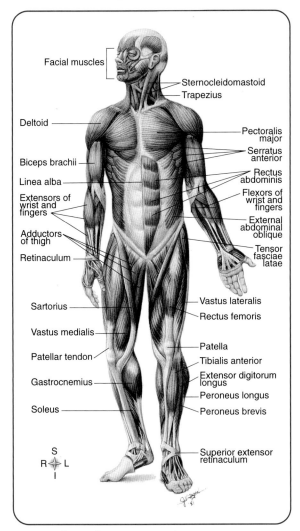

Facial muscles

Sternocleidomastoid
Trapezius

Deltoid

Pectoralis major
Serratus anterior
Rectus abdominis

Biceps brachii
Linea alba
Extensors of wrist and fingers

Flexors of wrist and fingers
External abdominal oblique

Adductors of thigh
Retinaculum

Tensor fasciae latae

Sartorius
Vastus lateralis
Rectus femoris

Vastus medialis

Patellar tendon
Patella
Tibialis anterior

Gastrocnemius
Extensor digitorum longus

Soleus
Peroneus longus
Peroneus brevis

S
R L
I

Superior extensor retinaculum

Overview of musculature – anterior view

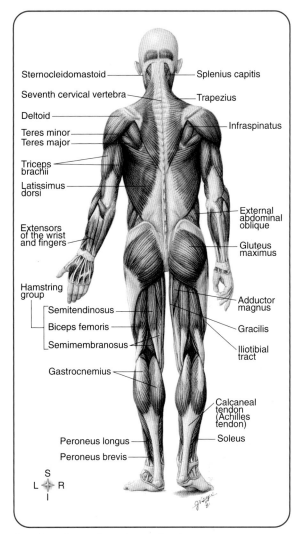

Sternocleidomastoid
Splenius capitis

Seventh cervical vertebra
Trapezius

Deltoid
Teres minor
Teres major
Infraspinatus

Triceps brachii

Latissimus dorsi

External abdominal oblique

Extensors of the wrist and fingers
Gluteus maximus

Hamstring group
Adductor magnus

Semitendinosus
Biceps femoris
Gracilis

Semimembranosus
Iliotibial tract

Gastrocnemius

Calcaneal tendon (Achilles tendon)

Soleus

Peroneus longus
Peroneus brevis

S
L R
I

Overview of musculature – posterior view

Exercise index

Chapter 1

Good posture and how it can be achieved

INTRODUCTION

Posture is an overall term comprising the relative disposition of all the many parts of the body, but particularly the shape and position of the spine. It cannot be considered in isolation but only in relation to the person's prevailing situation or environment, which may be static or dynamic.

In a static posture, whilst a person may be standing, sitting or lying still, this should really be regarded as temporarily suspended movement or dynamic posture, as even with so-called static posture there is always a tendency to change.

In dynamic posture there are constant changes in the relative positions and alignment of all the body parts, particularly against the integral structures of the spine, as most occur during activities such as walking, running, dancing, manual handling, etc. In fact, dynamic posture simply describes the constantly changing relationship between all the parts of the body that occur during movement.

Good posture, whether static or dynamic, is difficult to define, but as all the musculoskeletal components of the body – and not just those of the vertebral column – contribute and maintain posture, the term good posture might best refer to one that puts the least strain on bones, joints and their supporting structures. In practice, good posture should equate with standing, sitting, lying or moving comfortably.

The anatomical basis of good posture can be defined as a state of muscular and skeletal balance that protects the supporting structures of the body against injury, the effects of ageing, etc., irrespective of the activity or effort involved. This is best seen in manual handling techniques designed to keep the combined load and body mass over the feet as the supporting base. It enables the individual to work safely and comfortably. In less strenuous activities, such as walking or dancing, good posture reflects poise and an unselfconscious grace, ease or even economy of movement.

Bad posture, in contrast, implies inefficient use or frank misuse of joints and associated muscles and ligaments, with progressive and, ultimately, irreversible injurious effects, with associated physical, and possibly painful disability.

Posture when observed in others may be felt to range between good and bad, and these deviations are difficult to identify without a prescription for ideal, erect human posture. However, it must be noted that in reality normal posture and particularly good normal posture rarely exists, and when assessing and correcting posture it is essential to consider inherent physical features such as body type and proportions, together with ligament length and joint mobility. For example, people with

1

loose ligaments tend to stand with hyperextended knees and hips (resting on their iliofemoral ligaments) and with flexible, exaggerated curves of the spine that are much greater than those seen in people with tighter ligaments.

Posture can also reflect gender, personality, mood, age and state of health and can alter throughout the day, being related to stimulation or fatigue as individuals react with their environment.

Teaching good posture where it is lacking to a greater or lesser degree aims for an optimum relationship between all parts of the body at all times, so that the most effective musculoskeletal function prevails over the full range of an individual's activities.

Such teaching can only be effective through an understanding of the basic mechanics of static and dynamic posture, and combinations of the two, and the contributions of anatomical position and alignment, and of musculoskeletal function to overall good posture.

At the same time, it is necessary to consider skeletal abnormalities of bones and joints, whether inherent or acquired as in ageing or degenerative conditions, and problems of inadequate or inefficient muscle function following injury or in neurological conditions, leading to weakness, shortening or imbalance, and their mechanical consequences.

Furthermore, as teachers, good posture is something we should be able to see and feel in ourselves. This enhances our understanding of the basic components of good posture whilst maintaining our own good musculoskeletal function. Not only is this essential for safe, effective teaching through example, it also promotes and assists the achievements of better posture in our trainees.

Whether promoting overall good posture or correcting existing elements of bad posture in individuals or groups, each trainee should be helped to understand their specific postural faults or habits. This knowledge, together with tools and strategies for improving posture, will ensure that each trainee is equipped to gain the long-term benefits of good versus less good posture.

HOW THE MODERN HUMAN REMAINS ERECT

As humans evolved, the erect posture was adopted through the development of the bipedal gait. The upper limbs were thereby freed, allowing the functional use of the arms and hands to develop more complex activities. Naturally, the erect stance could only be achieved at the expense of a greatly reduced area and strength of base support, with inevitably less stability when the body had lost the support of what had become the upper limbs. At the same time, therefore, the lower limbs

gained strength and agility, and overall body mobility and stability were maintained and enhanced.

Gravity is constantly pulling the body as a whole towards the ground. This force is counteracted by the tone of the postural muscle group, a role that cannot be overestimated because the bones of the skeleton, especially the long limb bones, are too irregularly shaped to stand upon each other and maintain the upright position alone. However, muscles do not maintain the erect position alone and their ability to counteract gravity is under the control of the central nervous system which is implemented by information contributed by ligaments, tendons, joints and the muscles themselves, together with input from special senses, mainly visual and vestibular, which help to identify the position of the head in space. Other systems involved less directly by contributing to metabolic homeostasis include the respiratory, circulatory, excretory, digestive and endocrine systems (Thibodeau & Patton 1993).

Although the contributions that these systems make must be appreciated, they will not be considered here, as the topics for discussion in this chapter are posture, balance and the muscular activity involved in maintaining an erect posture.

Summary

Advantages of good posture

- It ensures that the progressive, but controlled, development of all the postural muscles is both promoted and maintained.
- It helps to maintain overall body fitness so that physical activity is efficient and well coordinated.
- It, therefore, also helps to protect the spine by aiding lifting and handling of loads efficiently.
- It helps to compensate for skeletal changes that occur, for instance in prolonged illness, as well as with advancing age.
- It helps to protect the back and prevent injury in pregnancy and during the postnatal period.
- Overall, it promotes a feeling of well-being, confidence and poise during sitting, standing, moving and general day-to-day activities.

Disadvantages of bad posture

- More rapid, and sometimes permanent, skeletal changes as age advances.
- Muscle imbalance and resulting injuries.
- Less efficient breathing and circulation.
- A sluggish digestive system.
- Lack of coordination and the ability to move with ease.
- An adverse effect on mood and well-being.

It is important to realize that bad posture, even when only temporary, as for instance with illness or pregnancy, etc., can lead to a long-term or even permanent loss of previously good posture with associated physical and sometimes psychological problems.

GOOD ERECT POSTURE

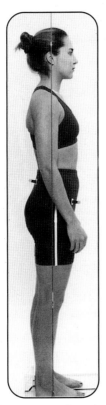

Figure 1.1   Good erect posture. Reproduced with permission from Sahrmann (2002).

Good erect posture (Fig. 1.1) requires an understanding of the vertebral column's structure and function as well as the basic principles of maintaining an upright stance. It also demands the ability to observe and assess posture so as to recognize common postural habits, faults and movement patterns.

These are discussed under the following headings:

■ Basic principles of maintaining an upright stance:
- Spinal anatomical structures
- Body mass and centre of gravity
- Base of support
- Line of gravity
- Centre of pressure
- Balance and stability.

■ Postural observational skills and assessment:
- Body types
- Assessment procedures
- Ideal alignment
- Easily recognized faulty postures
- Common faults in foot placement and leg alignment.

BASIC PRINCIPLES OF MAINTAINING AND UPRIGHT STANCE

Spinal anatomical structures

'The back' or 'the spine' comprises the vertebral column and associated ligaments and muscles, together with the intervertebral discs and the contents of the vertebral canal (Figs 1.2 & 1.3).

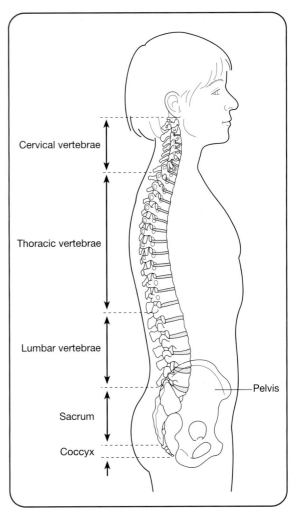

Cervical vertebrae

Thoracic vertebrae

Lumbar vertebrae

Pelvis

Sacrum

Coccyx

Figure 1.2   Side view of spine.

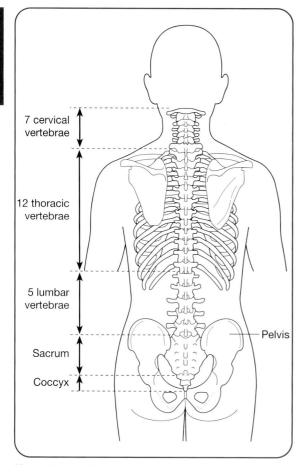

Figure 1.3   Back view of spine.

7 cervical vertebrae

12 thoracic vertebrae

5 lumbar vertebrae

Pelvis

Sacrum

Coccyx

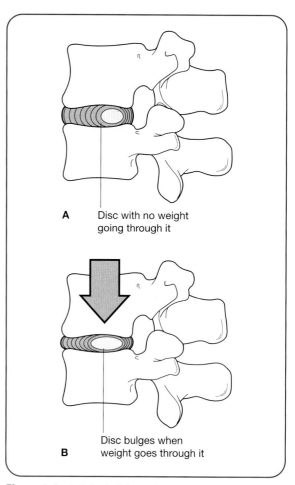

A   Disc with no weight going through it

B   Disc bulges when weight goes through it

Figure 1.4   **A** Unloaded disc: side view of spine. **B** Loaded disc: side view of spine.

The intervertebral discs cushion the bony vertebrae, providing shock absorption and giving flexibility for the spine to move. The shock absorption properties of the discs are essential in protecting the spine from trauma during everyday activities and are particularly effective for walking, going up or down steps or inclines, running, etc. In addition, the health and integrity of the intervertebral discs determine to a great extent the overall function of the spine as the discs allow movement to occur between each vertebra during bending, stretching and twisting, and movements comprised of combinations of these possibilities.

In a healthy disc, the spongy, jelly-like nucleus is enclosed within a fibrous ring (annulus) that allows the disc to change shape during movement but prevents the nucleus leaking out. The ability of the nucleus to change shape during loading and unloading of the spine is demonstrated in Figures 1.4–1.6.

As the disc nucleus contains a great deal of water, constant pressure exerted on the discs throughout the day will adversely affect their overall size, sponginess and shock-absorbing properties. As the day progresses, water leaks from the discs causing shrinkage of the nucleus. This leads to a loss of disc height that results in less effective disc function and overall mobility and function of the spine itself. However, these changes are reversed during periods of rest, especially when recumbent in bed at night, and varying the amount of pressure exerted on the discs throughout the day can also help to maintain and improve disc health and function (Fig. 1.7).

The intervertebral discs permit movement of the spine, and the range and types of movement are limited by the shape and structure of the different types of vertebra (compare the cervical and lumbar regions) and the strength and length of the ligaments. Movement is controlled by the muscles of the spine and trunk under the influence of motor nerve impulses from the brain.

In the normal spine, the small facet joints on the posterolateral aspects of the vertebrae fit neatly together, so that hyperextension and extreme twisting movements are limited. However, narrowing of the intervertebral space through an exaggerated lumbar lordosis or damage to the intervertebral discs places undue stress on the joints causing pain (Fig. 1.8).

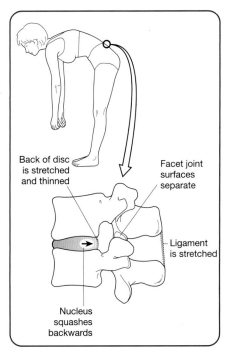

Back of disc is stretched and thinned
Facet joint surfaces separate
Ligament is stretched
Nucleus squashes backwards

Figure 1.5 Forward bending. Redrawn with permission from Oliver (1999).

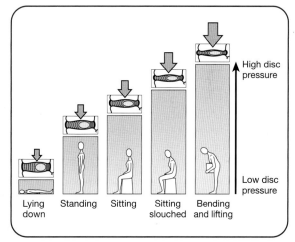

High disc pressure

Low disc pressure

Lying down | Standing | Sitting | Sitting slouched | Bending and lifting

Figure 1.7 How pressure on the discs is affected by different postures. Redrawn with permission from Oliver (1999).

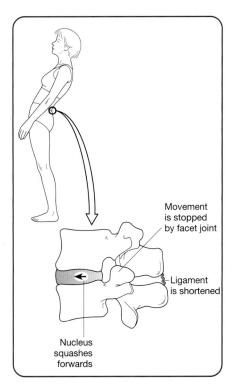

Movement is stopped by facet joint
Ligament is shortened
Nucleus squashes forwards

Figure 1.6 Backward bending. Redrawn with permission from Oliver (1999).

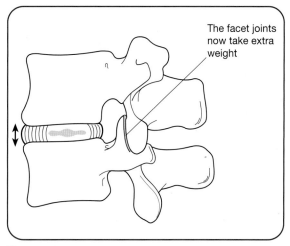

The facet joints now take extra weight

Figure 1.8 Narrowing of disc space increases pressure on facet joints. Redrawn with permission from Oliver (1999).

1

Muscles and ligaments supporting the vertebral column

Muscles

The erector spinae is a longitudinal mass of muscles ascending along the posterior aspect of the vertebral column from the sacrum to the skull (Figs 1.9 & 1.10A&B). This large and somewhat complex extensor of the spine is divided into three parallel columns termed deep, middle and superficial, each further subdivided into individually named components arranged in ascending series.

Deep layer – interspinales, intertransversarii, rotatores
- *Interspinales*: these small muscles, lying in series together with the interspinous ligaments, join adjacent spinous processes.
- *Intertransversarii*: these are a similar series of thin muscles that join adjacent transverse processes; they tend to be stronger in the upper part of the erector spinae.
- *Rotatores*: these join one transverse process to the spinous process of the vertebra above; they are confined to the thoracic spine, which is where the only true rotation of the vertebral column can occur.

These deep muscles are small and not individually strong; however, collectively, their close proximity to the vertebrae confers their important contribution to the integrity and correct function of the whole spine, possibly with respect to its more subtle postural adjustments.

Middle layer – multifidus, semispinalis, levatores costarum
- *Multifidus*: this has the deepest and shortest muscle fibres in this layer. Each extends from the laminae

and mamillary processes of one vertebra to the spinous process of a vertebra that is positioned two or three segments above. Multifidus extends in series from the sacrum to the upper part of the neck.
- *Semispinalis*: the fibres of this muscle lie superficial to multifidus, and extend over three levels from the lower thoracic region to the base of the skull, named in ascending order: semispinalis thoracis, cervicis and capitis:
  a. Semispinalis thoracis – extends from the transverse processes of the lower thoracic vertebrae to the spinous processes of the upper thoracic vertebrae (Last 1959, p. 612)
  b. Semispinalis cervicis – larger and more powerful than semispinalis thoracis, it originates above and in continuity with it. It is inserted into the spinous processes of the cervical vertebrae including the bifid spinous process of the axis or first cervical vertebra

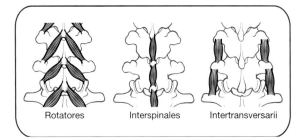

| Rotatores | Interspinales | Intertransversarii |

Figure 1.9   The deepest level of the spinal musculature demonstrates three primary patterns: spinous process to transverse process, spinous process to spinous process, and transverse process to transverse process. The more superficial muscles can be analysed as ever-longer express versions of these primary locals. Reproduced with permission from Myers (2001).

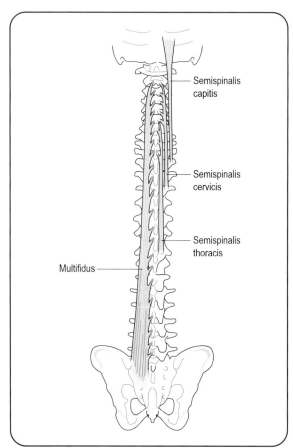

Semispinalis capitis

Semispinalis cervicis

Semispinalis thoracis

Multifidus

Figure 1.10A

c. Semispinalis capitis – the most powerful layer of semispinalis, it arises from the transverse processes of the upper thoracic and the articular processes of the lower cervical vertebrae and is inserted into the base of the skull around the midline of the occipital bone.

■ *Levatores costarum*: these are small, strong, triangular muscle pairs, 12 in number, found between the eleventh thoracic and seventh cervical vertebrae. Each of the 12 pairs descends from the transverse process of the vertebra above to the upper border of the rib below, near its tubercle. The fibres fan out as they pass downwards and laterally (Palastanga et al 2002, p. 481).

This whole middle layer constitutes a greater muscle mass than the deep layer and, together with the muscles of the anterior abdominal wall, makes a major contribution to the stabilization of the entire spine. Multifidus is the particular component thought to play an important role in establishing and maintaining good upright posture. Levatores costarum, on the other hand, is more concerned with assisting the inspiratory muscles of the thoracic ribcage.

Superficial layer – iliocostalis (lateral), longissimus (intermediate) and spinalis (medial)
Sacrospinalis is a collective term for this most superficial of the three layers and is itself subdivided into lateral, intermediate and medial columns lying in parallel. The whole extends from the back of the sacrum and inner edge of the iliac crest to the ribcage. It is a complex arrangement of muscle fibres and bundles, again subdivided into serial sections, of which the detailed origins and insertions are not of specific importance in the context of this manual:

■ *Iliocostalis*: the lateral column has three sections ascending in series: iliocostalis lumborum, thoracis and cervicis.
■ *Longissimus*: the intermediate and strongest column similarly has three sections: longissimus thoracis, cervicis and capitis.
■ *Spinalis*: is the relatively insignificant medial column, subdivided into spinalis thoracis, cervicis and capitis, of which spinalis thoracis is the most clearly defined. Spinalis cervicis and capitis are small, poorly defined and are frequently merged with adjacent sacrospinalis muscle columns.

All these long muscles of the back, together with those of the pelvic floor, the gluteal muscles, the adductors of the thigh and the muscles of the torso all help the erector spinae to stabilize the vertebral column and so provide the foundation of safe, effective movement of the whole body.

Body mass and centre of gravity

The centre of mass of an object is defined as the point about which the mass is evenly distributed and this definition cannot easily be applied to the irregularly shaped human body. However, by first considering the mass of the whole body and then assessing the percentage that the head, neck, trunk, upper and lower limbs individually contribute, allows an approximation of where the centre of gravity would lie when the body is standing upright (Table 1.1).

This is said to be approximately at the level of the second sacral vertebra within the pelvis but shifts according to body and limb movements. For example, flexing the shoulders and reaching both arms forward shifts the orientation of the body's centre of gravity relative to its base of support.

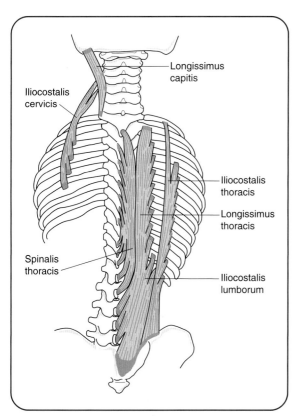

Iliocostalis cervicis

Longissimus capitis

Iliocostalis thoracis

Longissimus thoracis

Spinalis thoracis

Iliocostalis lumborum

Figure 1.10B The erector spinae muscle showing its constituent parts. Reproduced with permission from Palastanga et al (2006).

1

Table 1.1 Mass of each body segment in percentage of total body mass

Segment	% of body mass
Trunk	49.7
Head and neck	8.1
Upper arm	2.8 each
Lower arm	1.6 each
Hand	0.6 each
Total arm	5.0 each
Upper leg	10.0 each
Lower leg	4.7 each
Foot	1.4 each
Total leg	16.1 each

Reproduced with permission from Palastanga et al (2002).

Base of support

Any part of an object in contact with a surface that is, therefore, supporting it is described as its base of support. This can alter and depends on whether the object is static or in motion and, where the human body is concerned, will depend on the specific posture adapted at any particular time. For example, when standing upright both feet provide the base of support, but during walking, the base of support shifts from one foot to the other as each step is taken. When moving from standing to lying supine, the base of support is increased as more of the body is supported on a surface and, when moving from lying supine to four-point kneeling, the base of support is decreased as the whole of the body weight is supported by the hands, lower legs and feet.

Line of gravity

In the ideal upright static posture the line of gravity is described as a perpendicular line falling through the middle of the body's centre of gravity. When a body is viewed from the side it is imagined falling through the middle of the external auditory meatus, slightly in front of the shoulder joint, just behind the axis of the hip joint, in front of both the knee and ankle joints and just in front of the heel bone. When a body is viewed from in front or behind, the line divides the body into two equal parts and falls between the feet.

During postural assessment, observing the line of gravity is useful in that it defines ideal static alignment and confirms the enormous variations in human posture; however, it should be realized that it will not necessarily identify underlying biomechanical faults.

Centre of pressure

There is a force reflected from the ground as a result of the action of the body's weight onto the ground. The centre of this reflected force is described as the centre of pressure and, in the upright stance, it lies within the body's base of support.

Balance and stability

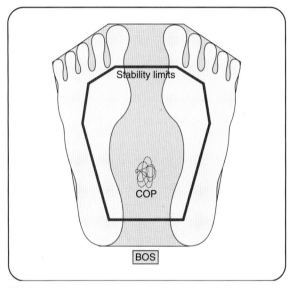

Figure 1.11 During quiet upright standing the contact area with the floor underneath the feet and the area in between the feet is the base of support (BOS). Because people cannot easily move their line of gravity to the outer edges of the BOS, the stability limit has been defined as the area within which people can move their line of gravity without losing balance. The centre of pressure (COP) of the ground reaction force is located well within those two areas. Because a person will always sway a bit, the COP oscillates with a certain amplitude. Reproduced with permission from Trew & Everett (2005).

A body's shape, mass and orientation in relation to the surface area, shape and position of its base of support determines where both its centre and line of gravity will lie (Fig. 1.11). All these factors contribute to overall balance and stability.

A stable body will have a stable centre of gravity lying sufficiently low above its base of support to ensure this. Additionally, its line of gravity should fall through the centre of pressure to lie within the base of support.

A stable body will be able to maintain both its centre and line of gravity whilst resisting a short duration of applied force, or will be able to be displaced by an applied force of short duration and yet return to its original, balanced position.

Conversely, an unstable body will lose both its centre and line of gravity when a force of short duration is applied, and will then continue to lose balance as it is further displaced so as to become subject to the influence of gravity.

POSTURAL OBSERVATIONAL SKILLS AND ASSESSMENT

As all individuals have unique anatomical profiles it is difficult to identify definitive attributes for describing normal posture. However, it is possible to identify the components of ideal alignment and posture and these are the standards used for observing and assessing the many postural variations that may be encountered.

Before assessing posture, personal details such as age, sex, medical history, psychological status and adaptive influences, such as occupation, lifestyle, etc., should be noted.

Body types

Classifying body type can also be helpful as inherent characteristics are commonly associated with specific postural faults. These underlying factors will also predetermine the outcome of an exercise programme for a particular person.

For example, a tall, slim individual with naturally poor muscle tone (ectomorph) may be inclined towards having a sway back or exaggerated kyphotic posture and be resistant to building and maintaining muscular strength. Although carefully designed exercise programmes may improve muscle tone and endurance, this would be lost without ongoing training.

The basic anthropometrics classifications are as follows:

- *Endomorphs* are inclined to be pear shaped with comparatively shorter limbs and extra subcutaneous fat around the hips and thighs.
- *Ectomorphs* tend to have slender, lean bodies with comparatively poor muscular development, do not gain body weight easily and may even be underweight.
- *Mesomorphs* have strong athletic bodies with broad shoulders and comparatively narrow hips and need regular exercise to maintain their musculature and prevent loss of muscle tone and weight gain.

Assessment procedures

Assessment of static standing posture

To begin, ask the subject to stand with the feet bare and approximately 8 cm apart (the examiner can place one foot between the subject's feet to achieve this correct position) and the body weight distributed evenly between the feet.

Considering the fall of the plumb line, observe posture from the side and back (initially one might use a plumb line but with experience exercise teachers learn to imagine such a line) and note the surface markings and underlying anatomical structures that would normally coincide with the plumb line as shown in 'Ideal alignment side view' and 'Ideal alignment back view'. Record any deviations from ideal alignment and note the overall balance of the whole body over the lower limbs and feet.

Next scan the body from the feet up to the head to identify obvious features associated with common postural faults such as flat feet, foot pronation or supination, bow legs or knock knees, exaggerated spinal curves or a forward-poking chin, etc.

Continue with a more careful study of segmental alignment beginning with the head, spine, pectoral girdle and upper limbs followed by the pelvis, hips, lower limbs and feet using the landmarks described in the following charts as guidelines.

Compare deviations from an ideal alignment with those identified as features of common postural faults to confirm specific problems and how to address them.

This same process is used to identify and address faults that occur during sitting, when moving from sitting to standing, and when mobilizing the spine.

Exercises to improve spine mobility should aim to provide continuous support for the intrinsic spinal structures whilst moving each vertebral joint through its optimum range of movement (see Chapter 4).

Assessment of sitting

This might also be formally assessed to confirm the effects that adaptive influences and habits have on a particular person.

To begin, ask the subject to sit on a chair or firm bed that allows the feet to rest on the floor with the upper thighs fully supported and the backs of the knees unrestricted. The feet are positioned approximately hip distance apart.

Scan the body from the feet up to the head to identify habits such as slouching with excessive rounding of the thoracic spine as well as other features associated with common postural faults – a forward-poking chin, incorrect pectoral girdle and pelvic alignment, foot pronation or supination, etc.

1

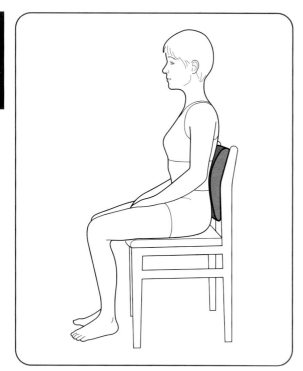

Figure 1.12   A backrest or cushion behind your low back helps to straighten it. Redrawn with permission from Oliver (1999).

Ideal sitting posture

In correct sitting posture the body weight is adjusted to balance over the ischial tuberosities so that, together with the thighs, they provide a stable base of support (Fig. 1.12). The knees are flexed approximately 90 degrees and the lower legs are perpendicular, with the heels aligned with the backs of the knees.

The lumbar spine is in approximately mid flexion with the lordotic curve intact but slightly reduced in comparison with standing, and the soft supporting structures in the lower back should appear comparatively relaxed. The whole spine is lengthened, with the crown of the head reaching towards the ceiling and the upper torso balanced above the pelvis. The position may be actively supported by gentle pelvic floor and lower abdominal muscle activation but ideally is maintained without conscious muscular effort.

Ideal supported sitting position

In ideal supported sitting the whole length of the spine rests against a firm surface that inclines very slightly backwards from the perpendicular.

Moving from sitting to standing

When moving from sitting to standing the knees are flexed between 90 and 110 degrees so that the feet lie directly below or slightly behind the knee joint. The spine remains stable whilst the hips increase flexion to about 55 degrees from the upright sitting position to move the body and its centre of gravity slightly in front of the ankle joints. Still seated, the shoulder joints flex up to around 50 degrees, bringing the arms and therefore the body's centre of gravity further in front of the ankle joints to lift the buttocks from the seat. As the body's weight is transferred from the seat to the legs, the hips and knees may extend slightly but still remain in flexion. At this stage the ankles are dorsiflexed to their maximum so the dorsiflexors as well as gluteus maximus and the hamstrings are strongly active.

Once the body's centre of gravity is well established over the feet, the hips and knees simultaneously begin extending and, as extension progresses, the trunk moves more vertically towards the upright position. At the same time plantarflexor activity at the ankle assists hip and knee extension, and slight cervical spine flexion occurs to ensure that the skull balances correctly on top of the spine. Hip, knee and trunk extension continue until standing is achieved.

Assessment of forward bending

Normal

Forward bending from a standing position is the most common movement occurring in daily activities. It begins with the pelvis swaying backwards as the hips flex, so allowing the body to remain balanced over its base of support. Ideally, during this initial hip flexion, the lumbar spine also begins to move into flexion, but only slightly. However, there are normal variations in movement patterns, especially in relation to gender, with men tending to flex more easily in the lumbar spine and women more so in the hips. Even so, the correctly functioning lumbar spine should still not have moved through more than 50% of its total range of flexion.

To progress forward bending, the lumbar spine continues to reduce its lordosis until the curve has just flattened. Once this has occurred, hip flexion continues the motion to the end of the range of forward bending. Ideally, the alignment at that stage should have remained balanced over the feet with the knees passively extended and with no exaggerated swaying back at the ankles, knees or hips. The hips will then be flexed by approximately 70–80 degrees, the lumbar spine just flattened and the thoracic spine forming a lengthened, gentle and smooth curve (Palastanga et al 2002, p. 58).

Variations in alignment at the end of forward bending

- Limited hip flexion causing lower thoracic spine flexion with a backwards sway of the hips, as may occur in individuals with a trunk that is long in relation to the lower limbs.

- Normal hip flexion (70–80 degrees) with a flattened lumbar spine but with excessive thoracic flexion, as may occur in individuals with impaired segmental spine mobility.
- Normal hip flexion but with the lumbar spine curve being actually reversed as opposed to only flattened, as may occur in individuals with a trunk that is short in relation to their lower limbs.
- Limited hip and spine flexion and with an exaggerated swaying back of the ankles, knees and hips, as may occur in individuals with restricted spine mobility and short or tight calf musculature, particularly gastrocnemius.
- Excessive lumbar flexion, as may occur in individuals with a flat back posture. The normal range of lumbar flexion is no more than approximately 50 degrees, and when moving into flexion from the normal lordotic position the first 20–35 degrees will only bring the lumbar spine into a neutral position, thereby allowing a further 15–20 degrees of lumbar flexion during forward bending. When an individual with a flat back posture flexes the lumbar spine from a neutral position, 50 degrees of lumbar flexion can still occur during forward bending. This could allow the lumbar spine a degree of flexion outside its safe anatomical range which might damage ligaments and other soft supporting structures at the back of the spine.

Assessment of return from forward bending

Normal
When returning from forward bending the initial part of the motion is hip extension, and then the hips and spine extend concurrently and smoothly, with the vertebral segments mobilizing in sequence to return to the upright position. A correct movement pattern demonstrates combined lumbar spine and hip extension, and, as the hips have the greatest overall range of movement, they can be seen to move the most. Once the upright position is achieved, the normal spinal curves are re-established to balance the body correctly over the lower limbs and feet (Palastanga et al 2002, p. 60).

Common faults in movement sequencing during flexion and return from flexion
During flexion:
- More than 50% of the total range of lumbar flexion occurring before the initiation of hip flexion occurs in individuals with excessive lumbar spine mobility and restricted segmental movement in other areas of the spine and who commonly have associated low back pain.
- Failure of each segment of the vertebral column to contribute its optimum range of movement can be

found in individuals with exaggerated spinal curves or where pathology or pain limits overall mobility. Some segments may then become hypermobile whilst others become correspondingly hypomobile.
- Lumbar flexion greater than 25–30 degrees at the end of forward flexion is a feature in some individuals with low back pain associated with excessive lumbar spine mobility and restricted movement in other areas of the spine.
- An exaggerated swaying back of the hips and ankles with restricted hip and spine flexion, as may be associated with calf muscle tightness and reduced spine mobility.
- Exaggerated thoracic spine flexion, limited hip flexion and bent knees towards the end of forward bending, as may be found in individuals with a trunk that is long relative to the lower limbs or in those with inflexible gluteal, hamstring or calf muscles.

During return from flexion:
- The motion initiates in, or is confined more to, the lumbar spine soon after the hips begin to extend, as may occur in individuals who have low back pain caused by extension, or who habitually use the lumbar spine rather the hips when performing everyday activities.
- During the motion the hips and ankles sway forwards markedly to reduce the load on the hips as found in those with swayback posture and weak hip flexors.
- The motion initiates in and remains confined more to the hips with minimal spine mobilization as found in individuals such as gymnasts who repeatedly hyperextend the lumbar spine and who possibly have strong, tight anterior abdominal wall muscles that may limit thoracic spine mobility.
- Failure of each segment of the vertebral column to contribute its optimum range of movement can be found in individuals with exaggerated spinal curves or where pathology or pain limits overall mobility. Some segments may then become hypermobile whilst others become correspondingly hypomobile. This can contribute to low back pain.

Assessment of lateral flexion or side bending

Normal
The total range of side bending motion may be greater than 75 degrees depending on the number of mobile thoracic spine segments involved. Movement occurs

1

most freely in the lower segments of the thoracic spine (approximately 8–10 degrees per segment) where the ribs do not restrict side bending. In the other thoracic and the lumbar spine segments side bending is comparatively restricted (approximately 6 degrees per segment) but fairly evenly distributed between them; however, at the lumbosacral junction only about 3 degrees of lateral movement is possible.

During side bending the lateral movement of the vertebral segments occurs concurrently with rotation. When the spine flexes to the right the thoracic vertebrae rotate to the right and the lumbar vertebrae rotate to the left; this coupling action results in restricted lateral flexion to the right, reducing spine mobility during rotation to the left, and vice versa.

When assessing side bending, the lumbar spine should appear to curve smoothly and gently from just above the lumbosacral junction, and this curve blends into a more obvious lateral curve along the lower thoracic spinal segments. The lower thoracic curve continues upwards as a more gentle curve formed by middle and upper spine segments so that, as the body folds over the iliac crest, the spine forms a lengthened, smooth, C-shape.

Table 1.2   Summary of ideal movement during bending forwards and returning from bending forwards

Movement sequencing into forward bending	Movement sequencing to return from forward flexion
1 The pelvis sways slightly backwards and the hips begin to flex to initiate forward bending	1 The hips extend to initiate the return from forward bending
2 The lumbar spine begins to reduce its curve to progress forward bending	2 The hips and spine extend concurrently, with the hips moving more than the spine to continue the motion
3 The lumbar spine continues to reverse its curve until it begins to flatten to and further progress forward bending	3 The hips and spine extend concurrently, with the hips moving more than the spine to continue the motion
4 The lumbar spine flattens and the movement continues as hip flexion to and further the end range of motion	4 The hips and spine extend concurrently, with the hips moving more than the spine to continue the motion
5 The lumbar spine has flattened, the hips are flexed approximately 70–80 degrees and the thoracic spine forms a lengthened, gentle curve at the end of the motion	5 The lumbar lordosis is re-established to return to a correctly aligned and balanced upright posture at the end of the motion

Table 1.3   Summary of ideal movement during spine lateral flexion and rotation*

Lateral flexion	Rotation
1 The greatest range of motion is in the lower thoracic spine. The whole thoracic spine has a total range of movement greater than 75 degrees (*the whole spine should form a smooth continuous curve*) As the spine flexes to the right the thoracic vertebrae rotate to the right	1 The movement initiates in the thoracic spine (*the movement should be cued to occur from above the waist, e.g. for 'rotate the chest'*)
2 The range of motion in the lumbar spine (L1–S1) is approximately 27 degrees. The range of motion at the lumbosacral junction is approximately 3 degrees (*the lumbar segments should form a smooth continuous curve*) As the spine flexes to the right the lumbar vertebrae rotate to the left	2 As the motion continues it should be confined more to the thoracic spine

*Based on data from Bobath (1978), Larson & Gould (1974), Sahrmann (2002), White 1969, White & Panjabi (1978).

Observable faults during the side bending motion

During side bending to the right:

- Failure of each segment of the vertebral column to contribute its optimum range of movement can be found in individuals with exaggerated spinal curves or where pathology or pain limits overall mobility. Some segments may then become hypermobile whilst others become correspondingly hypomobile. This can contribute to low back pain.
- Lumbar spine straightness as found in those individuals with very well-developed paraspinal muscles, the stiffness of which might inhibit lumbar vertebral movement, so that during side flexion the lumbar spine remains straight apart from one axis of rotation towards its base at the lumbosacral junction.
- To assess and correct this, the teacher may support the subject at the level of the iliac crest to stabilize the pelvis before side flexion and then cue for the lower ribs to be drawn in towards the waist on the side of flexion. If the above measures correct the problem, and the lumbar spine then curves during side flexion, the lumbar paraspinal muscles are probably stiff but not necessarily shortened.
- Lumbar spine straightness may also result from tensor fasciae latae tightness that may restrict lumbar spine mobility when side bending to the opposite side.
- Restricted side bending movement to one side, with comparatively free side bending to the other, can be attributed to the postural rotation of spinal segments occurring in conditions such as scoliosis. Should the spine habitually rotate to the right during side bending, its rotation to the left is limited, so restricting side bending to the right. Conversely, as the spine is already rotated to the right, side bending to the left is relatively free.

Assessment of spine rotation

The thoracic spine allows approximately 35 degrees of rotation in each direction, the lumbar spine approximately 13 degrees and at the lumbosacral junction there is normally about 5 degrees of motion, making it the most mobile single junction. The thoracic spine is where spine rotation should mostly occur, as the shape and orientation of each thoracic vertebra allow an optimum range of movement for each spinal segment. The lumbar spine and the lumbosacral junction are prone to injuries caused by excessive, repetitive rotary motions with the lumbar spine flexed, and therefore should be comparatively immobile during spine rotation (Tables 1.2 & 1.3).

Ideal alignment

Static postural observation from the side

In this position the imaginary plumb line represents the postural line of gravity and facilitates the observation of relative symmetry in the sagittal plane. Beginning with the spine, observe in relation to the plumb line the positions of the head, tips of the shoulders, hip and knee joints, and note unnecessary tension in associated muscles and soft tissue (Figs 1.13–1.15).

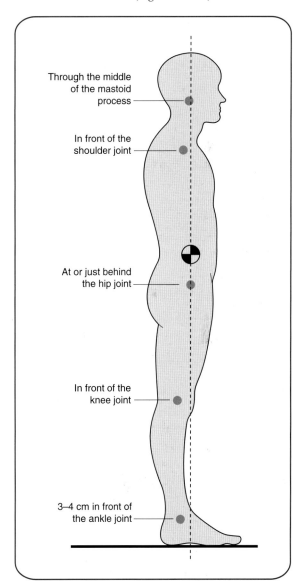

Through the middle of the mastoid process

In front of the shoulder joint

At or just behind the hip joint

In front of the knee joint

3–4 cm in front of the ankle joint

Figure 1.13 A line projected through the centre of gravity onto the floor is called the line of gravity. In the picture this line is shown on a person standing ideally upright. Some anatomical landmarks give a better indication of where the line is located. Reproduced with permission from Trew & Everett (2005).

1

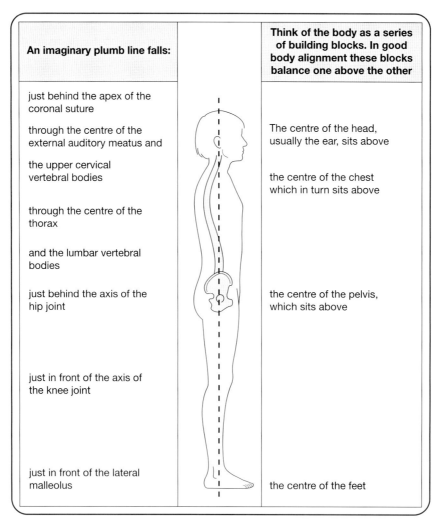

An imaginary plumb line falls:		Think of the body as a series of building blocks. In good body alignment these blocks balance one above the other
just behind the apex of the coronal suture		
through the centre of the external auditory meatus and		The centre of the head, usually the ear, sits above
the upper cervical vertebral bodies		the centre of the chest which in turn sits above
through the centre of the thorax		
and the lumbar vertebral bodies		
just behind the axis of the hip joint		the centre of the pelvis, which sits above
just in front of the axis of the knee joint		
just in front of the lateral malleolus		the centre of the feet

Figure 1.14 Ideal alignment side view: the subject stands upright in bare feet placed slightly apart to be directly below the hip joints. The feet are facing forward and parallel with each other. The knees are straight but relaxed, the arms hang freely so that the hands are just in front of the hips. The eyes look straight ahead and both hips and shoulders are unrotated. Reproduced with permission from Trew & Everett (2005).

When observing the lower legs and feet, note whether the line of gravity falls approximately through the lateral malleolus as well as the state of the knee joints and leg muscles which should appear comparatively relaxed. Also note the tone and development of the hamstring and gluteal muscles in relation to one another.

Static postural observation from behind

In this position the imaginary plumb line represents the postural line of gravity and facilitates the observation of relative symmetry in the coronal plane. Beginning with the spine, observe in relation to the plumb line the ana-

tomical landmarks including associated muscles and soft tissue (Fig. 1.16).

Next, look at the feet, noting their position and whether the medial longitudinal arch is present. With the subject standing barefoot, the feet should toe out slightly. Note the appearance of the Achilles tendons, and in particular whether they are of equal length and thickness and their development in relation to that of the calf muscles.

The calves should be observed for symmetry and over- or underdevelopment. The levels of the popliteal, gluteal and waist creases should be equal with the underlying anatomical features.

A subject demonstrating good alignment may be aware of some of the following:		For subjects with poor alignment the Pilates practitioner should consider the following questions:
The head balancing on top of the spine, the chest balancing over the pelvis and the legs	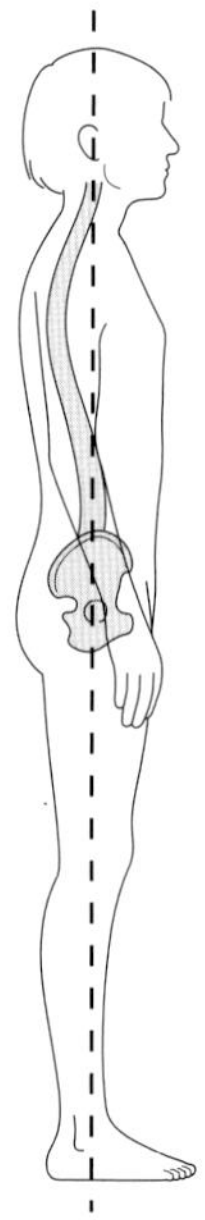	**Head:** is this forward, retracted, tilted or rotated?
The eye line is straight ahead		**Neck:** does this appear tense or shortened?
The neck is lengthened (both front and back)		
The chest is open whilst the lower ribs retain a sense of connection to the whole torso (i.e. not poking forward)		**Shoulders:** are these the same height? Do they appear rounded or unevenly rotated?
A lengthened lumbar spine, retaining a slight natural curvature, but supported by abdominal muscles, which draw back gently towards the spine		**Waist:** is this parallel with the floor?
		Hips: are these level?
The pelvis is neutral, neither arched backward nor tucked under, with a feeling of length in the groin		**Hands:** do these drop to the same height?
		Thighs: do these bow in or out?
Activitation of the inner thigh		**Legs:** is the muscle development even?
The knees relaxed but not bent		**Knees:** are these level/knocking together/bowing out/swaying back?
Weight evenly distributed between both feet		**Feet:** do they roll in/out? Are the arches dropped?

Figure 1.15 Postural alignment must be seen in regard to the force of gravity which seeks constantly to pull us down. A subject exhibiting ideal posture will feel an overall sense of well-being. With their postural muscles working effectively they will have a sense of ease and lightness and their muscle tone will be normal, unstrained and unstretched. Reproduced with permission from Trew & Everett (2005).

In an ideal subject you will observe the following:	An imaginary plumb line divides the body into two symmetrical halves, the plumb line following the line of the spine	Look for symmetry and even horizontal levels in the following surface landmarks
Head erect and balanced on top of the spine	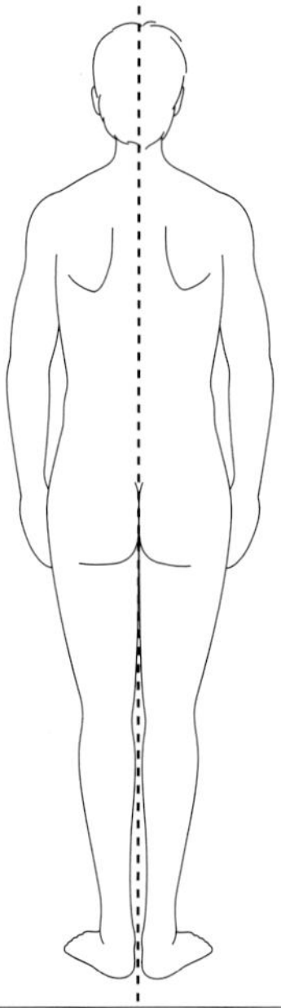	Earlobes Occipital protuberances Hairline
Shoulders level		
Scapulae lying flat against the back. The medial borders 3–4" apart with the medial and anterior angles equal		Shoulder blades Medial and inferior borders
Pelvic rims level		Waist creases
		Hips Sacroiliac joints
Hands level		Gluteal creases Greater trochanters Wrists
Legs neither bowing in nor out		
		Popliteal creases
Achilles tendons equally developed and of normal length and thickness		Calves
Feet toeing out slightly. The medial longitudinal arch is apparent		Achilles tendons
		Medial malleoli

Figure 1.16 Ideal alignment back view: the subject stands upright in bare feet placed slightly apart to be directly below the hip joints. The feet are facing forward and parallel with each other. The knees are straight but relaxed, the arms hang freely so that the hands are just in front of the hips. The eyes look straight ahead and both hips and shoulders are unrotated. Reproduced with permission from Trew & Everett (2005).

1

POSTURAL FAULTS

Easily recognized faulty postures

Sway back (Kendall et al 1993)

In sway back posture the mechanical efficiency of the posterior hip muscles is compromised by the altered relationships in their bony attachments to the pelvis and femur (Fig. 1.17). The gluteus maximus in particular is no longer able to generate its full force of contraction and the overall effect in sway back posture is an impaired control of the femoral head within the acetabulum. Over a period of time the gluteus maximus will undergo a degree of disuse atrophy thus limiting its normally dominant role in hip extension and lateral rotation, and compromising its action in the heel strike and stance phases of the gait.

Skeletal features of sway back

- Head: forward head position
- Upper thoracic spine: sways backwards with an exaggerated thoracic kyphosis
- Lumbar spine: the anterior curve is flattened, and the pelvis sways forward with a posterior tilt or in a neutral position
- Pelvis: sways forwards with a posterior pelvic tilt
- Hip joints: extended
- Knee joints: hyperextended
- Centre of gravity: shifted backwards

Gluteus maximus atrophy can usually be observed or palpated. During hip extension in the prone position, hamstring action may also be seen to precede rather than coincide with gluteus maximus activation, so that their contours no longer alter simultaneously.

Other problems
- Neck tension and cervical spine problems associated with the 'forward head' position
- Loss of spine mobility associated with impaired thoracic spine alignment and muscle function
- Shoulder problems associated with impaired scapular alignment and mobility
- Lower back problems associated with imbalance, weakness or tightness in the muscles of the anterior abdominal wall, the iliopsoas, the back extensors and the posterior hip muscles
- Hamstring problems associated with gluteus maximus atrophy and hamstring overuse
- Knee and ankle problems associated with faults in pelvic, lower limb and foot alignment, and in quadriceps and hamstring muscle performance (Table 1.4 – please turn to end of chapter).

Flat back (Kendall et al 1993)

Flat back posture may be skeletal with a flattened lumbar curve when the pelvis is in a neutral position, or it may be acquired by tilting the pelvis posteriorly and moving the hip joints into extension (Fig. 1.18). When flat back posture is acquired, the posterior pelvic tilt and reduced lordosis shift the line of gravity and body weight towards the front of the feet, impairing foot mechanics and muscle function. This weight shift also affects the tibialis anterior muscle, with an adverse effect on knee and hip function as well as ankle and foot mobility.

Skeletal features of flat back

- Head: forward head position
- Upper thoracic spine: an exaggerated thoracic kyphosis
- Lumbar spine: a markedly reduced lumbar lordosis
- Pelvis: if not in a neutral position, sways forwards with a posterior pelvic tilt (as in sway back posture)
- Hip joints: extended
- Knee joints: extended
- Body alignment: the whole body leans forward slightly so that the line of gravity is shifted towards the front of the feet

A markedly reduced lumbar curve compromises correct spinal function, and localized or overall stiffness of the vertebral column may limit flexion and/or extension.

Other problems
- Neck tension and cervical spine problems associated with the 'forward head' position
- Impaired spine function associated with poor thoracic spine alignment and spinal extensor muscle weakness; shortened anterior abdominal wall muscles; shortened or tight gluteal and/or hamstring muscles
- Shoulder problems associated with impaired pectoral girdle alignment and scapular mobility
- Lower back problems associated with lower back and gluteal muscle tightness
- Hip problems associated with impaired iliopsoas, posterior hip and quadriceps muscle performance
- Hamstring problems associated with shortened, tight hamstring muscles
- Knee and ankle problems associated with faults in pelvic, lower limb and feet alignment, and in quadriceps and hamstring muscle performance (Table 1.5 – please turn to end of chapter).

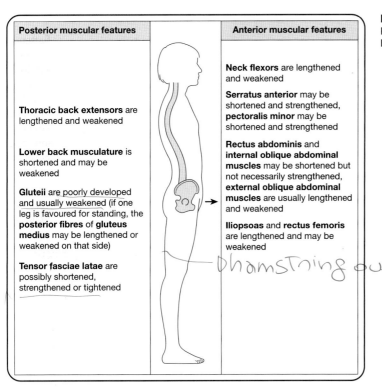

Posterior muscular features		Anterior muscular features
Thoracic back extensors are lengthened and weakened		**Neck flexors** are lengthened and weakened
Lower back musculature is shortened and may be weakened		**Serratus anterior** may be shortened and strengthened, **pectoralis minor** may be shortened and strengthened
Gluteii are poorly developed and usually weakened (if one leg is favoured for standing, the **posterior fibres** of **gluteus medius** may be lengthened or weakened on that side)		**Rectus abdominis** and **internal oblique abdominal muscles** may be shortened but not necessarily strengthened, **external oblique abdominal muscles** are usually lengthened and weakened
Tensor fasciae latae are possibly shortened, strengthened or tightened		**Iliopsoas** and **rectus femoris** are lengthened and may be weakened

(handwritten annotation) Ohamstring overuse

Figure 1.17 Posture in sway back. Reproduced with permission from Trew & Everett (2005).

1

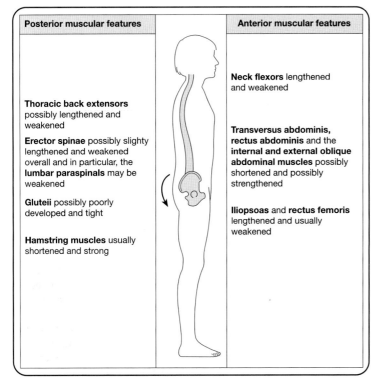

Posterior muscular features		Anterior muscular features
Thoracic back extensors possibly lengthened and weakened		**Neck flexors** lengthened and weakened
Erector spinae possibly slighty lengthened and weakened overall and in particular, the **lumbar paraspinals** may be weakened		**Transversus abdominis**, **rectus abdominis** and the **internal and external oblique abdominal muscles** possibly shortened and possibly strengthened
Gluteii possibly poorly developed and tight		**Iliopsoas** and **rectus femoris** lengthened and usually weakened
Hamstring muscles usually shortened and strong		

Figure 1.18 Posture in flat back. Reproduced with permission from Trew & Everett (2005).

Kyphosis (Kendall et al 1993)

Skeletal features of kyphosis

- Head: forward head position
- Thoracic spine: exaggerated posterior curve
- Ribs: exaggerated curvature
- Scapulae: more lateral position with the scapulae abducted, upwardly rotated and possibly winging or tilting

Kyphosis is an anatomical term referring to the primary posterior thoracic and sacral spinal curvatures, but as a clinical term it describes an exaggerated posterior thoracic curve when viewed from the side (Fig. 1.19). This exaggerated curve will alter the balance of the whole body over the lower limbs and feet and affect spine mobility by preventing each vertebral joint from moving through its optimum range of motion.

An impaired scapular alignment is also commonly associated with kyphosis, as the exaggerated curve of their ribs may abduct and upwardly rotate as well as possibly tilt the scapulae so that they wing to protrude their vertebral borders posteriorly from the ribcage. This faulty resting alignment will compromise shoulder joint function, as both scapular upward rotation during and scapular depression at the completion of shoulder flexion are affected.

Kyphosis may also be accompanied by lateral curvatures (scoliosis) that can be seen when viewed from the rear.

A kyphosis may be mobile, or it may become rigid and fixed. A mobile kyphosis is a persistently adopted kyphotic posture that has not become fixed and is therefore amenable to change. Adolescents and young adults are the most vulnerable to stresses that lead to the development of this particular postural fault, and it may also occur as a result of pregnancy and lactation, obesity, prolonged periods of inactivity or physical or depressive illness.

A fixed kyphosis, as the name implies, is not amenable to change, and it may occur as a result of trauma or the effects of underlying conditions such as osteoarthritis, osteoporosis, ankylosing spondylitis and Scheuermann's disease or it may occur in elderly people with age-related intervertebral degeneration.

Other problems
- Neck tension and cervical spine problems associated with the 'forward head' position
- Impaired spine function associated with poor thoracic spine alignment, overall spine mobility and erector spinae muscle weakness

- Shoulder problems associated with impaired scapular alignment and mobility
- Lower back problems associated with lower back or gluteal muscle tightness, faults in the muscles of the anterior abdominal wall or skeletal pathology such as intervertebral disc degeneration
- Hip problems such as degenerative disease or congenital dislocation of the hip
- Lower limb and foot problems associated with accompanying postural faults such as knock knees, flat feet, etc. (Table 1.6 – please turn to end of chapter).

Lordosis

Skeletal features of lordosis

- Lumbar spine: exaggerated anterior lumbar curve
- Sacral angle: more than 30 degrees
- Pelvis: increased anterior pelvic tilt
- Hip joints: in flexion
- Knee joints: possibly in flexion

In relaxed standing the sacral angle is approximately 30 degrees and the lumbar spine curves gently inwards to allow the pelvis to balance directly over the hip joints. This in turn allows the abdominal, spinal, posterior hip and hamstring muscles to achieve their optimum length to control the tilt of the pelvis and the balance of the whole body over the lower limbs and feet.

With a lordotic posture the sacral angle is more than 30 degrees, the anterior lumbar curve and pelvic tilt are markedly increased and the hip joints are slightly flexed (Fig. 1.20). The line of gravity is shifted towards the heels and the role individual muscles play in controlling the lumbar spine and pelvis is therefore altered to maintain the balance of the whole body over the feet and lower limbs.

The muscles of the anterior abdominal wall and the glutei, in particular the lower fibres of gluteus maximus, lengthen and weaken, and erector spinae, the iliopsoas and the hamstring muscles shorten, tighten and possibly strengthen.

These muscle faults impair hip, lumbar spine and sacroiliac function and subsequently affect vertebral column joint mobility and overall spine function. This in turn can lead to further muscle imbalances and biomechanical faults in the lower limbs and feet.

Other problems
- Hip problems due to faulty hip biomechanics as a result of shortened, tightened hip flexors,

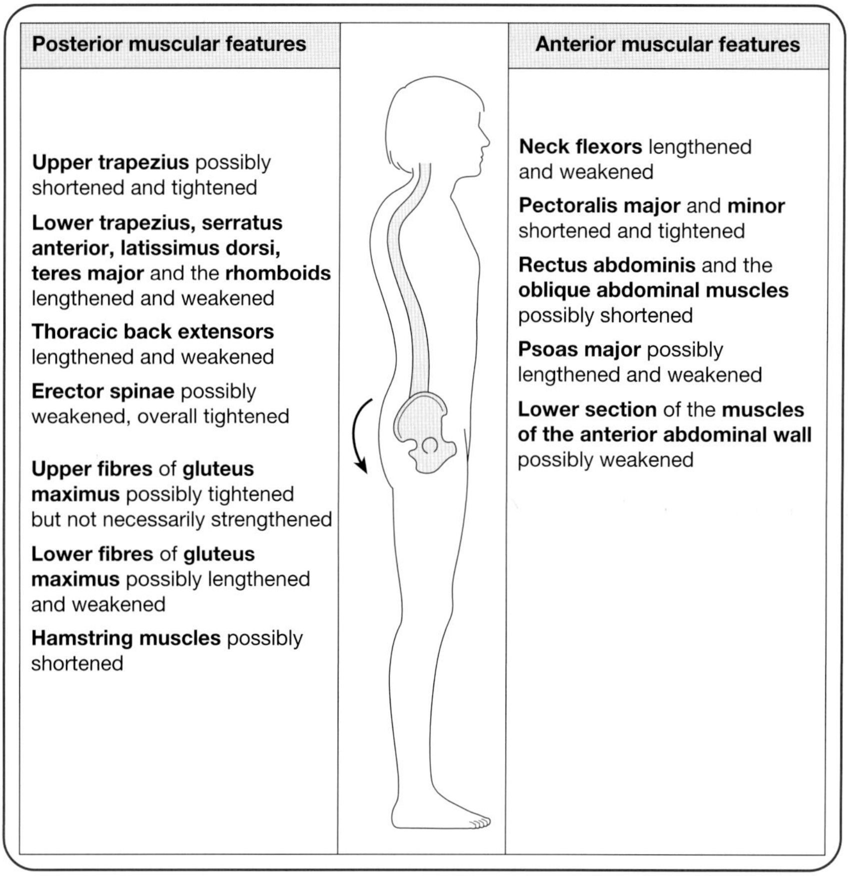

1

Posterior muscular features		**Anterior muscular features**
Upper trapezius possibly shortened and tightened		**Neck flexors** lengthened and weakened
Lower trapezius, serratus anterior, latissimus dorsi, teres major and the **rhomboids** lengthened and weakened		**Pectoralis major** and **minor** shortened and tightened
Thoracic back extensors lengthened and weakened		**Rectus abdominis** and the **oblique abdominal muscles** possibly shortened
Erector spinae possibly weakened, overall tightened		**Psoas major** possibly lengthened and weakened
Upper fibres of **gluteus maximus** possibly tightened but not necessarily strengthened		**Lower section** of the **muscles of the anterior abdominal wall** possibly weakened
Lower fibres of **gluteus maximus** possibly lengthened and weakened		
Hamstring muscles possibly shortened		

Figure 1.19 Posture in kyphosis. Reproduced with permission from Trew & Everett (2005).

degenerative disease or congenital dislocation of the hip
- Lower back problems associated with:
  - poor abdominal muscle tone and control
  - lower back or gluteal muscle tightness
  - skeletal pathology such as intervertebral disc degeneration
  - iliopsoas inflexibility and excessive tightness in the lower back muscles and ligaments
  - repetitive mobilization of the lumbosacral junction or specific lumbar vertebral joints
  - lumbar spine extension to assist hip extension as occurs with gluteal muscle weakness and hamstring muscle tightness and dominance
  - faulty lower limb, knee and foot alignments such as knock knees, flat feet, etc. (Table 1.7 – please turn to end of chapter).

Kypholordosis

With a kypholordotic posture both the posterior thoracic and the anterior lumbar curves are markedly increased, the hip joints are flexed and the knee joints are hyper-extended (Fig. 1.21). The head is the most anterior anatomical feature and the chin appears to jut forwards.

Skeletal features of kypholordosis

- Head: forward head position (it is perhaps the most forward anatomical feature)
- Thoracic spine: exaggerated posterior curve
- Ribs: exaggerated curvature
- Scapulae: a more lateral position with the scapulae abducted, upwardly rotated and possibly winging or tilting
- Lumbar spine: exaggerated anterior lumbar curve
- Sacral angle: more than 30 degrees
- Pelvis: increased anterior pelvic tilt
- Hip joints: in flexion
- Knee joints: possibly in flexion

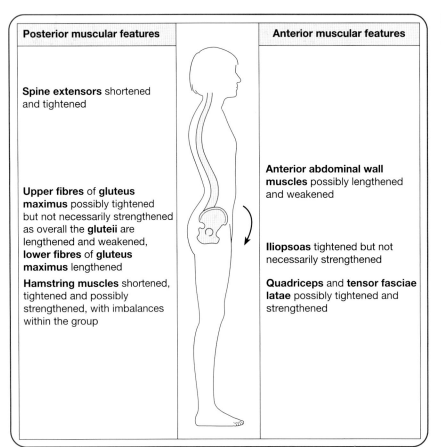

Posterior muscular features		Anterior muscular features
Spine extensors shortened and tightened		
		Anterior abdominal wall muscles possibly lengthened and weakened
Upper fibres of **gluteus maximus** possibly tightened but not necessarily strengthened as overall the **gluteii** are lengthened and weakened, **lower fibres** of **gluteus maximus** lengthened		**Iliopsoas** tightened but not necessarily strengthened
Hamstring muscles shortened, tightened and possibly strengthened, with imbalances within the group		**Quadriceps** and **tensor fasciae latae** possibly tightened and strengthened

Figure 1.20   Posture in lordosis. Reproduced with permission from Trew & Everett (2005).

The exaggerated spinal curves limit segmental spine mobility overall, but particularly impede atlanto-occipital and atlantoaxial joint mobilization in the cervical spine, thoracic spine mobilization into extension and lumbar spine mobilization into flexion.

In the upper torso the increased curvature of the ribs may impair scapular alignment, with the scapulae abducting, upwardly rotating and possibly tilting or winging to protrude their vertebral borders posteriorly from the ribcage. This will compromise shoulder joint function, as both scapular upward rotation during and scapular depression at the completion of shoulder flexion are affected.

In the lower torso the pelvis is tilted more anteriorly, the sacral angle is increased to more than 30 degrees, the hips are flexed, the knees are hyperextended and the line of gravity is shifted towards the heels. The muscles of the anterior abdominal wall and the glutei, in particular the lower fibres of gluteus maximus, lengthen and weaken, and erector spinae, the iliopsoas and the hamstring muscles shorten, tighten and possibly strengthen.

These muscle faults impair hip, lumbar spine and sacroiliac function and subsequently affect vertebral column joint mobility and overall spine function. This in turn can lead to further muscle imbalances and biomechanical faults in the lower limbs and feet.

Other problems

- Neck tension and cervical spine problems associated with the 'forward head' position
- Impaired spine function associated with poor spine alignment and mobility and erector spinae performance
- Shoulder problems associated with impaired scapular alignment and mobility
- Hip problems due to faulty hip biomechanics as a result of shortened, tightened hip flexors, degenerative disease or congenital dislocation of the hip

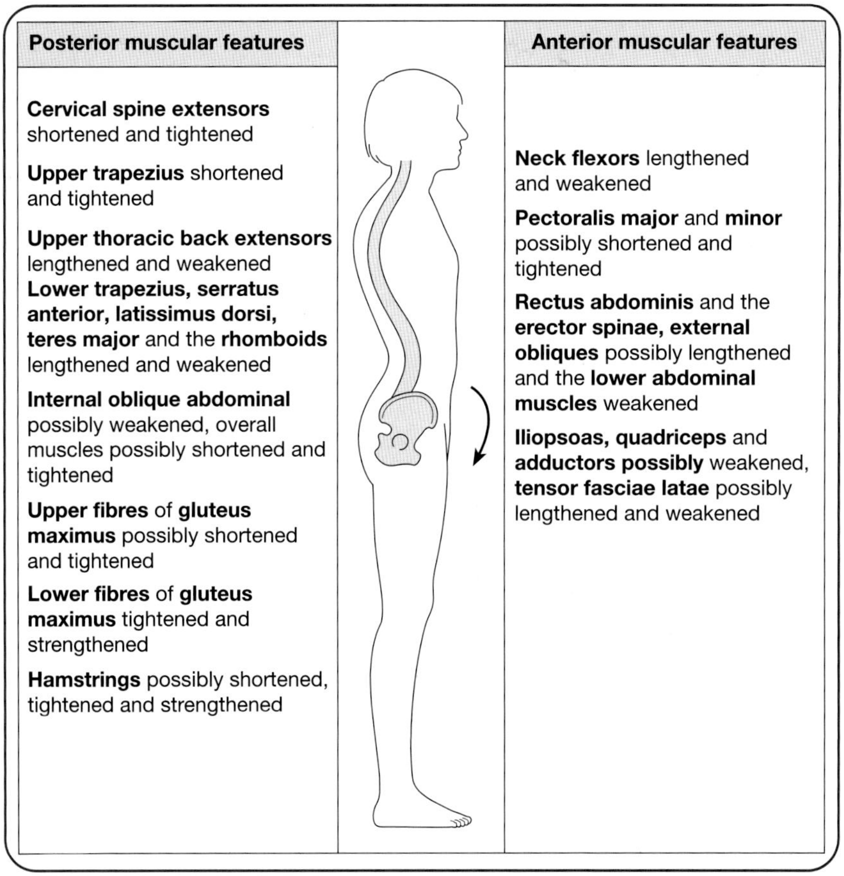

Posterior muscular features		Anterior muscular features
Cervical spine extensors shortened and tightened		
Upper trapezius shortened and tightened		**Neck flexors** lengthened and weakened
Upper thoracic back extensors lengthened and weakened		**Pectoralis major** and **minor** possibly shortened and tightened
Lower trapezius, serratus anterior, latissimus dorsi, teres major and the **rhomboids** lengthened and weakened		**Rectus abdominis** and the **erector spinae, external obliques** possibly lengthened and the **lower abdominal muscles** weakened
Internal oblique abdominal possibly weakened, overall muscles possibly shortened and tightened		**Iliopsoas, quadriceps** and **adductors possibly** weakened, **tensor fasciae latae** possibly lengthened and weakened
Upper fibres of **gluteus maximus** possibly shortened and tightened		
Lower fibres of **gluteus maximus** tightened and strengthened		
Hamstrings possibly shortened, tightened and strengthened		

Figure 1.21 Posture in kypholordosis. Reproduced with permission from Trew & Everett (2005).

- Lower back problems associated with:
  - poor abdominal muscle tone and control
  - lower back or gluteal muscle tightness
  - skeletal pathology such as intervertebral disc degeneration
  - iliopsoas inflexibility and excessive tightness in the lower back muscles and ligaments
  - the repetitive mobilization of the lumbosacral junction or specific lumbar vertebral joints
  - lumbar spine extension to assist hip extension as occurs with gluteal muscle weakness and hamstring muscle tightness and dominance
  - faulty lower limb, knee and foot alignments such as knock knees, flat feet, etc.
- Hip problems such as degenerative disease or congenital dislocation of the hip
- Lower limb and foot problems associated with accompanying postural faults such as knock knees,

flat feet, etc. (Table 1.8 – please turn to end of chapter).

Scoliosis

'Scoliosis refers to an appreciable lateral deviation from the normally straight vertical line of the spine' (White & Panjabi 1978) (Fig. 1.22).

Idiopathic scoliosis

This is commonly found in otherwise healthy children but in up to 90% of cases there is no obvious aetiology. As these children often come from families with a history of scoliosis there appears to be a strong genetic factor in its incidence.

Scoliosis involves deformities in the bones, muscles and ligaments of the spine and these may be difficult to recognize in childhood. Faults in alignment and posture tend to become more observable as the child progresses through puberty into adolescence.

Posterior muscular features		Anterior muscular features
Cervical spine extensors possibly shortened and tightened **Intercostal** and **thoracic paraspinals** on the side of the concavity probably shortened and tightened and on the side of convexity lengthened and weakened Faults in the length and muscle tone of **upper, middle** and **lower trapezius, serratus anterior, latissimus dorsi, teres major** and **rhomboids** may occur as a result of faulty pectoral girdle alignment **Lumbar paraspinals** shortened and tightened on the side of concavity and lengthened and weakened on the side of convexity **Gluteii** and **hamstring muscles** possibly lengthened and weakened on the side of lumbar spine concavity and shortened and tightened on the side of convexity **Gluteus maximus** may be weakened bilaterally	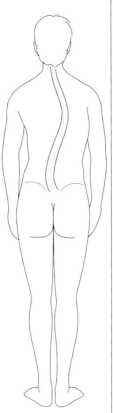	**Cervical spine flexors** possibly lengthened and weakened **Pectoralis major** and **minor** possibly shortened and tightened **Rectus abdominus** possibly shortened and tightened and other individual anterior abdominal wall muscles possibly also have faults in length and/or strength. Overall muscle lengthening to accommodate the relative lengthening of the anterior components of the spine may occur **Iliopsoas** possibly shortened but not neccessarily strengthened **Lower fibres** of **tensor fasciae latae** possibly lengthened and weakened on the side of lumbar spine concavity and strengthened and tightened on the side of convexity **Adductors** possibly weakened with imbalances between the muscles within the adductor group

Figure 1.22 Posture in scoliosis. Reproduced with permission from Trew & Everett (2005).

The bony deformities occur within and between each vertebra and cause the lateral deviations that arise within the normally straight vertical alignment of the spine. These subsequently alter the dimensions, orientation and, therefore, the mechanical effects of the associated muscles and connective tissues and so greatly compromise their normal function, making it unlikely that the use of exercise alone could permanently correct the deformity.

The lateral vertebral column deviations are usually associated with rotation of one or two vertebrae at the point of curvature, the vertebral bodies rotating towards, and the spinous processes rotating away from, the convex side of the curve. These changes alter the orientation of the ribs and sternum, depressing the ribs on the concave side. At the same time the sternum is drawn towards the convexity and the ribs are pushed posteriorly and laterally, also on the convex side. Both ribcage mobility and breathing efficiency are therefore compromised.

Skeletal features of scoliosis

- Thoracic spine: exaggerated lateral curvature in the frontal plane (should a very slight right thoracic curvature occur in an otherwise well-aligned spine, it may be associated with right handedness or the position of the aorta); reduced thoracic kyphosis
- Sternum: drawn in towards the convexity
- Ribs: bulging both laterally and posteriorly on the side of the convexity, depressed on the side of the concavity
- Shoulder girdle: orientated to adapt to the ribcage deformity with the scapulae possibly abducted, upwardly rotated, winging or tilting
- Lumbar spine: lateral curvature contralateral to the thoracic lateral curve
- Pelvis: rotated and/or tilted
- Lower limbs: length discrepancy with weight bearing more on one leg

The deformities also affect the length and tone of the trunk muscles, those on the side of the concavity tending to be contracted and those on the side of the convexity to be stretched and lacking normal tone.

Acquired scoliosis as a result of disease
This may a feature of certain diseases that alter the material properties of bone, such as rickets, or the shapes of bones, as in asymmetric spina bifida, or that affect the intrinsic structure of ligaments, as in Marfan's syndrome.

It also occurs in association with neuromuscular disorders such as cerebral palsy where faulty musculoskeletal function affects postural alignment as well as static and dynamic control and balance of the body.

Other known causes are injuries, physical disabilities and surgical procedures such as rib resection or spinal surgery.

Functional scoliosis
Functional scoliosis (acquired scoliosis as a result of postural habits or handedness) also involves alterations to the intrinsic structures and surrounding tissues of the spine. Initially these changes may be small and appear comparatively harmless, but over time permanent faults in spine structure and function will occur with associated ribcage deformities that affect breathing efficiency.

With functional scoliosis the initial or primary lateral deviation develops in the lumbar spine and is compensated by a secondary lateral deviation to the opposite side in the thoracic spine. The normal kyphotic and lordotic curves are also affected and are commonly reduced.

Corrective exercises during the early stages of functional scoliosis may appear to improve the deformity but it is doubtful that exercise alone can permanently correct scoliosis. As the tone and behaviour of the spinal muscles have been considerably affected, a vigorous and thoroughly supervised exercise programme should be carried out under the direction of a suitably qualified medical professional.

Initially the aim of an exercise programme would be to reduce the primary lateral deviation, restore the normal kyphotic and lordotic curves and improve overall spine mobility and function.

Scoliosis prevention and treatment
Whilst little is known about how to prevent scoliosis, the severity of the condition may be modified by early diagnosis. Screening programmes to identify scoliosis in childhood and educational programmes to increase awareness of adaptive influences that affect health and posture will assist prevention and early treatment.

Conventional treatments include orthotics, traction, surgery, electrical stimulation of muscles and exercise administered under the direction of a suitably qualified clinician.

Orthotics is the application of a body brace (e.g. the Milwaukee brace) to correct the deformity. This works by supporting, splinting and stretching the spine to gradually correct alignment. Exercises to improve breathing efficiency and pelvic alignment as well as other active exercises are prescribed whilst the individual is in the brace.

Traction is applied to lengthen the spinal structures over a period of approximately 3 weeks through the use of head halters and/or ankle straps. Traction is used to treat more severe cases of scoliosis and is not normally prescribed for people under the age of 20 years. Internal fixation may be by Harrington rods that are inserted surgically into the bones of the spine. Electrical muscle stimulation is achieved through electrodes implanted in erector spinae on the convex side of the curve.

Exercises
It is doubtful that exercises alone correct scoliosis. A vigorous and thoroughly supervised exercise programme may re-educate patient and muscles so as to correct a functional curve. The muscle forces that can be applied are of a relatively low amplitude and frequency and usually of short duration, and they are rarely working at a significant mechanical advantage for correction of the scoliotic spine. Exercise should not be relied upon to hold or correct a curve when used alone.

(White & Panjabi 1978)

Other problems associated with idiopathic and acquired scoliosis
- Neck tension and cervical spine problems
- Upper back problems associated with the loss of the normal thoracic kyphosis and faults in the strength and performance of the intercostals and thoracic paraspinal muscles
- Compromised respiratory function associated with the loss of the normal thoracic kyphosis
- Shoulder problems associated with impaired pectoral girdle alignment and scapular mobility
- Lower back problems associated with the pelvis being rotated and/or tilted, and faults in and between right and left iliopsoas muscles as well the right and left side of the anterior abdominal wall muscles
- Non-specific back pain possibly associated with loss of spine mobility and erector spinae muscle performance

1

- Loss of hip mobility associated with poor pelvic alignment and impaired iliopsoas, gluteal and quadriceps muscle performance
- Knee, ankle and foot problems associated with faults in pelvic, lower limb and feet alignment, and in length and performance of the quadriceps and hamstring muscles.

Exercise programmes to treat scoliosis should be thoroughly supervised and carried out under the direction of a suitably qualified clinician.

The following is only a guideline for a Pilates approach to ongoing management:

- Improve awareness of postural habits, handedness, carrying books on one shoulder, standing on one leg with one hip more to one side, etc.
- If possible, aim to re-establish the normal kyphotic and lordotic curves and correct the balance of the whole body over the lower limbs and feet.
- Improve ribcage mobility and breathing efficiency.
- Improve postural alignment, pectoral girdle alignment and erector spinae performance.
- Improve performance of the pelvic floor and transversus abdominis muscles.
- Improve performance and flexibility of rectus abdominis and the oblique abdominal muscles.
- Improve performance of the posterior hip muscles (Table 1.9 – please turn to end of chapter).

Common faults in foot placement and leg alignment

Eversion of the foot

The sole of the foot is twisted at the ankle away from the midline so that the body weight is balanced more over the medial aspect of the sole (Fig. 1.23).

Measures to help correct lower limb and foot alignment
- Enhance awareness of leg alignment.
- Centre the body weight more over the second and third toes.

Improve the performance of:
- the hip adductors
- the small, deep lateral hip rotators
- gluteus maximus during hip extension
- the lower fibres of gluteus maximus
- hamstrings
- iliopsoas and soleus, particularly during eccentric contraction
- peroneus longus, brevis and tertius
- the foot inverters – tibialis posterior and anterior
- the intrinsic foot muscles, including toe flexors and extensors.

Inversion of the foot

The sole of the foot is twisted at the ankle towards the midline so that the body weight is balanced more over the lateral aspect of the sole (Fig. 1.24).

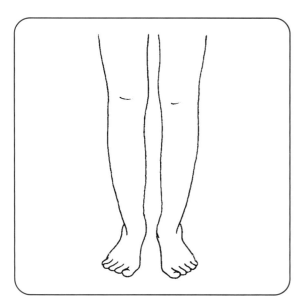

Figure 1.23

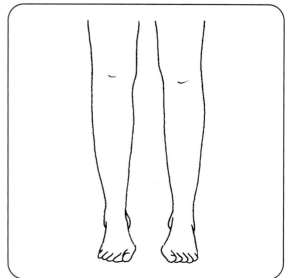

Figure 1.24

Measures to help correct lower limb and foot alignment

- Enhance awareness of leg alignment.
- Centre the body weight more over the second and third toes.

Improve the performance of:
- tensor fasciae latae, gluteus medius and minimus
- iliopsoas and soleus, particularly during eccentric contraction
- the calf muscles overall
- the intrinsic foot muscles, including toe flexors and extensors.

Medial rotation of the femur

The thighs rotate medially from a neutral alignment (Fig. 1.25).

Measures to help correct lower limb alignment
- Enhance awareness of leg alignment.
- Cue to send the knees forwards over the second and third toes during hip/knee flexion.
- Perform specific hip mobilization and strengthening exercises with the hip joints in lateral rotation.

Release excessive tightness in:
- iliopsoas
- rectus femoris
- hip adductors.

Improve the performance of:
- the pelvic floor and transversus abdominis muscles
- iliopsoas, particularly during eccentric contraction
- lower fibres of gluteus maximus
- gluteus maximus, piriformis and iliopsoas
- hip adductors
- hamstrings.

Lateral rotation of the femur

The thighs rotate laterally from a neutral alignment with pronounced outward toeing of the feet (Fig. 1.26).

Measures to help correct lower limb alignment
- Enhance awareness of leg alignment.
- Perform specific hip mobilization and strengthening exercises with the hip joints in neutral and the feet parallel to each other.

Release excessive tightness in:
- gluteus maximus, piriformis and the small, deep, lateral hip rotators
- iliopsoas
- rectus femoris
- hamstrings
- hip adductors.

Improve the performance of:
- the pelvic floor and transversus abdominis muscles
- lower fibres of gluteus maximus

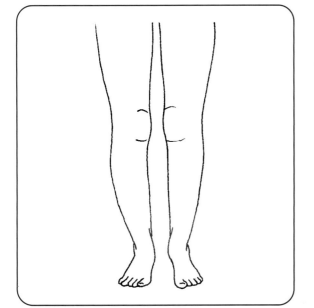

Figure 1.25

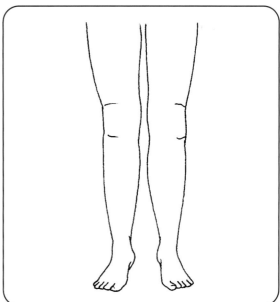

Figure 1.26

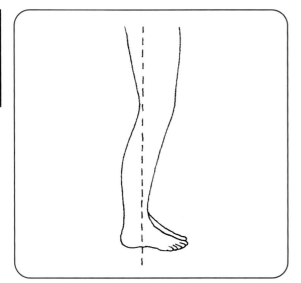

Figure 1.27

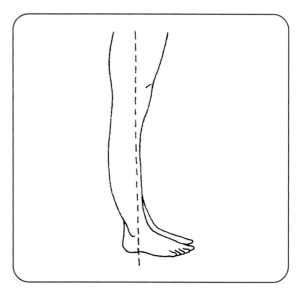

Figure 1.28

- hamstrings, iliopsoas and rectus femoris so as to act synergistically during hip flexion and extension
- gluteus medius
- gluteus minimus
- tensor fasciae latae.

Knee joints that do not fully extend

During standing the knee joints remain observably in flexion and are not able to fully extend (Fig. 1.27). Flexion increases in both knees during standing on one leg with the opposite hip flexed and its leg extended in front of the body. This limited range of knee joint extension motion is associated with lumbar spine and lower back stiffness, hamstring tightness, quadriceps weakness and reduced ankle joint mobility.

Measures to help improve knee function

- Enhance awareness of alignment during knee mobilization.
- As the knee joints move towards extension, cue for the thighs to 'pull up' and for vastus medialis to perform fully during the final 20 degrees of extension motion.

Release excessive tightness in:

- lower back muscles and ligaments
- sacroiliac area
- iliopsoas
- rectus femoris
- hamstrings – consider each muscle within the group individually

- calf muscles and soft structures at the back of the knee
- hip adductors.

Improve:

- lumbar spine mobility and stability.

Improve the performance of:

- the pelvic floor and transversus abdominis muscles
- lower fibres of gluteus maximus
- tensor fasciae latae
- iliopsoas
- quadriceps, in particular vastus medialis
- hamstrings – ensure all muscles within the group are fully involved during knee mobilization.

Knee joint hyperextension

During knee extension the knee joints push backwards (Fig. 1.28). When standing the legs form an observable backwards bow and the lumbar spine lordosis is increased to shift the body's centre of gravity back to be more over the heels. The increased range of knee joint extension is also associated with pelvic instability, weakened hamstrings and quadriceps and excessively long ligaments and muscles that are at or cross the back of the knee.

Measures to help improve knee function

When standing, cue for the knee joints to remain very slightly flexed and for the body's weight to come forwards more over the centre of the feet. Also encourage awareness of knee alignment to help prevent them being allowed to lock backwards. During knee extension, cue for the thighs to 'pull up' without pushing the knee joint backwards.

Improve:
- the alignment, balance and stability of the pelvis
- hip joint stability
- subtalar mobility.

Release excessive tightness in:
- lower back muscles and ligaments
- sacroiliac area
- upper fibres of gluteus maximus
- hip abductors
- calf muscles
- sole of the foot.

Improve the performance of:
- the pelvic floor and transversus abdominis muscles, particularly during hip mobilization
- iliopsoas
- lower fibres of gluteus maximus
- gluteus maximus and the hamstrings during hip extension
- the hamstrings and quadriceps during knee mobilization
- adductors
- gastrocnemius
- soleus
- tibialis anterior and posterior
- peroneus longus and brevis
- flexor digitorum longus
- flexor hallucis longus
- extensor digitorum longus
- extensor hallucis longus
- lumbricals.

Outwards bowing of the legs

The thighs rotate medially and bow outwards, possibly with hyperextension of the knees (Fig. 1.29). The patellae may be orientated laterally instead of centrally along the axis of the lower leg. The lumbar spine lordosis is possibly increased, shifting the body's centre of gravity back to be more over the heels.

Measures to help improve knee function

When standing, cue for the knee joints to remain very slightly flexed and for the body's weight to come in more over the medial aspect of the feet and through the second and third toes. Also encourage awareness of knee alignment to help prevent them being allowed to lock backwards.

Improve:
- the alignment, balance and stability of the pelvis
- hip lateral rotation
- subtalar mobility.

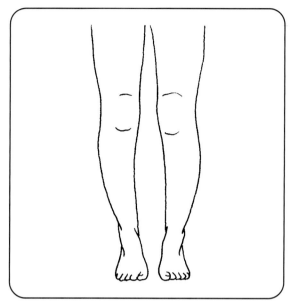

Figure 1.29

Release excessive tightness in:
- lower back muscles and ligaments
- sacroiliac area
- upper fibres of gluteus maximus
- hip abductors
- calf muscles
- sole of the foot.

Improve the performance of:
- the pelvic floor and transversus abdominis muscles, particularly during hip mobilization
- iliopsoas
- lower fibres of gluteus maximus
- gluteus maximus, piriformis, deep rotators and iliopsoas together with the adductors during hip lateral rotation
- hamstrings – address imbalances within the group
- gastrocnemius
- soleus
- tibialis anterior
- peroneus longus and brevis
- flexor digitorum longus
- flexor hallucis longus
- extensor digitorum longus
- extensor hallucis longus
- lumbricals.

The knees are orientated medially from a neutral position

The knees knock together when the feet are placed hip distance apart (Fig. 1.30). The body's weight is more over the medial aspect of the feet.

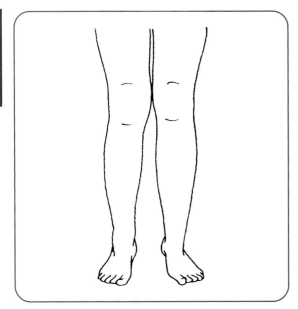

Figure 1.30

Measures to help improve knee function

When standing, encourage awareness of knee alignment. Cue for the knee joints to remain very slightly flexed, the knees to align with the second and third toes and for the lateral borders of the feet to make firm contact with the ground.

Improve:
- the alignment, balance and stability of the pelvis
- hip lateral rotation
- subtalar mobility.

Release excessive tightness in:
- lower back muscles and ligaments
- sacroiliac area
- posterior hip muscles
- tensor fasciae latae
- vastus lateralis
- calf muscles
- the peronei
- sole of the foot.

Improve the performance of:
- the pelvic floor and transversus abdominis muscles, particularly during hip mobilization
- gluteus maximus, piriformis, deep rotators and iliopsoas together with the adductors during hip lateral rotation
- adductors
- quadriceps, especially vastus medialis
- hamstrings – address imbalances within the group

- gastrocnemius
- soleus
- tibialis anterior and posterior
- flexor digitorum longus
- flexor hallucis longus
- extensor digitorum longus
- extensor hallucis longus
- lumbricals.

USEFUL TESTS

Gait assessment

Normal gait

Gait (walking) is a complex process comprising separate, sequential activities that alternately move the right and left lower limbs progressively in the same direction.

For easier understanding, gait can be seen as a cycle of events that begins when the heel of the foot strikes the ground and ends when the opposite leg swings through in preparation for the other heel strike.

Heel strike during a normal gait pattern

This is when the leading leg makes initial contact with the ground whilst the following leg is still in contact with the ground, so increasing the body's base of support. This contributes to the body's achieving its lowest centre of gravity within the gait cycle and therefore being its most stable state.

Moving into the stance phase

This occurs as the leading leg becomes the supporting leg for the whole of the body's weight. The foot swiftly moves from dorsiflexion towards plantarflexion until both the forefoot and heel are in contact with the ground and the foot and leg can receive the body's weight.

Middle-stance phase

The whole of the body's weight continues to move forwards to balance over the supporting leg whilst the following leg leaves the ground and swings through. This contributes to the body's achieving its least stable state within the gait cycle, as its base of support is reduced whilst its centre of gravity is at its highest as it moves from behind to in front of the supporting foot During the stance phase the hip abductors of the supporting limb contract concentrically to maintain the pelvis level as the leg moves through the middle of its swing.

1

End of the stance phase moving into the propulsive phase of gait

This occurs as successive events propel the body forwards towards the next heel strike. With the body continuing to move forwards, the heel of the supporting foot lifts from the ground, initiating plantarflexion that progresses until the forefoot and toes lift from the ground sequentially. During the latter part of this phase the calf muscles act so that the forefoot and toes push against the ground to propel the body forwards.

Swing phase

After the following leg has progressed through the propulsive gait phase, its foot continues to clear the ground, allowing it to swing through and become the leading leg ready for the next heel strike.

The swing phase comprises the acceleration, mid-swing and deceleration components.

During acceleration the hip and plantarflexors are assisted by momentum and gravity as they act to accelerate the forward motion of the swinging leg. To allow the toes of the swinging foot to clear the ground, the ankle moves the foot swiftly towards dorsiflexion.

The mid-swing component occurs simultaneously with the mid-stance phase and is when the body is least stable. To maintain the toes sufficiently clear of the ground, both the hip and knee joints remain in flexion although the foot may have lowered slightly towards plantarflexion.

The hip abductors on the supporting leg, already contracted to maintain the pelvis level for the mid-swing component, then act eccentrically to control the lowering of the pelvis towards the swinging leg side.

During deceleration the hip joint remains in flexion as the knee extends and the ankle joint dorsiflexes ready for the next heel strike. Knee extension occurs not as a result of quadriceps action but as a consequence of the momentum generated by the forward motion of the leg. It is then resolved towards the end of deceleration by eccentric hamstring action (Fig. 1.31).

During walking, hip extension is accompanied by lumbar spine rotation towards the extending leg and this is reversed as the leg swings through to take the next step. To allow the head to keep facing forwards there are also compensatory thoracic and cervical spine motions away from the side of lumbar rotation. Also during walking each shoulder joint normally flexes as the opposite hip flexes to bring about a swinging motion of the arms that accompanies the thoracic spine rotation. Without this unconscious and easy arm motion walking is stiff and more laborious.

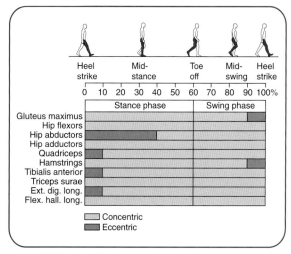

Figure 1.31 Muscle activity, as indicated by EMG, is variable between subjects. It also varies with velocity and the faster the velocity, the more muscle input will be required. This figure shows the type and duration of muscle activity that might be expected in moderate velocity walking. Ext. dig. long., extensor digitorum longus; flex. hall. long., flexor hallucis longus. Reproduced with permission from Trew & Everett (2005).

In addition, when observing gait, noting the speed of walking, as well as an individual's ability to readily alter that speed, can give an indication of joint stiffness, muscle weakness and pain. In slow walking the number of steps is around 40–50 steps per minute and in moderate walking 110 steps per minute. The former would normally be able to be progressed towards faster walking and running as required but this would be affected by musculoskeletal disease and pain (Fig. 1.32).

To help assess the speed of walking, consider the following: stride length – the distance between successive heel strikes with the same foot; step length – the distance between successive heel strikes with opposite feet; step width – the distance maintained between the legs and feet.

Also observe whether the feet toe in or out with each step as this relates mainly to hip joint mobility and may also indicate abnormal rotation between the tibia and fibula. It is more common for the feet to turn slightly outwards at about a 30-degree angle from a facing forwards direction.

Abnormal or pathological gait

Faulty gait patterns may be noticed when patrons initially enter the exercise studio and may be confirmed during a more detailed assessment by a suitably qualified person such as a physiotherapist or podiatrist.

However, it is important for all exercise teachers to be able to recognize the more obvious abnormal

1

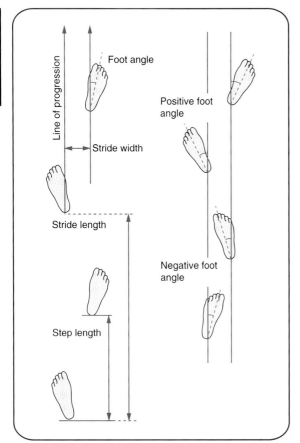

Figure 1.32 Characteristics of gait that can be measured from footprints. Reproduced with permission from Trew & Everett (2005).

gait patterns and to know when exercise would be inappropriate.

Trendelenburg gait

Hip abductor weakness is commonly associated with a pathological gait as the abductors control pelvic stability during walking. During the stance phase of gait they act on the supporting side to maintain the hips level with each other and they then control the slight dropping of the hip on the unsupported side as the leg swings through.

However, weakened or lengthened abductors may allow the hip on the unsupported side to drop during the stance phase, thus producing early sideways tilting. This particular feature is associated with a 'Trendelenburg gait' and is easily recognized, particularly in more severe cases. There may also be an accompanying lateral flexion of the whole trunk towards the supporting leg

that shifts the body's centre of gravity more over the supporting leg, thus helping to prevent the pelvic tilting and physical discomfort.

High stepping gait

Neurological disorders that involve the lower limb and foot will also affect normal gait patterns. For example, should nerve damage prevent or markedly reduce dorsiflexion, the toes could not clear the ground as the unsupported leg swings through. The hip and knee must therefore flex further to keep the foot away from the ground (a high stepping action). Such cases can be identified by the toes making contact with the ground first and the heel slapping down quickly afterwards.

Other causes for abnormal gait patterns

Injuries involving back, hip, knee, ankle or foot pain will also affect gait as strategies to avoid weight bearing on painful joints occurs subconsciously. Even a temporary abnormal gait pattern can lead to ongoing poor posture with particular associated faults in muscle function and this should be considered when planning exercise programmes.

Ongoing bony changes that continue to reduce joint mobility as in hallux valgus of the great toe, chondromalacia of the patella or arthritis of the hip will lead to global changes in musculoskeletal function and therefore gait. Here, local as well as overall muscle function should be optimized to allay more progressive deterioration.

Assessment of prone hip extension for related muscle imbalances

Hamstring recruitment dominance during hip extension

Normal function

Gluteus maximus and the hamstring muscles contract simultaneously to extend the hip by approximately 10 degrees whilst the lumbar spine extends slightly.

Abnormal function

The change in the contour of the contracting gluteus maximus muscle occurs after the initiation of hip extension; should this occur, it is an indication of dominant hamstring recruitment over that of gluteus maximus.

Assessment of iliopsoas muscle length and iliotibial band flexibility

Normal function

The hip extends by approximately 10 degrees whilst the lumbar spine extends slightly.

Abnormal function

The hip extends by only approximately 5 degrees and is accompanied by normal or excessive lumbar spine extension; this occurs when the iliopsoas and rectus femoris muscles are shortened and stiff and there is possibly also insufficient abdominal muscle control over lumbar spine stability.

Assessment of abdominal muscle control over lumbar spine stability

Normal function

As the hip achieves approximately 10 degrees of extension the lumbar spine extends only very slightly.

Abnormal function

Hip extension is accompanied by an anterior pelvic tilt and excessive lumbar spine extension; this occurs when there is insufficient abdominal muscle control over lumbar spine stability and/or stiffness in rectus femoris and iliopsoas.

Assessment of femoral glide

Normal function

The lumbar spine extends slightly whilst the axis of the hip joint remains stable as the hip extends by approximately 10 degrees.

Abnormal function

The greater trochanter moves anteriorly during hip extension; this occurs when the anterior joint capsule is overstretched and is commonly associated with dominant hamstring recruitment over that of gluteus maximus and with shortness and tightness of tensor fasciae latae.

Assessment of hip flexor length and strength (seated hip flexion test)

Normal function

During sitting the lumbar spine and pelvis remain in a neutral position when the hip is flexed to 120 degrees against maximum resistance.

Abnormal function

During sitting the lumbar spine and pelvis lose their stable, neutral position when the hip is flexed against resistance; should this occur within a range of up to 105 degrees of hip flexion, the iliopsoas muscle is weakened.

Assessment of iliopsoas muscle function

Whilst maintaining the correct sitting position, resistance is tolerated at 105–110 degrees of hip flexion but not at 120 degrees of hip flexion; should this occur the iliopsoas muscle is lengthened but not necessarily weakened.

Thomas test (Sahrmann 2002)

The Thomas test is performed with the subject lying supine at the end of a table so that one leg can drop over the edge (Fig. 1.33). The other knee is gently held over the abdomen and the back is relaxed with the lumbar spine flattened. The thigh of the extended leg rests on the table, its femur aligned with the axis of its hip joint. The hip joint remains neutral in abduction, adduction and rotation whilst it extends 10 degrees. The knee joint is able to flex approximately 80 degrees whilst the tibia neither abducts nor rotates.

Assessment of abdominal muscle function

Normal function

The lumbar spine remains in neutral when the hip is extended 10 degrees.

Abnormal function

Pelvic tilting or rotation accompanies hip extension. This may indicate intrinsic abdominal muscle weakness with insufficient abdominal muscle control over lumbar spine stability or lumbar spine hypermobility: should pelvic tilting occur, pelvic floor and transversus abdominis muscle function may be inadequate; should pelvic rotation occur there might be insufficient oblique muscle control.

Assessment of hip joint function

Normal function

The hip joint remains neutral in abduction, adduction and rotation whilst it extends 10 degrees and the knee

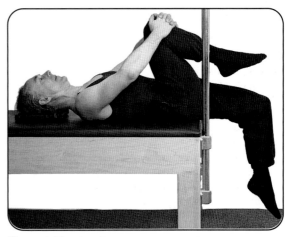

Figure 1.33 The 'Thomas test'.

1

joint is able to flex approximately 80 degrees whilst the tibia neither abducts nor rotates.

Abnormal function

- As the hip extends it abducts and the knee extends passively; this occurs when the rectus femoris muscle is shortened.
- Hip extension is restricted, and the hip abducts whilst the knee extends; this occurs when the iliopsoas muscle is shortened
- Hip extension is increased by medially rotating and/or abducting the hip; this occurs when the tensor fasciae latae muscle is shortened and tight.
- Hip extension comprises an anterior glide of the femoral head; this occurs when the anterior joint capsule is stretched and the iliopsoas muscle is lengthened and weakened.

Assessment of knee joint function

Normal function

The knee joint flexes relatively easily to 80 degrees whilst the tibia neither abducts nor rotates.

Abnormal function

- Hip extension involves lateral rotation of the tibia; this occurs when the tensor fasciae latae muscle is shortened and the iliotibial band is tight.
- Hip extension involves a lateral shift of the tibia; this occurs when the iliotibial band is shortened and tight.
- Hip extension with adduction brings about discomfort or pain in the knee; this occurs when a shortened tensor fasciae latae muscle and tight iliotibial band cause a lateral shift of the patella.

Assessment of lumbar spine stability and function (supine test with bilateral hip/knee extension)

Normal function

Whilst lying supine the lumbar spine and pelvis remain in neutral when the hips and knees fully extend.

Abnormal function

- The lumbar spine extends and the pelvis tilts anteriorly; this can occur when the abdominal muscles are underperforming and the hip flexors are possibly shortened and tightened. Should back pain or discomfort brought about by the assessment be relieved by simultaneous hip and knee flexion, this would confirm poor abdominal and hip flexor muscle performance.
- The lumbar spine flexes and the pelvis tilts posteriorly; this can occur when the back extensors

are lengthened and the abdominal muscles are shortened. Should back pain or discomfort that occurs during the assessment be relieved by simultaneous hip and knee flexion, this would confirm that the back extensors are lengthened and the abdominal muscles are shortened.

Assessment of lumbar spine, pelvis and hip and lower limb alignment and stability (standing on one leg test)

Normal function

The pelvis is in neutral with the anterior superior iliac spines lying in the same horizontal plane (Fig. 1.34). The spine is lengthened with the normal spinal curves intact, the upper body balances over the pelvis and the pelvis balances over the supporting leg and foot. The supporting leg is correctly aligned so that the femur and the knee are neutral in rotation whilst the tibia maintains constant relationships with both femur and ankle.

Abnormal function

- The trunk bends sideways towards the supporting leg; this feature is associated with hip adductor weakness on the side of the supporting leg.

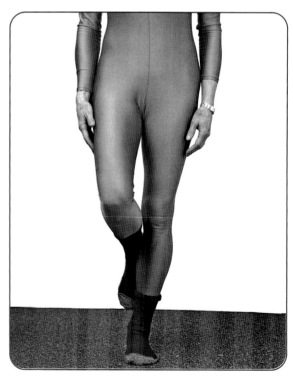

Figure 1.34 Standing on one leg.

- The pelvis rotates downwards away from the supporting leg; this feature is associated with hip adductor weakness on the side of the supporting leg.
- The pelvis rotates downwards towards the supporting leg; this feature is associated with lengthened lateral hip rotator and shortened medial hip rotator muscles.
- The femur of the supporting leg rotates medially; this feature is associated with lengthened and weakened lateral hip rotator muscles.
- The femur is correctly aligned whilst the knee rotates; this feature is associated with abnormal rotational forces between the tibia and femur.
- The femur and tibia maintain a constant relationship whilst the ankle pronates, everting the foot; this feature is associated with underlying pathology such as a shortened peroneus brevis muscle.

Assessment of resting scapular alignment

Normal alignment
The scapulae are applied to the posterior aspect of the thorax overlying the second to seventh thoracic vertebrae with their vertebral borders parallel and approximately 7.5 cm from the midline (Figs 1.35–1.37). To

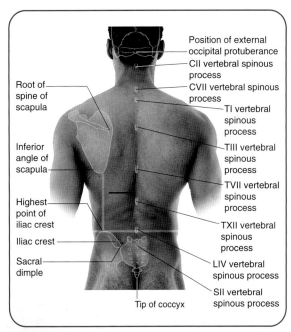

Figure 1.35 The back with the positions of vertebral spinous processes and associated structures indicated in a man. Reproduced with permission from *Gray's Anatomy for Students* (2005).

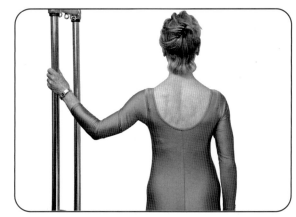

Figure 1.36

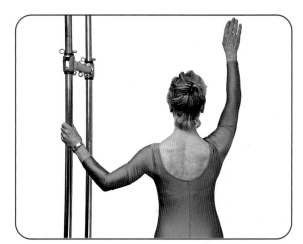

Figure 1.37

accommodate the curvature of the ribs they must rotate forwards by approximately 30 degrees.

Abnormal alignment
- The scapula wings so that the vertebral border projects away from the posterior aspect of the thorax; this may occur with the loss of the normal thoracic kyphosis as seen in some ballet dancers and yoga practitioners or in other postural faults such as scoliosis and exaggerated thoracic kyphosis. It is commonly associated with serratus anterior weakness but may also be an indication of other pectoral girdle muscle imbalances brought about by strenuous upper body activities. In these latter cases the whole scapula may have lost contact with the posterior aspect of the thorax.
- The scapula is tilted so that its inferior border projects away from the ribcage; this is most commonly associated with a shortened, tightened pectoralis minor muscle but may also be an

1

indication of other faults in the upper arm and pectoral girdle muscles.

■ The scapula is downwardly rotated; this is when the scapula's medial border lies obliquely rather than parallel to the vertebral column, orientating the scapula's inferior angle more medially. This is a feature seen in individuals with an exaggerated thoracic kyphosis and has associated faults in muscles such as shortened, tightened levator scapulae and rhomboid muscles and lengthened, weakened upper fibres of trapezius and serratus anterior.

■ The scapula is upwardly rotated; this is when the scapula's medial border lies obliquely rather than parallel to the vertebral column, orientating the scapula's inferior angle more laterally. This may also be a feature associated with an exaggerated thoracic kyphosis, as the exaggerated curve of the ribs may abduct and upwardly rotate, as well as tilt, the scapulae. Shortening and tightening of the upper fibres of trapezius is a probable fault when the scapulae are upwardly rotated.

■ The scapulae are adducted; this is when they are drawn towards each other so that their vertebral borders are less than 15 cm apart. This may be associated with shortening and tightening of the rhomboids and the middle and lower fibres of trapezius, and lengthening and weakening of serratus anterior.

■ The scapulae are abducted; this is when their medial borders lie more than 15 cm away from each other. Therefore to accommodate the shape of the ribs they also rotate further than 30 degrees anterior to the frontal plane and orientate the glenoid fossa more anteriorly. The upper arm may also appear to be medially rotated but this apparent alignment is due to the rounded shoulder position rather than rotation of the glenohumeral joint itself. This may be a feature seen in individuals with an exaggerated thoracic kyphosis or in those who regularly perform strenuous upper body activities. Normally the main faults in muscles would be shortness and tightness in serratus anterior and pectoralis major.

■ The scapulae are elevated so that the neck appears shortened; this refers to the elevation of the whole scapula when the upper fibres of trapezius are markedly shortened – the elevation of the superior angle but not the acromion process of the scapula when levator scapulae may be shortened. In addition, should elevation be accompanied by apparent adduction, there may be shortness and tightness of the upper fibres of

trapezius and levator scapulae as well as the rhomboids.

■ The scapulae are depressed so that the neck appears lengthened; this is when the scapulae are orientated on the posterior aspect of the thorax overlying vertebrae below the second to seventh thoracic vertebrae. Associated faults in muscles may be a lengthening of the upper fibres of trapezius, together with shortening and/or strengthening of latissimus dorsi and pectoralis major.

Assessment of shoulder joint range of motion

Normal function
The shoulder joint flexes through a range of 180 degrees whilst the inferior angle of the scapula upwardly rotates through a range of 60 degrees to approximately the mid axillary line. During this motion the spine remains well aligned and stable, the pectoral girdle remains correctly orientated over the ribs with relatively little shoulder elevation or depression, and the scapula abducts no more than 3 cm beyond the posterolateral border of the ribcage. At the end of the 180 degrees of shoulder joint motion the scapula depresses.

Abnormal function
■ Loss of spine alignment and stability; this is associated with insufficient awareness and/or core control when independently mobilizing the upper limbs.

■ The abdominal muscles sag and the lumbar spine extends; these features are associated with insufficient strength within or control over the muscles of the pelvic floor, anterior abdominal wall and back when independently mobilizing the upper limbs.

■ The pectoral girdle elevates during shoulder flexion; this occurs when the upper fibres of trapezius are overactive and dominant over the middle and lower fibres of trapezius, and other associated pectoral girdle muscles are comparatively weak.

■ The shoulder joint flexes through less than 180 degrees of range of motion; this is associated with shortening and stiffening of the pectoral muscles, shortening of latissimus dorsi and weakness of the shoulder flexors, pectoralis major and the anterior fibres of the deltoid. Painful shoulder pathology may also limit range of flexion motion.

■ The inferior angle of the scapula does not upwardly rotate and abduct to reach approximately the mid axillary line; this is associated with shortened, stiffened rhomboids and lengthened serratus anterior muscles.

- Scapular rotation is less than 60 degrees; this is associated with shortened, tightened rhomboid muscles and lengthened, underperforming serratus anterior and trapezius muscles.
- The scapula does not depress at the end of shoulder flexion motion; this occurs when pectoralis minor is shortened and tightened and the lower fibres of trapezius are lengthened and weakened.

Test for pectoral girdle alignment and torso stability when weight bearing through the upper extremities

Normal function

The body is in a prone position, raised away from the floor and supported by the upper and lower limbs (Fig. 1.38). The hands are in line with the glenohumeral joint and the elbow joints are extended. The little fingers press lightly into the floor to assist engagement of the pectoral girdle stabilizing muscles. The knees are extended and the legs reach behind the body. The toes are dorsiflexed and the body's weight is balanced between the flexed toes and the hands. The spine is lengthened and normal spinal curves are intact, with the back of the neck lengthened and the crown of the head reaching forward. The gaze is between the thumbs.

The upper body and pectoral girdle are correctly aligned with the scapulae lying flat over the ribs, adducting, winging, tilting or abducting no more than 4 cm beyond the posterolateral borders of the ribcage.

Abnormal function

- The scapulae excessively adduct, wing, tilt or excessively abduct: should the scapula adduct, wing or tilt, this is associated with serratus anterior weakness and underperformance; should the scapula abduct more than 3 cm beyond the posterolateral borders of the ribcage, serratus

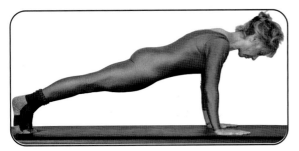

Figure 1.38

anterior is shortened and dominant over lengthened and weakened rhomboid and trapezius muscles.

- The abdominal muscles sag and the lumbar spine extends; these features are associated with insufficient strength within, or control over, the muscles of the pelvic floor, anterior abdominal wall and back.
- Pain occurs in the wrists, elbows or shoulder; this could be associated with muscle imbalances or other underlying pathology such as rheumatoid arthritis.

Assessment of abdominal muscle tone in standing

Normal function

When standing upright the abdomen is flat and the abdominal muscles are their normal length and relatively relaxed.

Abnormal function

- The lumbar lordosis is exaggerated and the abdomen sags; this occurs when the muscle tone of the anterior abdominal wall is poor overall.
- The anterior abdominal wall below the umbilicus lacks tone in comparison with the rest of the abdomen, and during a deep abdominal contraction that narrows and tightens the waist this area remains comparatively relaxed; this can occur in individuals who regularly train the rectus abdominis and oblique abdominal muscles without addressing faults in transversus abdominis performance.
- The thoracic kyphosis is exaggerated and the chest is depressed; this may be associated with one of the common faulty postures such as kypholordosis or be due to training the rectus abdominis rather than the transversus abdominis and oblique abdominal muscles. In the latter the increase in the thoracic kyphosis may be slight but the recti noticeably bulge forwards, particularly during abdominal exercises such as 'sit-ups'.

Assessment of dynamic lower limb and spine alignment and function in standing during knee flexion and extension with the feet parallel and in line with the hip joints (Trew & Everett 2005)

Normal function

- *During flexion*: the knees flex a minimum of 45 degrees and the heels maintain contact with the floor whilst the longitudinal arch of the foot is

1

reduced (Fig. 1.39). As the knees bend they move directly forwards to align approximately with the second and third toes. The soft tissues at the front of the ankle appear comparatively relaxed without overactivity in either tibialis anterior or extensor digitorum longus.

■ *During extension*: as the *hips* extend, the movement is confined to the hip joints so the spine remains stable with its normal curves intact (Fig. 1.40). As the *knees* extend, the patellae move upwards along the axis of the lower leg and during the final 20 degrees of extension vastus medialis acts strongly to pull the patellae medially so as to allow the medial femoral condyles to slide posterolaterally on the medial tibial condyles, thus bringing the knee joint structures into perfect alignment.

■ *At the end of extension*: the thigh muscles including vastus medialis on the inferior medial aspect of the thigh are fully pulled up and the knees neither push nor lock backwards.

Abnormal function

■ During flexion the knees orientate medially from a neutral position and the body's weight shifts towards the medial aspect of the feet; this occurs when posterior hip muscle function, and in particular that of the lateral hip rotator muscles, is impaired, and when ankle and subtalar joint mobility as well as overall foot mobility and function are compromised, as in hallux valgus.

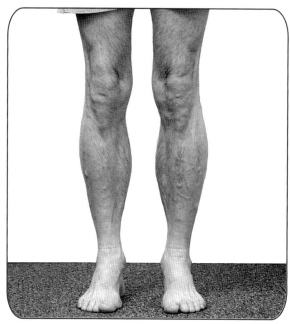

Figure 1.40

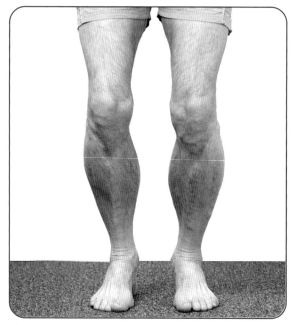

Figure 1.39

Associated features are tightness in soft tissue structures of the lower back, the posterior hip, the lateral aspects of the thigh and lower leg, and the sole of the foot, and impaired performance of the hip adductors, knee flexors and extensors, as well gastrocnemius, soleus, tibialis anterior and posterior, flexor digitorum longus, flexor hallucis longus, extensor digitorum longus, extensor hallucis longus and the lumbricals. Function may be further impaired as lack of awareness and poor proprioception allow poor postural habits to progress.

■ During extension the hips rotate medially and the knee joints push backwards to form an observable backwards bow. At the same time the lumbar lordosis is increased to shift the body's centre of gravity to move back over the heels. This increased range of knee joint extension is specifically associated with pelvic instability, weakened lateral hip rotators, hamstrings and quadriceps, and ligaments and muscles at, or crossing, the back of the knee that are excessively long.

It also commonly involves tightness in soft tissue structures of the lower back and upper fibres of gluteus maximus, the hip abductors, the calf muscles and the sole of the foot.

A lack of awareness or poor proprioception may help to further impair knee function as it allows the development of the unconscious habit of pushing back and locking the knee joints.

- As the knees extend, the patella tracks more obliquely and laterally; this is associated with quadriceps overloading and tensor fasciae latae tightness as seen in keen leisure sports participants, runners, etc. It is also associated with vastus medialis weakness and knee pathology that prevents the knee joint fully extending.

Assessment of spine mobility and muscle action from supine to the upright sitting position

Normal function

Starting position – lying supine with the legs extended and the arms by the sides of the body. To initiate flexion the head nods forwards on top of the spine (cranioatlantal flexion) and this progresses into sequential flexion of the cervical and thoracic vertebrae as the pelvis tilts posteriorly, flattening the lumbar spine. At the same time the shoulder joints are flexed approximately 90 degrees, reaching the arms forwards (Fig. 1.41). The thoracic spine and lumbar spine continue to flex until their combined actions reach the end range of flexion and at this point the hips are flexed to approximately 80 degrees. The rest of the motion into the upright sitting position is hip flexion and spine extension. In the sitting position the pectoral girdle is correctly aligned and the arms reach forwards (Fig. 1.42).

During flexion the iliopsoas and abdominal muscles act together, helping to prevent rectus abdominis hyperactivity (i.e. they bulge anteriorly) and assisting sequential mobilization of the vertebral column.

Abnormal function

- As the cervical and thoracic spine flex, the lumbar lordosis remains intact or reduces insufficiently to flatten the lumbar spine; this occurs when the iliopsoas muscle is shortened and tight or there is

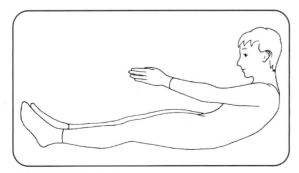

Figure 1.41

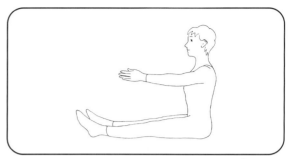

Figure 1.42

underlying spine pathology restricting lumbar vertebral column mobility.

- Thoracic and lumbar flexion occur simultaneously but overall flexion is limited; this may be due to oblique abdominal muscle weakness or underlying spine pathology that restricts vertebral column mobility.
- The vertebrae mobilize sequentially through a full range of flexion but there is insufficient strength to continue moving towards the sitting position; iliopsoas and/or abdominal muscle strength is insufficient.
- The vertebrae mobilize sequentially but with lumbar spine flexion the recti bulge anteriorly; this indicates rectus abdominis dominance over transversus abdominis and the oblique abdominal muscles.
- The vertebrae do not mobilize in sequence and the abdominal muscles bulge; this is commonly associated with malfunction of iliopsoas and the oblique abdominal muscles and may also be due to underlying spine pathology that restricts vertebral column mobility.

Return from the sitting position

Normal function

To initiate this motion the pelvis tilts posteriorly and this is followed by cranioatlantal flexion as lumbar flexion progresses. The posterior pelvic tilt is maintained and overall flexion of the spine increases as the vertebrae continue to mobilize in sequence. This allows the lumbar spine to flatten and make contact with the floor as the thoracic and lumbar vertebrae move through flexion and then extension towards the supine position (Fig. 1.43).

At the end of the movement the posterior pelvic tilt is reduced and reversed so that the pelvis achieves a neutral alignment whilst the body lies supine with the legs extended. The shoulder joints remain flexed to approximately 90 degrees so that the arms are able to reach towards the ceiling without elevating or protract-

1

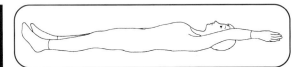

Figure 1.43

ing the shoulders. The arms may then reach over the head before being returned to rest beside the body.

During flexion the iliopsoas and abdominal muscles act together to control the position of the torso and assist vertebral column mobilization.

At the end of the motion the upper back muscles are relaxed so as to prevent spine extension and ensure a correct relationship between the ribs and the pelvis. This allows the trunk muscles to achieve their normal resting length.

Abnormal function

- To initiate the motion, the pelvis does not move into a posterior pelvic tilt; this occurs when lumbar spine mobility is compromised and abdominal muscle control is insufficient.
- To progress flexion, the lumbar spine remains flattened whilst the thoracic kyphosis is markedly increased; this occurs when lumbar spine mobility is compromised and possibly the iliopsoas muscles are shortened and tight.
- The vertebrae do not mobilize in sequence and the abdominal muscles bulge; this is commonly

associated with malfunction of iliopsoas and the oblique abdominal muscles and may also be due to underlying spine pathology that restricts vertebral column mobility.

References

Bobath B 1978 Adult hemiplegia: evaluation and treatment, 2nd edn. Heinemann, London

Gray's Anatomy for Students 2005 Churchill Livingstone, Edinburgh

Kendall FP, McCreary EK, Provance PG 1993 Muscles: testing and function, 4th edn. Lippincott Williams & Wilkins, Philadelphia

Larson CB, Gould M 1974 Orthopaedic nursing, 8th edn. Mosby, St Louis

Last RJ 1959 Anatomy: regional and applied, 2nd edn. Churchill, London

Myers TW 2001 Anatomy trains: myofascial meridians for manual and movement therapists. Churchill Livingstone, Edinburgh

Oliver J 1999 Back in line. Butterworth-Heinemann, Oxford

Palastanga N, Field D, Soames R 2002 Anatomy and human movement, 4th edn. Butterworth-Heinemann, Oxford

Palastanga N, Field D, Soames R 2006 Anatomy and human movement, 5th edn. Butterworth-Heinemann, Oxford

Sahrmann SA 2002 Diagnosis and treatment of movement impairment syndromes. Mosby, St Louis

Thibodeau GA, Patton KT 1993 Anatomy and physiology, 2nd edn. Mosby, St Louis

Trew M, Everett T 2005 Human movement: an introductory text, 5th edn. Churchill Livingstone, Edinburgh

White AA 1969 Analysis of the mechanics of thoracic spine in man, an experimental study of autopsy specimens. Acta Orthop Scand Suppl 127:1

White AA, Panjabi MM 1978 Clinical biomechanics of the spine. Lippincott, Philadelphia

TABLES OF EXERCISES FOR ADDRESSING POSTURAL FAULTS

Table 1.4 Swayback posture – what to do

For improved	Increase mobility (M)/flexibility (F)	Improve strength/performance	Exercises
Breathing efficiency	Ribs, sternum and thoracic spine	Diaphragm and abdominal muscles	Diaphragmatic breathing series
Cervical spine alignment and function	(M) Atlanto-occipital joint – flexion and extension; atlantoaxial joint – rotation (F) Cervical spine extensors and sternocleidomastoid	Cervical spine flexors	Quadriped series: BCS13, BCS14 Stretching series: ST10–ST12
Thoracic spine alignment and function	(M) Thoracic spine in lateral flexion, rotation, extension	Thoracic spine extensors	Spine mobilization series: *Side lying* SLM27 *Prone* PSM25, PSM26 Quadriped series: BCS16
Pectoral girdle alignment and function	(F) Upper trapezius and pectoral muscles (M) Scapula (M) Upper limbs whilst maintaining scapular stability	Middle and lower fibres of trapezius Serratus anterior, latissimus dorsi, teres major and rhomboids	Upper body series: *Supine* UBE1–UBE5 *Sitting* UBE6, UBE7 *Prone* UBE11, UBE12 *Side lying* UBE13 Stretches: ST14–ST16, ST18.1, ST18.2
Lumbar spine alignment and function	(F) Rectus abdominis and oblique abdominals (M) Lumbar spine in flexion and extension (M) Whole spine in flexion and extension	Pelvic floor and transversus abdominis, especially lower fibres Oblique abdominals, especially external obliques Iliopsoas – during eccentric and concentric contraction	Basic core strengthening (select in order as appropriate): BCS1, BCS2, BCS3, BCS4, BCS5, BCS6, BCS7 (BCS8 if appropriate) Stretches: ST13, ST15 Spine mobilization series: *Quadriped* BCS19

Continued

1

Table 1.4 Swayback posture – what to do—cont'd

For improved	Increase mobility (M)/flexibility (F)	Improve strength/performance	Exercises
Hip alignment and function		Gluteus maximus – lower fibres and during hip extension Hamstrings during knee flexion/extension Erector spinae	*Supine* SSM20–SSM22 Quadriped series: BCS16–BCS18
Hip alignment and function	(M) Hip joint (F) Tensor fasciae latae, possibly more on one side than the other (F) Gluteus maximus, especially upper fibres	Gluteus medius, especially lower fibres and possibly more on one side than the other hip adductors Quadriceps, especially rectus femoris during knee flexion and vastus medialis during knee extension Hip medial and lateral rotators	Side lying posterior hip muscle strengthening: BCS9–BCS12 Quadriped series: BCS15
Knee	(F) Hamstrings	Knee joint stabilizers (as required)	Knee strengthener: KS28 Stretches (select as appropriate): ST1–ST4.3, ST7
Lower limb/foot alignment and function	(F) Calf muscles (M) Subtalar joint (M) Feet	Soleus, especially during eccentric contraction Tibialis anterior and posterior Peroneus longus and brevis Intrinsic foot muscles	Stretches (select as appropriate): ST1–ST4.3, ST7 Exercising the ankle and forefoot (select as required): FM1.1, FM1.2, FM3.2
	Progress to . . .		Original mat exercises

Table 1.5 Flat back posture – what to do

For improved	Increase mobility (M)/flexibility (F)	Improve strength/performance	Exercises
Breathing efficiency	Ribs, sternum and thoracic spine	Diaphragm and abdominal muscles	Diaphragmatic breathing series
Cervical spine alignment and function	(M) Atlanto-occipital joint – flexion and extension; atlantoaxial joint – rotation (F) Cervical spine extensors and sternocleidomastoid	Cervical spine flexors	Quadriped series: BCS13, BCS14 Stretching series: ST10–ST12
Thoracic spine alignment and function	(M) Thoracic spine in lateral flexion, rotation, extension	Thoracic spine extensors	Spine mobilization series: *Side lying* SLM27 *Prone* PSM25, PSM26 *Quadriped series:* BCS16
Pectoral girdle alignment and function	(F) Upper trapezius and pectoral muscles (M) Scapula (M) Upper limbs whilst maintaining scapular stability	Middle and lower fibres of trapezius Serratus anterior, latissimus dorsi, teres major and rhomboids	Upper body series: *Supine* UBE1–UBE5 *Sitting* UBE6, UBE7 *Prone* UBE11, UBE12 *Side lying* UBE13 Stretches: ST18.1, ST18.2
Lumbar spine alignment and function	(F) Rectus abdominis and oblique abdominals (M) Lumbar spine in flexion and extension	Pelvic floor and transversus abdominis, especially lower fibres Iliopsoas	Basic core strengthening (select in order as appropriate): BCS1, BCS2, BCS3, BCS4, BCS5, BCS6, BCS7 Stretches: ST15–ST17

Continued

1

Table 1.5 Flat back posture – what to do—cont'd

For improved	Increase mobility (M)/flexibility (F)	Improve strength/performance	Exercises
	(M) Whole spine in flexion and extension	Gluteus maximus – lower fibres and during hip extension Erector spinae	Spine mobilization series: *Quadriped* BCS19 *Supine* SSM20–SSM22 Quadriped series: BCS15, BCS17, BCS18
Hip alignment and function	(M) Hip joint (F) Tensor fasciae latae (F) Gluteus maximus, upper fibres	Hip medial and lateral rotators Hip adductors Quadriceps, especially rectus femoris during hip flexion and vastus medialis during knee extension	Side lying posterior hip muscle strengthening: BCS9–BCS12 Stretches (select as appropriate): ST1–ST4.2, ST6
Knee	(F) Hamstrings	Knee joint stabilizers (as required)	Knee strengthener: KS28 Stretches: ST2.1, 2.2
Lower limb, foot alignment and function	(F) Calf muscles (M) Subtalar joint (M) Feet	Soleus, especially during eccentric contraction Tibialis anterior and posterior Peroneus longus and brevis Intrinsic foot muscles	Stretches: ST1 Exercising the ankle and forefoot (select as required): FM1.1, FM1.2, FM3.2
	Progress to . . .		Original mat exercises

Table 1.6   Mobile kyphosis – what to do

For improved	Increase mobility (M)/flexibility (F)	Improve strength/performance	Exercises
Breathing efficiency	Ribs, sternum and thoracic spine	Diaphragm and abdominal muscles	Diaphragmatic breathing series
Cervical spine alignment and function	(M) Atlanto-occipital joint – flexion and extension; atlantoaxial joint – rotation (F) Cervical spine extensors and sternocleidomastoid	Cervical spine flexors	Quadriped series: BCS13, BCS14 Stretching series: ST10–ST12
Thoracic spine alignment and function	(M) Thoracic spine in lateral flexion, rotation, extension	Thoracic spine extensors	Spine mobilization series: *Side lying* SLM27 *Prone* PSM25, PSM26 Quadriped series: BCS16, BCS18
Pectoral girdle alignment and function	(F) Upper trapezius and pectoral muscles (M) Scapula (M) Upper limbs whilst maintaining scapular stability	Middle and lower fibres of trapezius Serratus anterior, latissimus dorsi, teres major and rhomboids	Upper body series: *Supine* UBE1–UBE5 *Sitting* UBE7 *Prone* UBE11, UBE12 *Side lying* UBE13 Stretches: ST4.3, ST18.1, ST18.2
Lumbar spine alignment and function	(F) Sacroiliac region (M) Lumbar spine in flexion (M) Whole spine in flexion	Pelvic floor and transversus abdominis, especially lower fibres Iliopsoas	Basic core strengthening (select in order as appropriate): BCS1, BCS2, BCS3, BCS4, BCS5, BCS6 (BCS7–BCS12 as required)

Continued

Table 1.6 Mobile kyphosis – what to do—cont'd

For improved	Increase mobility (M)/flexibility (F)	Improve strength/performance	Exercises
	(F) Rectus abdominis and oblique abdominals (F) Hamstrings and gluteus maximus, especially upper fibres	Erector spinae Gluteus maximus, especially lower fibres Hamstrings	Stretches: ST15–ST17 Spine mobilization series: *Quadriped* BCS19 *Supine* SSM20–SSM22 Quadriped series: BCS15–BCS18
Hip alignment and function	(M) Hip joint (F) Tensor fasciae latae, iliopsoas and rectus femoris (as required)	Hip medial and lateral rotators (as required)	Side lying posterior hip muscle strengthening (select as required): BCS9, BCS11 Prone hip muscle strengthening: BCS8 Stretches (select as appropriate): ST1–ST4.2, ST6
Knee	(F) Hamstrings	Knee joint stabilizers (as required)	Knee strengthener: KS28 Stretches: ST2.1, 2.2
Lower limb/foot alignment and function	(F) Calf muscles (M) Subtalar joint (M) Feet	Soleus Tibialis anterior and posterior Peroneus longus and brevis Intrinsic foot muscles (as required)	Stretches: ST1 Exercising the ankle and forefoot (select as required): FM1.1, FM1.2, FM3.2
Progress to . . .			Original mat exercises

Table 1.7 Lordosis – what to do

For improved	Increase mobility (M)/flexibility (F)	Improve strength/performance	Exercises
Lumbar spine alignment and function	(M) Lumbar spine in flexion (M) Whole spine in lateral flexion, rotation, extension (F) Erector spinae (F) Iliopsoas and rectus femoris (F) Gluteus maximus, especially upper fibres (F) Hamstrings (F) Sacroiliac region (M) Whole spine in flexion	Pelvic floor and transversus abdominis, especially lower fibres Oblique abdominal muscles Abdominal muscles in controlling lumbar spine stability during hip flexion Iliopsoas, especially during eccentric contraction Lower fibres of gluteus maximus Gluteus maximus so as to act synergistically with the hamstrings during hip extension	Basic core strengthening: BCS1–BCS13, BCS16–BCS18 Spine mobilization series: *Side lying* SLM27 *Quadriped* BCS19 *Supine* SSM20–SSM22 Quadriped series: BCS18 Stretches: ST4.3
Hip alignment and function	(M) Hip joint whilst maintaining lumbar spine stability (F) Rectus abdominis and oblique abdominals (F) Tensor fasciae latae, iliopsoas and rectus femoris	Adductors Quadriceps, especially vastus medialis during knee extension	Stretches: ST12–ST17 Quadriped series: BCS15
Knee	(F) Hamstrings	Hamstrings during knee flexion, especially during eccentric contraction	Knee strengthener: KS28 Stretches: ST2.1, 2.2
Lower limb/foot alignment and function	(F) Calf muscles (M) Subtalar joint (M) Feet	Soleus, especially when contracting eccentrically Tibialis anterior and posterior Peroneus longus and brevis Intrinsic foot muscles	Stretches: ST1–ST4.2, ST5–ST7 Exercising the ankle and forefoot: FM.1.1–FM3.3

Table 1.8 Kypholordosis – what to do

For improved	Increase mobility (M)/flexibility (F)	Improve strength/performance	Exercises
Breathing efficiency	Ribs, sternum and thoracic spine	Diaphragm and abdominal muscles	Diaphragmatic breathing series
Cervical spine alignment and function	(M) Atlanto-occipital joint – flexion and extension; atlantoaxial joint – rotation (F) Cervical spine extensors and sternocleidomastoid	Cervical spine flexors	Quadriped series: BCS13, BCS14 Stretching series: ST10–ST12
Thoracic spine alignment and function	(M) Thoracic spine in lateral flexion, rotation, extension	Thoracic spine extensors	Spine mobilization series: *Side lying* SLM27 *Prone* PSM25, PSM26 Quadriped series: BCS16, BCS18
Pectoral girdle alignment and function	(F) Upper trapezius and pectoral muscles (M) Scapula (M) Upper limbs whilst maintaining scapular stability	Middle and lower fibres of trapezius Serratus anterior, latissimus dorsi, teres major and rhomboids	Upper body series: *Supine* UBE1–UBE5 *Sitting* UBE7 *Prone* UBE11, UBE12 *Side lying* UBE13 Stretches: ST4.3, ST18.1, ST18.2
Lumbar spine alignment and function	(M) Lumbar spine in flexion (M) Whole spine in lateral flexion, rotation, extension (F) Erector spinae (F) Iliopsoas and rectus femoris	Pelvic floor and transversus abdominis, especially lower fibres Oblique abdominal muscles Abdominal muscles in controlling lumbar spine stability during hip flexion	Basic core strengthening: BCS1– BCS13, BCS16–BCS18 Spine mobilization series: *Side lying* SLM27 *Quadriped* BCS19

1

Table 1.8 Kypholordosis – what to do—cont'd

	Gluteus maximus, especially upper fibres (F) Hamstrings (F) Sacroiliac region	Iliopsoas, especially during eccentric contraction Lower fibres of gluteus maximus Gluteus maximus so as to act synergistically with the hamstrings during hip extension	*Supine* SSM20–SSM22 Quadriped series: BCS18 Stretches: ST4.3
Hip alignment and function	(M) Hip joint whilst maintaining lumbar spine stability (F) Rectus abdominis and oblique abdominals (F) Tensor fasciae latae, iliopsoas and rectus femoris	Adductors Quadriceps, especially vastus medialis during knee extension	Stretches: ST12–ST17 Quadriped series: BCS15
Knee	(F) Hamstrings	Hamstrings during knee flexion, especially during eccentric contraction	Knee strengthener: KS28 Stretches: ST2.1, 2.2
Lower limb/foot alignment and function	(F) Calf muscles (M) Subtalar joint (M) Feet	Soleus, especially when contracting eccentrically Tibialis anterior and posterior Peroneus longus and brevis Intrinsic foot muscles	Stretches: ST1–ST4.2, ST5–ST7 Exercising the ankle and forefoot: FM1.1–FM3.3

1

Table 1.9 Functional scoliosis – what to do

For improved	Increase mobility (M)/flexibility (F)	Improve strength/performance	Exercises
Breathing efficiency	Ribs, sternum and thoracic spine, particularly on more contracted side	Diaphragm and abdominal muscles	Diaphragmatic breathing series
Cervical spine alignment and function	(M) Atlanto-occipital joint – flexion and extension; atlantoaxial joint – rotation (F) Cervical spine extensors and sternocleidomastoid	Cervical spine rotators Cervical spine flexors	Quadriped series: BCS13, BCS14 Stretching series: ST10–ST12
Thoracic spine alignment and function	(M) Thoracic spine in lateral flexion, rotation, extension	Thoracic spine extensors – address imbalances	Spine mobilization series: *Side lying* SLM27 *Prone* PSM25, PSM26 Quadriped series: BCS16, BCS18
Pectoral girdle alignment and function	(F) Upper trapezius and pectoral muscles (M) Scapula (M) Upper limbs whilst maintaining scapular stability	Middle and lower fibres of trapezius Serratus anterior, latissimus dorsi, teres major and rhomboids	Upper body series: *Supine* UBE1–UBE5 *Sitting* UBE7 *Prone* UBE11, UBE12 *Side lying* UBE13 Stretches: ST4.3, ST18.1, ST18.2
Lumbar spine alignment and function	(M) Lumbar spine in flexion (M) Whole spine in lateral flexion, rotation, extension (F) Erector spinae (F) Iliopsoas and rectus femoris (F) Gluteus maximus, especially on more contracted side	Pelvic floor and transversus abdominis, especially lower fibres Oblique abdominal muscles – address imbalances Abdominal muscles in controlling lumbar spine stability during hip flexion	Basic core strengthening: BCS1–BCS13, BCS16–BCS18 Spine mobilization series: *Side lying* SLM27 *Quadriped* BCS19 *Supine* SSM20–SSM22 Quadriped series: BCS18

Table 1.9 Functional scoliosis – what to do—cont'd

	(F) Hamstrings	Erector spinae overall – address imbalances
	(F) Sacroiliac region, especially on more contracted side	Iliopsoas – address imbalances
		Lower fibres of gluteus maximus – address imbalances
		Gluteus maximus during hip extension – address imbalances
		Stretches: ST4.3, ST12–ST17
Hip alignment and function	(M) Hip joint whilst maintaining lumbar spine stability	Adductors, abductors and quadriceps – address imbalances
	(F) Rectus abdominis and oblique abdominals, especially on more contracted side	
	(F) Tensor fasciae latae, iliopsoas and rectus femoris, especially on more contracted side	Quadriped series: BCS15
Knee	(F) Hamstrings	Hamstrings during knee flexion – address imbalances
		Knee strengthener: KS28
		Stretches: ST2.1, 2.2
Lower limb/foot alignment and function	(F) Calf muscles	Soleus, especially when contracting eccentrically
	(M) Subtalar joint	Tibialis anterior and posterior
	(M) Feet	Peroneus longus and brevis
		Intrinsic foot muscles – address imbalances
		Stretches: ST1–ST4.2, ST5–ST7
		Exercising the ankle and forefoot: FM1.1–FM3.3

Chapter 2

Common medical conditions and problems

Many health professionals recommend Pilates as a suitable form of exercise for individuals who are recovering from illness or injury or have a specific ongoing medical condition. Therefore, over a period of years, Pilates' teachers are likely to encounter a variety of disease processes and problems when teaching.

The following common conditions are covered to assist client assessment and exercise programme development, as well as appropriate onward referral so that health and safety are not compromised:

- Eating disorders
- Obesity
- Chronic fatigue syndrome
- Epilepsy
- Multiple sclerosis
- Parkinson's disease
- Diabetes mellitus
- Thyroid disease
- Osteoporosis
- Osteoarthritis
- Rheumatoid arthritis
- Other forms of arthritis
- Hypertension
- Cardiovascular disease
- Cerebrovascular disease
- Chronic obstructive pulmonary disease
- Asthma
- Gastrointestinal problems
- Neck problems

- Shoulder problems
- Back problems
- Hip problems
- Knee problems
- Lower leg problems
- Ankle and foot problems.

GENERAL POINTS APPLICABLE IN ALL CASES

- Understand the significance of coexisting medical and other problems, always liaising with the person's medical and other health professionals.
- Review the current situation before each exercise session.
- Be aware that analgesic and anti-inflammatory medication could be masking physical deterioration.
- Always begin by correcting postural faults and associated muscle malfunction.
- Always focus on correct spine alignment and stability in preparation for exercising the extremities.
- Ultimately provide an exercise programme appropriate to the individual's level of fitness, so as to progressively increase strength and stamina and thereby build on the individual's trust and confidence.

Specific points follow each medical condition.

EATING DISORDERS

These constitute a form of behavioural problem associated with physiological changes that may lead to physical disability. There is a disturbance of eating habits and of weight control behaviour.

Anorexia nervosa and *bulimia nervosa* comprise the vast majority of cases in the context of fitness for exercise. They are an important cause of morbidity in girls and young women but are much less common in men. The aetiology is complex and poorly understood but involves social, psychological and biological factors, and there is a genetic predisposition. Subjects have an exaggerated perception of their size and shape that they feel the need to reduce and control, either by starvation or by other less obvious means.

In *anorexia nervosa* there is self-starvation leading to marked weight loss. Subjects may be physically overactive to a punishing degree and develop various ruses to distract attention from their behaviour. They may wear voluminous clothing in the pockets of which they can conceal heavy objects when attending weight checks. There may be misuse of laxatives and diuretics to com-plement a regimen of strict dieting, or even frank starvation. Subjects may be seriously underweight with low muscle bulk and weakness, and low bone density with progressive osteoporosis. Thyroid underactivity, with cold extremities, cardiovascular depression with hypotension and bradycardia, constipation and amenorrhoea may develop. Many are chronically unwell, but even marked changes can usually be reversed, with the possible exception of reduced bone density. However, some may die from the physical complications or, ultimately, from suicide.

In *bulimia nervosa* self-starvation alternates with self-induced vomiting after eating large amounts of food. Weight may be normal but the bouts of vomiting may lead to dehydration and metabolic disturbances, including alkalosis and electrolyte depletion with cardiac arrhythmias and kidney damage. There may also be obvious dental damage from the frequent passage of gastric acid over the teeth during vomiting.

Management

Those with these eating disorders may see Pilates as an additional contribution to image control and to their overactive exercise regimens, and it is important to identify these motivating factors as well as the extent of any underlying physical abnormalities when initially assessing the suitability of such clients for Pilates exercise programmes, whether bulimic or, especially, anorexic.

Faults in posture and muscles

These may include:

- kyphosis with forward head position
- slouched position and overall muscle weakness; the spinal and posterior hip muscles in particular may be affected due to prolonged periods of inactivity
- muscles of the upper and lower limbs due to overactive exercise regimens.

Good teaching practice

This would include:

- awareness of risks such as dehydration and electrolyte imbalance
- avoidance of overactive regimens
- a gradual building of strength and endurance.

OBESITY

This is an increasing problem in much of the developed world. In the United Kingdom, for example, 50% of the population is overweight and 20% is obese, as judged

2

by body mass index (BMI) which is calculated by dividing body weight by height squared (kg/m^2). If the normal BMI range is 18.5–24.9, then 25 or more is overweight, 30 or more is obese, 40 or more is extremely obese, and so on. Most weight gain occurs between the ages of 20 and 40. Whilst there may be specific causal factors in some cases, the aetiology generally involves behavioural and genetic factors.

Whilst obesity has become much more prevalent in the last 20 years, actual food intake has not been shown to increase over the same period, whereas there seems to have been an overall decrease in physical activity. However, it is important to realize that, although food intake may not have increased, its composition has been changing towards energy-dense foods that combine high fat and sugar content with low bulk. Increased appetite for food, and also alcohol, may also follow cessation of smoking. Such behavioural factors have now come to be regarded as of prime importance in the trend towards obesity.

Genetics factors may also operate and, whilst felt to be relatively much less common, may underlie the difference between abdominal (apple-shaped) and generalized hip and thigh (pear-shaped) body weight distribution.

Specific causes of weight gain should always be borne in mind, such as endocrine abnormalities of the thyroid and of the pituitary–adrenal systems. The numerous complications of weight gain – in particular, non-insulin dependent diabetes mellitus, hypertension, stroke, coronary heart disease, breathing problems, weight-related musculoskeletal disorders and arthritis, and urinary stress incontinence – are important factors to be taken into account when assessing clients for, and designing, their exercise programmes.

Faults in posture and muscles

These may include any of the postural faults described in Chapter 1.

Good teaching practice

This would include:

- understanding that moving too quickly from supine to standing could result in postural hypotension, a possible side effect of antihypertensive agents
- considering side lying, sitting or standing positions to avoid compromising the breathing effort, gastric reflux syndrome or general discomfort when exercising
- improving pelvic floor muscle tone to reduce stress incontinence as required

- building strength and endurance gradually
- supporting a weight loss regimen as required.

CHRONIC FATIGUE SYNDROME

This is the term now given to a loosely defined condition, other names for which include post-viral fatigue syndrome, myalgic encephalomyelitis (ME), epidemic neuromyasthenia and Icelandic disease.

There is an abnormal degree of muscle fatigue after (often minimal) physical or even mental exercise that may readily reach the point of exhaustion, following which recovery may be very slow. In addition to abnormal fatigability, there is a wide variety of features including headache, dizziness, poor concentration, impaired memory, irritability and sleep disturbance, together with muscle aches and, in some cases, fever and enlarged lymph glands. There may also be various cardiac or gastrointestinal symptoms such as palpitations, chest pain and tightness, abdominal pain and cramps, etc. Whilst there are often symptoms of anxiety and depression, women get chronic fatigue syndrome much more commonly than men, but for unknown reasons.

As much of this may occur after a viral illness, particularly influenza, and is normally short lived, a diagnosis of chronic fatigue syndrome is now made only after a duration of some 6 months, without necessarily any history of viral illness, but infectious mononucleosis (glandular fever), epidemic myalgia (Bornholm disease), hepatitis A (with or without clinical jaundice) and a wide variety of relatively mild viral illnesses have been implicated. Laboratory tests are usually normal, even though there may be a clear history typical of viraemia. Whilst the whole notion of this condition remains controversial, most medical authorities accept its existence, although it is still considered by some to constitute a wholly psychiatric disorder.

Management

This is based on behavioural and cognitive approaches aimed at gradually consistently increasing activity (graded exercise), and discouraging the tendency to rest rather than to exercise so as to improve confidence as well as stamina. The subject is encouraged to accept the need for exercise as the key to physical recovery. Some subjects respond to antidepressants of the serotonin reuptake inhibitor type such as fluoxetine (Prozac).

Not surprisingly, subjects with chronic fatigue syndrome may present, or be referred, for Pilates exercises and these can be expected to confer real benefit if the programme is carefully paced, depending on the severity of the features which must, of course, be regarded as very real to the subjects concerned. It is essential for the subject's medical advisers to be aware of and to approve of what is proposed.

Faults in posture and muscles

These may include slouched position and overall muscle weakness. In particular, the spinal and posterior hip muscles may be affected due to prolonged periods of inactivity.

Good teaching practice

This would include:

- understanding that relapse can occur, particularly after overexertion
- building stamina through the promotion of shorter rest periods between exercises
- assisting a gradual return to normal everyday activities.

EPILEPSY

In epilepsy there is a tendency to recurrent seizures that are the effect of an electrical discharge in the brain and therefore a symptom of, rather than actual, brain disease. A single seizure is not epilepsy, although the recurrence rate after the first seizure is 70% in the first year, usually within the first couple of months.

In some cases it is only necessary to identify and eliminate certain triggering factors to control the condition. In others, only complex anticonvulsant medication programmes, or even brain surgery, can achieve adequate control. Triggering factors may include lack of sleep or other causes of fatigue, alcohol, or alcohol withdrawal, substance abuse, lights flickering at some critical frequency, as from a television screen or in a nightclub, and so on. Intercurrent infections or metabolic disturbances may also destabilize even well-controlled epileptics.

The aetiology of epilepsy covers an enormous variety of factors, congenital and acquired. In some disorders, seizures are the only symptoms, in others they are only one of several features. *Primary generalized epilepsy* usually develops in childhood or adolescence and is not associated with any structural, as opposed to functional, nervous system abnormality.

Secondary generalized epilepsy may be related to many factors, including a wide variety of drugs and metabolic disturbances, and certain uncommon genetic disorders.

Partial seizures arise from some abnormal focus in the cerebral cortex in the surface layer of the brain and affect first a limb or other localized area that will often prog-

ress to *generalized seizures*. Causes in otherwise fit people include previous head injury or following essential brain surgery. There may be a history of meningitis, encephalitis or certain tropical diseases, or genetic or degenerative conditions.

Major seizures, as classically associated with epilepsy, cause loss of consciousness with the patient falling to the ground with a history of 'blackouts', although this term often refers also to minor seizures without loss of consciousness.

A typical major seizure with tonic–clonic features may begin with a partial phase or aura that the patient may not subsequently recall. Rigidity with loss of consciousness follows, and injuries may occur if the patient falls to the ground or against something, especially if out of doors in traffic, etc. Breathing ceases and cyanosis may follow. This rigid tonic phase should soon give way to the clonic phase, with alternating muscular contractions and relaxations so that the whole body jerks violently. There follows a flaccid relaxed phase, breathing is resumed and the colour and general appearance improve. After a few more minutes, consciousness begins to return, but confusion and disorientation may persist for over half an hour or more and memory of the event may not return for several hours.

There may be headache and generalized malaise, and tongue biting and urinary, or even bowel, incontinence may have occurred. Such major seizures can be most alarming to a casual observer.

A partial seizure, much less dramatic or even obvious, comprises an episode of altered consciousness without physical collapse. A form of 'blackout' or 'absence' occurs, with blank staring, with or without involuntary movements of the eyes, lips, limbs, etc., all lasting a few minutes. Consciousness returns but again there may be residual confusion, drowsiness, etc. As with major seizures, there may be an aura that the patient can usually recall. An aura may comprise a variety of features, including alterations of mood, memory and perception, visual hallucinations, nausea and abdominal pain, etc. Such phenomena may also be familiar to migraine suffers.

Many other forms of seizure may be encountered involving only motor or sensory features of one side of the body or a limb.

Late onset epilepsy in older people is common and the incidence in those over 60 years is rising. The difference between fits and faints may be less clear and the condition may present as a cause of confusion in the elderly. Minor simple absences may recur several times in a day. More recently, they have become easier to control with specific anticonvulsant medication.

Little can be done for a person whilst a major seizure is occurring, except first aid and common sense

2

2

manoeuvres to prevent injury and other secondary complications.

First aid

- Move the person away from danger (fire, water, machinery, furniture).
- After convulsions cease, turn the subject into the 'recovery' position (semi-prone).
- Ensure the airway is clear.
- *Do not insert anything in the mouth* (tongue biting occurs at seizure onset and cannot be prevented by observers).
- If convulsions continue for more than 5 minutes or recur without the person regaining consciousness, summon urgent medical attention.
- The person may be drowsy and confused for some 30–60 minutes and should not be left alone until fully recovered.

Status epilepticus, which exists when a series of seizures occurs without a subject regaining consciousness, can constitute a life-threatening medical emergency. First aid, as described, is appropriate whilst awaiting urgent medical attention.

Non-epileptic attacks (psychogenic attacks, 'pseudo-epilepsy') superficially resemble epileptic seizures, but the basis is psychological rather than one of an abnormal epileptic discharge. Attacks may be difficult to differentiate and may even take the form of *apparent status epilepticus* but movements may be exaggerated, perhaps with marked arching of the back (opisthotonos). Whilst cyanosis and tongue biting will be absent, urinary incontinence may still occur. Such episodes may be associated with other aspects of complex personality disorders that, whilst commoner in women, do not carry the dangers of epileptic attacks.

Management

Before assessing an epileptic for an exercise programme, it is essential to obtain the approval of the patient's medical advisers, taking into account the incidence of seizures and the likelihood of encounterable known triggering factors, and to have then fully appraised the doctors of the nature of any proposed Pilates exercise regimen. Even with informed medical consent, it would, on balance, seem inadvisable to take on any other than a well-controlled epileptic with a low incidence of, certainly, major seizures, although good control will have been obtained in around 80% of cases. Even so, staff must always be prepared for a possible seizure and should know what reaction is appropriate. Well-controlled patients may succumb to destabilizing factors such as fatigue, or the onset of a respiratory or other viral infection, and at those times their sessions should generally be cancelled as a precaution.

In practice, however, most epileptics understand their condition well enough to predict such eventualities and take any measures necessary to avoid loss of control.

Faults in posture and muscles

These may include any of the postural habits and faults described in Chapter 1.

Good teaching practice

This would include:

- a knowledge of specific 'trigger points'
- considering hunger, fatigue, stress or the onset of a viral infection as potential destabilizing factors
- understanding 'first aid' procedures in the event of seizure
- providing an exercise programme appropriate to the individual's level of fitness – the person could otherwise be well and extremely fit.

MULTIPLE SCLEROSIS

In multiple sclerosis (MS), the most common neurological cause of long-term disability, the body may be setting up an immune or antibody–antigen reaction to its own tissues, an autoimmune condition in which the cells of the central nervous system (CNS) concerned with the production of myelin are attacked. Myelin occurs, and has a protective and nutrient effect, in relation to nerve fibres throughout the CNS, comprising the brain and spinal cord but not the peripheral nerves. A basic immune reaction could create an inflammatory response leading to loss of the myelin-producing cells that occur throughout the CNS and result in areas of demyelination. Electrical insulation of nerve fibres is impaired, impulse conduction is affected and ultimately nerve fibres are destroyed and areas of scarring result. The brain stem, optic nerve and the spinal cord tend to be the first areas affected.

The condition starts with a relatively acute phase of inflammation that begins the process of nerve damage. This initial acute phrase often responds to corticosteroids, but in the established condition nerve fibres are destroyed both by inflammation and by the loss of their myelin sheaths. However, the whole notion of MS as an autoimmune condition has recently come back into question so it has to be accepted that, at present, its real cause remains unknown.

The majority of subjects have a relapsing and remitting course, others have a slowly progressive course, and some progress rapidly and severely to early death. Onset is rare before puberty or after the age of 60, and is commoner in women. Drug treatment, however, continues to be based on beta-interferon and other immunomodulating agents, although their effectiveness is disputed.

The demyelinating lesions cause features that come on over days or weeks and may resolve over weeks or months. Different patterns of progress are encountered and in some cases there may be years or decades between attacks that range between mild visual and sensory deficits to more disabling motor deficit, but significant intellectual impairment is unusual until late in the disease.

Common features clinical of MS

- Fatigue and depression (common, and respond to medication)
- Motor weakness or spasticity
- Altered sensation: numbness or paraesthesiae
- Paroxysmal or dysaesthetic pain
- Urinary frequency, urgency, incontinence (common)
- Constipation
- Impotence
- Swallowing disorders
- Visual disorders: optic neuritis, diplopia, nystagmus
- Cerebellar effects: ataxia, intention tremor
- Cognitive impairment: amnesia, euphoria, dementia
- Vertigo.

Management

Management during an acute relapse will usually require hospital inpatient treatment involving high dose steroids and immunosuppressive drugs. Longer term complications and disabilities require a range of measures involving occupational and physiotherapy, together with a possible array of medications targeting specific disabilities.

Those in lengthy remission with minimal established disability may present themselves for Pilates exercises, or may be referred by physiotherapists once remission is underway. Regular exercise can assist recovery of muscle strength, promote confidence building and create well-being.

Faults in posture and muscles

These may include any of the postural habits and faults described in Chapter 3. In addition, as the disease progresses, balance and posture deteriorate according to the individual's specific disabilities.

Good teaching practice

This would include:

- designing a flexible programme of exercises appropriate to the individual's current level of fitness – during early disease there may be no obvious functional deficits
- strengthening muscle groups that help to maintain independence during everyday activates
- allowing the individual sufficient time to complete each exercise sequence
- ensuring torso muscle control is adequate for safe spine mobilization
- avoiding overexertion and fatigue
- using props, supports and specialized Pilates' equipment to increase exercise efficiency by reducing any unwanted gravitational effects on posture and balance.

PARKINSON'S DISEASE

This is the commonest of a group of degenerative neurological conditions. Its main features include slowness of movement, rigidity, loss of postural reflexes and the well-known tremors.

The classic features may be absent initially, there being only tiredness, aches and pains, mental slowness and depression. Later, tremor appears, usually unilaterally at first, perhaps in an upper limb, but later becoming generalized, affecting limbs, mouth, tongue, etc. Slowness of movement may develop gradually, as may rigidity, causing stiffness and a flexed posture. Impaired postural reflexes may lead eventually to a tendency to falls. Muscle strength, reflexes and sensation remain normal. Intellectual faculties also remain normal, at least initially, belying the physical appearance.

Management

This is based on drug therapy that can benefit especially the slowness of movement and rigidity. Neurosurgical intervention may be used to treat tremor that has not been helped by drug therapy. Physiotherapy benefits Parkinson's disease subjects at all stages by helping to reduce rigidity and abnormal posture.

Although postural improvement is of great importance, it must performed under the guidance of the person's health care professionals.

Faults in posture and muscles

These may include any of the postural faults described in Chapter 3. In addition, as the disease progresses, posture becomes flexed and rigid, and there is a tendency to fall.

Good teaching practice

This would include:

2

- designing a flexible programme of exercises appropriate to the individual's current level of fitness – during early disease there may be no obvious functional deficits
- strengthening muscle groups that help to maintain independence during everyday activates
- allowing the individual sufficient time to complete each exercise sequence
- ensuring torso muscle control is adequate for safe spine mobilization
- improving core strength and balance over the lower limbs and feet
- avoiding overexertion and fatigue
- using props, supports and specialized Pilates' equipment to increase exercise efficiency by reducing any unwanted gravitational effects on posture and balance.

DIABETES MELLITUS

Diabetes mellitus is a clinical syndrome characterized by a raised blood sugar level (hyperglycaemia) due to an absolute or relative deficiency of the hormone insulin. The mechanism of action and the effects of deficiency of insulin are complex and involve the metabolism not only of glucose and other carbohydrates, but also of protein and fat, with secondary effects on water and electrolyte balance.

Whilst death may follow an acute diabetic metabolic derangement, a more long-standing chronic derangement associated with poor metabolic control may cause irreversible cell damage, affecting the vascular system in particular, with a wide variety of manifestations that comprise the complications of diabetes.

Blood glucose levels are normally tightly regulated within a narrow range which represents a balance between, on the one hand, entry of glucose into the circulation from storage forms in the liver, together with intestinal absorption after meals, and, on the other hand, uptake of glucose by the tissues, mainly the skeletal muscles, but also, most importantly, the brain, for which glucose is the principal fuel that must therefore be continuously supplied.

Whilst *glucagon* and *adrenaline* are the hormones that act to maintain hepatic glucose output, if required, between meals, it is *insulin* that counteracts the marked rise in blood glucose that would otherwise follow immediately upon a meal, by suppressing liver glucose output and stimulating its uptake by muscle and fat.

Insulin is secreted by special *pancreatic beta cells* directly into the pancreatic vein, as also is *glucagon* from the *pancreatic alpha cells*. These are distinct from the main pancreatic glandular cells, which secrete digestive juices into the duodenum, together with bile from the liver via the pancreatic and common bile ducts. *Adrenaline*, from the *suprarenal medulla*, is secreted directly into the adrenal veins.

The *hyperglycaemia* of diabetes develops because of an absolute (*Type 1 diabetes*) or relative (*Type 2 diabetes*) deficiency of insulin. In Type 1 diabetes, the absolute deficiency of insulin is due to either immunological or unknown factors. In Type 2 diabetes one or more of a variety of widely differing factors may operate to create a state of resistance to the action of insulin. These range from pancreatic disease affecting the entire gland, genetic defects, drug-induced effects, hormonal antagonism from various glands such as the pituitary, adrenal cortical, thyroid, etc., and from the placenta in pregnancy. *Gestational diabetes* refers to hyperglycaemia diagnosed for the first time during pregnancy in predisposed individuals. It may or may not resolve after delivery.

Glycosuria, the appearance of sugar in the urine, occurs when blood glucose levels exceed a certain level, the *renal threshold* for a particular individual. The excretion of glucose requires an obligatory increased excretion of water leading to the classic features of thirst and the passing of large volumes of urine (polyuria). These features may be less dramatic in Type 2 diabetes as it develops slowly over months or years, during which the renal threshold also rises and the symptoms of thirst and polyuria are mild so that detection of the condition tends to be delayed.

Testing of urine for glucose at routine medical examinations is the usual procedure that first detects diabetes but glycosuria may then be due merely to a low renal threshold when it is termed *renal glycosuria*, is relatively harmless and often occurs during normal pregnancy. However, the diagnosis depends ultimately on measurement of blood glucose levels. Sometimes an unduly rapid rise in blood glucose levels after a meal may exceed the renal threshold causing a so-called *alimentary glycosuria* that, like renal glycosuria, is benign. However, glycosuria in pregnancy should always be followed up with blood glucose measurements to distinguish it from an actual gestational diabetic state.

Testing of urine for *ketones* is also a routine procedure. *Ketonuria* is not necessarily associated with diabetes unless combined with hyperglycaemia when the diagnosis of diabetes becomes highly likely. When diabetes is suspected, confirmatory blood testing for glucose is required. Random raised levels may be misleading and must always be supplemented by measurement of fasting levels or a glucose tolerance test where levels are measured serially after an intake of a standard amount of glucose.

The major clinical features of diabetes are therefore due initially to hyperglycaemia and include, in addition to thirst, dry mouth and polyuria, nocturia (passage of urine during the night), fatigue, nausea, headache, weight change and a preference for sweet foods. The glycosuria, together with a lowered resistance to infection, also predisposes to genital thrush. These features are all more common in Type 1 diabetes compared with Type 2 in which symptoms may be absent or comprise only chronic fatigue or malaise.

Physical signs, other than perhaps weight loss, may be absent in Type 1 diabetes, but over 70% of Type 2 diabetics are overweight, at least in developed countries, and hypertension is present in around 50%. Other contrasting features are outlined in Table 2.1.

Ketones are organic compounds of which the best known is acetone with its characteristically pungent smell. They are acidic by-products of fat metabolism that are normally completely broken down in the liver. Ketone production is increased when fat is broken down during the general catabolism that results from a relatively acute insufficiency of insulin, perhaps during an infection or other form of stress when requirements rise even if loss of appetite, vomiting, diarrhoea, etc., might suggest the opposite. Hyperglycaemia with heavy glycosuria leads to a loss of water and electrolytes, particularly sodium and potassium, and a state of *ketoacidosis* that may lead ultimately to so-called 'diabetic coma', an unhelpful term as coma may only supervene at a relatively late, even terminal, stage. However, polyuria and thirst, with significant weight loss, weakness, nausea and vomiting, cramps and abdominal pain with dehydration, hypotension, tachycardia, air hunger and a smell of acetone in sweat and breath are combined in an acute medical emergency requiring insulin, fluids, electrolytes and treatment of any infection present.

Hypoglycaemia, in contrast, is an effect of the treatment of diabetes, commonly in insulin dependent, compared with non-insulin dependent, cases (controlled with oral medication). Features are due to an ensuing autonomic, mainly sympathetic, stress response comprising sweating, tremor, tachycardia and anxiety, together with confusion, drowsiness or even true coma (so-called 'insulin coma') and convulsions due to acute falls in brain glucose levels.

Complications of diabetes

Even with relatively good control of long-standing Type 1 diabetes, or a long-standing but undetected Type 2 diabetes, a variety of complications may slowly develop, for which the underlying mechanisms are basically vascular and ultimately highly disabling:

- Retinopathy and cataracts leading to impaired vision
- Nephropathy with renal failure
- Peripheral neuropathy with sensory loss and motor weakness
- Autonomic neuropathy with postural hypotension and impaired gut motility, etc.
- Foot problems, especially pain and ulceration due to neuropathy and peripheral circulatory impairment
- Coronary circulatory inadequacy with myocardial ischaemia and infarction
- Cerebrovascular inadequacy with ischaemic attacks and strokes.

Management of ongoing diabetes

This is commonly based on diet plus insulin in Type 1 cases and diet plus one or more types of oral agent (monotherapy) or perhaps two types of oral agent with the possible addition of insulin (combined therapy). Of new cases, around 50% can be controlled adequately by diet alone, a further 20–30% will require an oral hypoglycaemic drug and 20–30% will require insulin.

Lifestyle changes, especially regular exercise and a healthy diet with weight control, contribute to successful management, but may be difficult to sustain in older people.

The ultimate aim is therefore to achieve as near normal metabolism as is practicable, especially in terms of ideal body weight and blood glucose levels so

Table 2.1 Contrasting features between Type 1 and Type 2 diabetes

	Type 1	Type 2
Age of onset	< 40 years	> 50 years
Duration of symptoms	Weeks	Months to years
Body weight	Normal or low	Obese
Ketonuria	Yes	No
Fatal without insulin	Yes	No
Family history	Uncommon	Yes
Complications (vascular etc.) present at diagnosis	No	25%

2

as to lower the incidence of vascular disease and specific complications. Whilst a few people die from the acute complications of ketoacidosis or hypoglycaemia, it is the serious morbidity and the excess mortality of the long-term complications that are of most significance to the individual and the economy of the community.

Dietary management aims to provide an appropriate energy content so as to facilitate glycaemic control with oral agents or insulin. Of the two types of oral agent in use, both require the presence of endogenous insulin and are therefore ineffective in Type 1 diabetes. However, *muscular exercise* has been shown to increase sensitivity to endogenous insulin in the muscle vascular beds, thereby enhancing the effects of diet and oral agents.

Sulphonylureas, of which several are in use, depending on duration of action, etc., act mainly by stimulating increased levels of insulin from the pancreatic beta cells and can therefore cause hypoglycaemia. *Biguanides*, of which only one is now in use, may act by increasing tissue sensitivity to endogenous insulin, but do not actually stimulate insulin secretion and therefore cannot cause hypoglycaemia. Other types of oral agent have been, or are being, developed for use in specific regimens.

Insulin, discovered in 1921, transformed the management of diabetes, previously a fatal disorder. Originally only of animal origin, insulin can now be synthesized that is identical with the human form and a large variety of insulins is available for structured individual regimens comprising preparations of differing durations and rates of onset following subcutaneous injection. Inadvertent intramuscular injection may occur in children and in thin adults and may lead to more rapid absorption and exaggerated effects.

An important new development is that of *inhaled insulin* that would appear to be as effective as the injected form. Combined with a single daily injection of long-acting insulin, it would replace additional injections of short-acting insulin otherwise required during the day. This is likely to appeal to children and others unable to come to terms with multiple daily injections.

People with diabetes generally learn to handle all aspects of their management, including prediction and awareness of the effects of losing control. Acute decompensation leading to diabetic ketoacidosis is normally predicable in that it tends to develop over hours or even a day or two following some stressful episode such as a chest infection or a gut infection with vomiting and diarrhoea, a mild myocardial infarction, etc. An acute illness ensues and emergency hospital management is generally unavoidable.

Hypoglycaemia occurs far more often in insulin-dependent diabetics compared with those controlled by sulphonylureas. It is potentially fatal from ensuing coma, convulsions, cardiac arrhythmias or infarction, together with accidents, especially when driving. It is the most important complication of diabetes that could arise during the course of an exercise session and diabetics are taught that strenuous or protracted exercise should be preceded by a reduced dose of insulin and that all those taking insulin should always carry glucose tablets.

The condition is usually amenable to first aid, depending on the severity of the episode and how acutely it has developed. If the person is conscious, glucose should be swallowed as soon as possible and is usually rapidly effective. If consciousness is (or has been) lost, intravenous glucose, involving medical or paramedical attention, will be required. Further glucose should be given orally as soon as consciousness and the ability to swallow are recovered as hypoglycaemia can return in those using long-acting insulins or oral agents.

In addition to providing glucose, basic first aid with attention to posture, airway management and avoidance of injury apply.

The most experienced and basically well-controlled diabetics may still succumb to hypoglycaemia, even during exercise that is not particularly strenuous, so that the key is not to delay before the ability to swallow is lost, or before nausea and vomiting complicate the picture.

In general, diabetics, unless their condition has invariably been well controlled, should be assumed to have to greater or lesser degree manifestations of the complications of diabetes. This must always be borne in mind when planning exercise programmes that may impose on the cardiovascular system in particular, even at times when such diabetics seem to display general good health and well-being.

Faults in posture and muscles

These may include any of the postural habits and faults described in Chapter 3.

Good teaching practice

This would include:

- awareness of destabilizing factors such as hunger, fatigue, stress or the onset of a viral infection
- awareness of any visual impairment
- ensuring that minor injuries such as cuts to the legs could not occur whilst using props or specialized Pilates' equipment (poor peripheral circulation delays healing)

- understanding 'first aid' procedures in the event of a 'hypoglycaemic event'
- providing an exercise programme appropriate to the individual's level of fitness – the person could otherwise be well and extremely fit.

THYROID DISEASE

Disorders of this endocrine gland, in the front of the neck, comprise mainly *hyperthyroidism* (overactivity), *hypothyroidism* (underactivity) and *goitre* (enlargement). The thyroid is also susceptible to malignancy as well as to various rare inflammatory conditions. *Iodine* is a key component of thyroid hormone (thyroxine) and the gland is the site of dietary iodine uptake and metabolism in the body. Dietary iodine deficiency usually underlies the development of goitre and may be endemic in certain parts of the world. Low-dose iodine is routinely added to some brands of table salt in this country.

Thyroid disorders generally occur more commonly in middle age and in females, but abnormal thyroid function test results may be discovered on routine screening in the absence of any clinical abnormality.

In *hyperthyroidism* the commonest clinical features comprise weight loss, with a normal or increased appetite, heat intolerance, tremor and irritability. There may be palpitations, signifying atrial fibrillation. Thyroid function tests will confirm the diagnosis and help to quantify the degree of functional derangement. In the classic and commonest form of the condition (Graves' disease), regarded as having an immunological basis, there is a diffuse enlargement of the gland, an overproduction of thyroid hormone and, eventually if not initially, the development of the well-known abnormal eye features of thyroid overactivity: protrusion of the eyeballs and eyelid retraction leading to conjunctivitis, corneal ulceration and impaired vision, these changes being more common in cigarette smokers.

Management options in hyperthyroidism comprise antithyroid drugs such as carbimazole, surgery in the form of subtotal thyroidectomy, or oral radioactive iodine. Beta-adrenergic blocking drugs such as propranolol will quickly alleviate symptoms of hyperthyroidism and, whilst not suitable for long-term use, may be useful in, for example, those awaiting or experiencing some stressful life event. In less than well-controlled individuals, participation in exercise sessions is likely to aggravate the tremor, palpitations, irritability and the effects of heat intolerance.

In *hypothyroidism*, the commonest clinical findings comprise tiredness and sleepiness, weight gain, cold intolerance, bradycardia, hypertension and angina,

anaemia, hoarseness, dry skin, aches and pains, and muscle stiffness. There may be *myxoedema*, a non-pitting oedema most marked in the skin of the hands, feet and eyelids. However, in many cases, few of these features are well developed or obvious.

Hypothyroidism should be treated with hormone replacement therapy, using thyroxine in gradually increasing doses over a period of 3–6 weeks. Ischaemic heart disease may be present in hypothyroidism, but angina does not always occur until activity levels rise during replacement therapy, the scope of which may therefore become curtailed. In inadequately controlled individuals, participation in exercise sessions is likely to be limited by tiredness, cold intolerance, stiffness, etc., and the possibility of angina during excessive effort.

Faults in posture and muscles

These may include any of the postural habits and faults described in Chapter 3.

Good teaching practice

This would include:

- awareness of symptoms indicating the treatment is insufficient
- providing an exercise programme appropriate to the individual's level of fitness – the person could otherwise be well and fit.

OSTEOPOROSIS

This is a systemic skeletal disease with low bone mineral density and structural deterioration giving rise to a high risk of fractures. Diagnosis is generally based on bone mineral density thresholds set by the World Health Organization for spine, hip or forearm in postmenopausal women. However, it is probably appropriate to use the same criteria for men and premenopausal women (although not adolescents or children).

Peak bone mass is achieved by the age of 30 in the axial skeleton and earlier at peripheral sites. After skeletal maturity, about 1% of bone may be lost per year in both sexes but there is an accelerated bone loss in women for 3–5 years after the menopause. Bone loss leads to thinning of trabeculae more than cortical bone so that osteoporotic fractures tend to occur more at sites where this relatively weakened bone structure predominates: the lumbar vertebrae, neck of femur and distal radius.

Primary osteoporosis, which is predominantly postmenopausal, results from accelerated bone loss due to

2

oestrogen deficiency. Secondary osteoporosis, related to a larger variety of possible causes, accounts for 40% of cases in women and 60% in men. In addition to rheumatoid arthritis and ankylosing spondylitis, endocrine and gastrointestinal conditions affecting nutrition and calcium metabolism may be associated. Risk factors, in addition to heredity, include female sex, increasing age or early menopause, hypogonadism, smoking, high alcohol intake, physical inactivity and low body weight. Prevention of osteoporosis aims to increase peak bone mass and reduce the rate of bone loss by regular weight bearing exercise such as walking and aerobics; on the other hand, excessive exercise may also lead to bone loss. Dietary calcium and avoidance of smoking and alcohol excess are important, together with investigation and treatment of possible secondary causes.

Management

Osteoporosis is a serious public health issue that is now benefiting from progressive advances in assessment and management.

Reduction of any environmental factors leading to falls will obviously lead to fewer fractures and their socioeconomic effects.

Treatment centres on *pain relief* where required following injury as well as drug therapy that is based on prevention of bone resorption on the one hand and promotion of bone formation on the other.

Antiresorptive agents include calcium, fluoride and vitamin D, used singly or in combination, but the relative benefit of each remains undetermined.

Female hormone replacement therapy is now no longer recommended in osteoporosis, unless essential to control menopausal symptoms. Studies covering oestrogen alone and combined with progesterone have both shown reductions in subsequent osteoporotic fractures but the effects upon the incidence of strokes, cardiovascular effects and breast cancer have been difficult to quantify.

Bisphosphonates have constituted the biggest advance in bone antiresorption, although their inconvenient dosing regimen and gastrointestinal side effects have been limiting factors, and long-term adherence to treatment is needed for optimum effect. These drugs remain in the skeleton for decades and the long-term effects of this are not clear.

Selective oestrogen receptor modulators are being developed that can exert agonist effects upon oestrogen-sensitive tissues in bone, thereby benefiting osteoporosis, without unwanted effects on cardiovascular disease and breast tissue, etc. The effects on bone mineral density appear to be less than with bisphosphonates and there is still a risk of venous thrombosis, as there is with hormone therapy itself.

Promotion of bone formation by *anabolic therapy* using parathyroid hormone has proved effective but prolonged use is contraindicated and the benefits wane after withdrawal unless combined with bisphosphonates.

Newer agents include strontium salts that have been used with promising results that compare with bisphosphonates.

Faults in posture and muscles

These may include:

- kyphosis
- kypholordosis
- scoliosis

(see Chapter 3).

Good teaching practice

This would include:

- understanding the degree of bone density loss – severe disease carries a greater risk of spontaneous vertebral fracture
- being aware of the limitations of exercise when dealing with spinal deformities
- avoiding tripping or falling
- assisting bone health through specific weight bearing exercises – for example, providing core control is efficient, leg weights may be used to increase exercise demand during leg muscle strengthening
- avoidance of spinal flexion – this not only carries the risk of vertebral fracture, but studies have also shown that exercise programmes using mainly flexion or a combination of flexion and extension exercises may deplete rather than promote bone density; therefore, practically, hip mobilization would always occur with the lumbar spine neutral and stable
- exercising erector spinae through well-aligned and controlled back extension exercises
- avoiding loaded lumbar spine extension – this could cause vertebral fracture leading to spondylolysis and spondylolisthesis.

OSTEOARTHRITIS

This, by far the commonest form of arthritis, shows a strong association with ageing and becomes a major cause of pain and disability in the elderly.

The prevalence rises steadily from as early as 30 years of age so that, by 65, some 80% of people show radiological changes even though less than half of these have any associated symptoms.

Osteoarthritis (OA) affects synovial joints and leads to characteristic focal loss of the hyaline articular cartilage. At the same time, there is a proliferation of new bone so that the joint undergoes some remodelling with a resulting degree of alteration of the shape of adjacent bone. Inflammation is not a prominent feature, in contrast to rheumatoid arthritis. The knees and hips are principally affected, together with the fingers, toes and the clavicular joints, with resulting disability and reduced mobility. Although much less common, OA of the shoulder, elbow and ankle are still the main forms of arthritis occurring in this condition.

Generalized constitutional and localized biochemical factors may combine to predispose towards development of what is then best viewed as a dynamic damage and repair process of synovial joints that may have been triggered by a variety of insults, some of which may have resulted in irreversible changes. Whilst mechanical, metabolic, genetic or constitutional factors may initiate this damage and trigger the need for repair, the actual insult most often remains unclear unless it is something obvious like a ruptured ligament, menisceal tear or a fracture involving a joint. It should therefore be regarded as disease of the whole joint and adjacent structures, not just the cartilage The resulting osteoarthritic process then involves all the interdependent joint tissues: bone, cartilage, synovium, capsule, ligaments and muscles. Repair involves new tissue production and remodelling of joint shape that may succeed in compensating for the original insult or injury. The result may then be a pain-free, fully functioning, if somewhat deformed, joint. At the other extreme, severe or chronic changes, together with a poor tissue repair response, may result in progressive irreversible damage with pain and disability in addition to deformities.

The presenting clinical features of OA are pain and functional restriction but for many people the latter is an equal or greater problem than pain.

Common characteristics of pain in osteoarthritis

- Patient over age 45 (often over age 60), common in females
- Insidious onset over months or years
- Variable or intermittent over time (good days, bad days)
- Mainly related to movement and weight bearing, relieved by rest
- Only brief (<15 minutes) morning stiffness and brief (<1 minute) 'gelling' after rest
- Usually only one or a few joints painful

Common physical features underlying functional restriction in osteoarthritis

- Restricted movement (capsular thickening, blocking by osteophytes)

- Palpable, sometimes audible, coarse crepitus (rough articular surfaces)
- Bony swelling (osteophyte) around joint margins
- Deformity, usually without instability
- Joint-line or periarticular tenderness
- Muscle weakness, wasting
- Synovitis (effusion, increased warmth) mild or absent compared with rheumatoid arthritis.

Investigations

The diagnosis and assessment of OA are commonly purely clinical. However, plain radiographs, although not essential, may be useful in demonstrating some of the typical features of the condition. These may include narrowing of the joint space, osteophytes, loose bodies, deformity, etc., which may help to assess the overall severity of the structural changes, especially when surgery is being considered. As there is no acute inflammatory process, biochemical and haematological investigations are not especially indicated, but unexplained young onset OA requires more thorough investigation to identify factors such as haemochromatosis, acromegaly or a neuropathic mechanism.

Generalized nodal OA is a common form presenting typically in middle-aged women with pain, stiffness and swelling of a few finger joints with gradual proximal spread. Heberden's and Bouchard's nodes develop in affected joints. Symptoms may often subside with time, and function may remain relatively intact; however, thumb OA may in practice cause significant functional impairment. Generalized nodal OA, which has a strong genetic disposition, is associated with later involvement of other joints, especially the knee, so there may be a clear family history, especially in female relatives. Sometimes nodal OA has a more prolonged inflammatory course with more severe joint damage seen on radiography as erosive OA.

In *hip OA*, the superior pole of the joint is commonly affected in both men and women, often unilateral at first but of relatively poor prognosis. The less common medial aspect involvement, found more in women and usually bilateral, has a better prognosis.

Hip pain is felt deep in the groin and radiates to the buttock and front of the thigh, knee or shin. Lateral hip pain, especially when lying on the affected side, suggests trochanteric bursitis.

In addition to restricted movement, there will be a jerky, uneven gait, together with quadriceps and gluteal muscle wasting, limitation of movement (especially of internal rotation with the hip flexed) and anterior groin tenderness over the joint. There may be fixed flexion and external rotation deformities and even leg shortening on the more severely affected side. Obesity is an additional risk factor for a poor prognosis.

Knee OA may be isolated or a feature of nodal OA. Trauma is a more important factor in men and results in unilateral OA but most knee OA, particularly in women, is bilateral. Pain is commonly felt in the vicinity of the kneecap on stairs and slopes. Prolonged walking, getting in and out of a chair or a car, and bending may all pose difficulties. Examination shows avoidance of weight bearing on the painful joint and painful side of the joint with a jerky, uneven gait, abnormal alignment (especially a varus or bow-legged deformity), tenderness over the joint line and weakness and wasting of the quadriceps muscles, limitation of movements, crepitations and bony swelling. Sometimes crystal depositions of calcium phosphate may be associated with marked inflammation with stiffness and effusion, rather like the synovitis of gout.

In the context of *young onset OA*, young tends to mean under 45 years. Commonly only one joint is affected and there is a history of trauma. When, rarely, several joints are affected in young people, more obscure causes must be excluded.

Management

Whilst there is no cure, and having excluded the possibility of early rheumatoid disease, management centres on education, exercise and adjustments to lifestyle to minimize disability and limit further structural progression, and pain control.

Education

A full, preferably written, explanation of the nature OA with emphasis on risk factors such as obesity, heredity and previous or ongoing trauma, especially occupational, should be provided. Although structural changes are permanent, pain and function can improve, and the prognosis, which is good for hands and better for knees and hips, is in fact amenable to some degree of improvement in almost all joints, especially if adverse mechanical factors, particularly weight loss, can be remedied.

Exercise

Randomized controlled trials have shown that both aerobic and strengthening exercises – especially walking, cycling and swimming – produce modest but long-term improvements in pain, disability and function with large joint OA, even in older subjects. Ageing is no contraindication to such exercise regimens as the reduced muscle strength and proprioception and the impaired balance of ageing all contribute to the pain and disability of large joint OA which comprise the main musculoskeletal problems of the elderly.

Pain control

This can be implemented initially by a trial of paracetamol to which may be added topical *non-steroidal anti-inflammatory drugs* (NSAIDs) such as ibuprofen. Analgesics may be upgraded to paracetamol–opiate combinations such as co-codamol or to oral non-selective NSAIDs, bearing in mind possible side effects on gastric and kidney function, especially in the elderly. COX2 selective inhibitors have now been largely withdrawn because of the increased risk of cardiovascular problems. Topical 'counter irritants' such as capsaicin may be useful for knee and hand OA. There is no convincing evidence that glucosamine is of benefit over placebo.

Moderate or severe pain may derive temporary benefit from intra-articular injections of *corticosteroids*, and ultimately *surgery* should be considered if conservative measures fail and there is progressive disability, functional impairment and uncontrolled pain, especially at night. However, general fitness for surgery and anaesthesia must be taken into account as well as age, and as the prostheses have a limited life span of approximately 15 years, the older the better so far as the person's age is concerned.

Faults in posture and muscles

These may include:

- kyphosis
- kypholordosis
- scoliosis

(see Chapter 3).

Good teaching practice

This would include:

- awareness of the degree of pain and disability
- planning exercise sessions for when joint swelling and pain are least problematic – commonly this is in the morning
- spine mobilization, providing there is no painful spine pathology
- referring specific pains back to a health professional
- exercising the muscles supporting affected joints
- mobilizing affected joints as advised through a comfortable range of motion – usually around mid-range of possible joint movement
- improving proprioception and balance
- avoidance of aggravating activities.

RHEUMATOID ARTHRITIS

In contrast to OA, rheumatoid arthritis (RA) is an inflammatory condition. As the commonest form of inflammatory arthritis, it constitutes a potentially controllable, or even preventable, cause of a physical disabling disease of considerable socioeconomic significance.

There is a symmetrical, deforming, small and large joint arthritis that may be accompanied by systemic disturbance and extra-articular features. Whilst the disease is life long, it may range between mild and severe in degree, together with successive exacerbations and remissions. RA occurs throughout the world but no single aetiological factor has been identified, although female sex is a risk factor and this susceptibility is increased postpartum and with breast feeding. Cigarette smoking is also a risk factor, but whatever triggers the condition, there is a predominating inflammatory process with a strong autoimmune basis leading to chronic inflammatory joint destruction.

The earliest change is swelling and congestion of the synovial membranes with effusions into the joints. Adjacent articular cartilage is eroded and destroyed, muscle adjacent to the inflamed joint atrophies and some joints may eventually ankylose. Rheumatoid nodules may occur subcutaneously and in pleurae, lungs and pericardium. As irreversible damage occurs early, diagnosis and treatment must not be delayed.

Involvement begins gradually and symmetrically, typically in the small joints of the hands, wrists and feet, although onset in older people can be rapid and dramatic. There is morning and inactivity stiffness, and actively inflamed joints will be tender and painful to move. The process invariably extends to knees, elbows, hips and shoulders.

There are numerous possible extra-articular features of what is in fact a systemic disease with, commonly, fever, anorexia, weight loss, fatigue, anaemia and other more complex haematological problems.

There may be greater or lesser degrees of muscle wasting, small vessel arteritis, and ocular and neurological effects, together with the local effects of rheumatoid nodules in subcutaneous and other tissues.

Atlantoaxial subluxation is a common finding in long-standing RA due adjacent atlantoid transverse ligament erosion. Neck flexion can cause acute and potentially fatal compression of the cervical cord, which possibility must always be borne in mind during exercise routines. A history of occipital headache and of upper limb paraesthesiae, etc., occurring in relation to neck flexion should raise awareness of the possibility.

Management

The key objectives are relief of symptoms, suppression of inflammation, preservation of function in affected joints and lifestyle changes if practicable. In more severe cases domestic and personal aids such as wrist splints may also be needed.

Functional capacity decreases most rapidly at the start of the disease so it is essential to establish control as soon as possible. In the older age groups, osteoporosis and NSAID gastro and renal toxicity, especially in the presence of corticosteroid therapy, pose additional problems.

Physical rest, together with passive exercises and anti-inflammatory drug therapy, form the basis of acute stage treatment. There is the ultimate possibility of surgery in the form of synovectomies of the wrist joints and finger tendon sheaths for pain relief and the prevention of tendon rupture. There is now also the possibility of finger joint replacements, as well as the established large joint replacement arthroplasties.

Inflammation should be suppressed as early as possible, using *specific disease modifying antirheumatic drugs* (DMARDs) and the new *biological agents*, as well as the long-established NSAIDs and corticosteroids. Of these, the biological agents offer the greatest suppression of structural damage. It may even be possible to withdraw this therapy if inflammation can be suppressed adequately and for sufficient time.

Although for long a standard treatment, NSAIDs – whilst improving symptoms – do not alter the progress and long-term disability of the disease. DMARDs, in contrast, act to limit structural damage as well as to control symptoms. Agents such as gold, hydroxychloroquine, penicillamine, sulfasalazine, ciclosporin and methotrexate have all been used to effect, but toxicity has usually limited long-term use for most of these. Again in the older age groups, osteoporosis and NSAID gastro and renal toxicity, especially in the presence of corticosteroid therapy, also pose problems.

More recently, therapy has been revolutionized by the possibility of blocking the action of biochemical agents such as tumour necrosis factors (TNFs) active in RA. Used in combination with DMARDs such as methotrexate, anti-TNF biological agents have been shown to be highly effective and could be withdrawn after remission periods of 6 months or more. Although these agents, of which there are now several, are not without problems such as increased susceptibility to infections, including reactivation of latent tuberculosis, combining anti-TNF and DMARD therapy to induce remission and then continuing with DMARDs alone is a potentially safer approach, providing there is adequate screening to exclude active tuberculosis.

Regularity of exercise is important and treatment should specifically include occupational and physiotherapy together with an appropriate drug regimen. Joint swelling and pain are frequently worse in the morning so exercise sessions may be more effective later in the day.

JOINT REPLACEMENT SURGERY

There are now established and successful joint replacement arthroplasty procedures available for hip, knee, shoulder and elbow for both RA and OA, as well as digital and knuckle joints in rheumatoid arthritis. There is a failure rate in lower limb procedures of about 15% at 15 years for hip and 10% at 15 years for knee replacements. Arthroplasty will normally restore a full range of movement with compete safety, although in some cases hip dislocation may recur from time to time (e.g. when legs are crossed), or in the shoulder where rotator cuff integrity has been compromised before or during surgery.

PSORIATIC ARTHRITIS

This inflammatory arthritis usually presents in persons with current or previous psoriasis, but in some cases it predates the skin condition. There are several types of presentation, the commonest of which may affect upper and lower limb joints. Usually only one or two large joints are involved, mainly the knees, with often very large effusions. In others, there is a rheumatoid picture, or a close resemblance to ankylosing spondylitis.

The prognosis is generally better than for RA and treatment centres on simple analgesics, oral and topical NSAIDs and the same exercise regimens and attention to posture as for those with spondylitis. In some more resistant cases, DMARDs may benefit both the arthritis and the skin condition.

GOUT

This is a condition in which joints and periarticular tissues are inflamed and damaged by the presence of urate crystals derived from uric acid, with an inflammatory arthritis, tenosynovitis, cellulitis or nodular crystal deposits ('tophi'). There may be associated atheroma and insulin resistance. *Primary gout* is almost exclusively a male disease, in contrast to *secondary gout* due to kidney disease or drug therapy, usually seen in women.

Whilst an acute attack of gout, with pain more severe than almost any other form of arthritis, is likely to be incapacitating, requiring analgesia with colchicine, high-dose NSAIDs and oral or intra-articular corticosteroids, perhaps even for 2 or 3 weeks, there may be very little disability in remission. Management centres on diet, avoiding offal and other purine-containing ingredients of which uric acid is a metabolite. Drugs that promote the excretion of uric acid may be used to reduce the incidence of acute attacks.

Faults in posture and muscles

These may include:

- kyphosis
- kypholordosis
- scoliosis

(see Chapter 3).

Good teaching practice

This would include:

- awareness of the degree of pain and disability
- planning exercise sessions for when joint swelling and pain are least problematic – commonly this is in the morning
- referring specific pains back to a health professional
- spine mobilization, providing there are no contraindications such as osteoporosis or painful spine pathology
- avoidance of spinal flexion where there is a degree of osteoporosis or painful spine pathology; therefore, practically, hip mobilization would always occur with the lumbar spine neutral and stable
- exercising erector spinae through well-aligned and controlled back extension exercises
- exercising the muscles supporting affected joints
- mobilizing affected joints as advised through a comfortable range of motion – usually around mid-range of possible joint movement
- improving proprioception and balance, particularly after acute episodes requiring bed rest
- using props, supports and specialized Pilates' equipment to assist in creating comfortable and correctly aligned preparatory or rest positions
- avoiding overexertion and fatigue.

HYPERTENSION

High blood pressure features in a variety of conditions and situations. Blood pressure rises with age and, whilst the incidence of cardiovascular disease, especially of the coronary arteries and of cerebrovascular accidents or 'strokes', is closely related to the average blood pressure, regardless of age, antihypertensive therapy has been shown to reduce the incidence of both these problems. The cardiovascular effects of the blood pressure in a particular person are dependent on a number of identifiable risk factors, especially age, sex, weight, physical inactivity, smoking, family history, blood cholesterol, diabetes mellitus and pre-existing vascular disease.

Management therefore centres not only on lowering blood pressure, but also on tackling as many of those

2

identifiable risk factors that may be operating in the particular person.

Hypertension exerts adverse effects on blood vessels, particularly the CNS, the retina, the heart and kidneys.

In *blood vessels* the walls become thickened and the lumina narrowed by fibrous tissue causing arteriosclerosis and by lipid-based atheromatous deposits, together termed 'atherosclerosis', which may lead to coronary and cerebrovascular disease, especially in the presence of the above-listed risk factors. At the same time, narrowing may be accompanied by weakening of the vessel walls so that an aneurysm may develop, with the possibility of rupture and dissection, especially of the aorta. The narrowing and hardening of the blood vessels increase their resistance to blood flow, so perpetuating and aggravating the hypertension.

In the *CNS*, stroke is a common complication due to a cerebral haemorrhage when a vessel ruptures, or an infarct when narrowing and atheroma lead to blockage, with ischaemic damage to brain tissue in both cases.

Retinal vessels may undergo the changes seen elsewhere in the vascular system and these can be viewed during retinoscopy as a simple and highly informative clinical procedure.

In the *heart*, the increased cardiac morbidity and mortality are largely related to the higher incidence of coronary artery disease and myocardial damage. Hypertension places a pressure load on the heart so that left ventricular hypertrophy (LVH) develops, the degree of which can be assessed by electrocardiographic (ECG) and radiological imaging studies. When present, LVH is highly predictive of cardiovascular complications and provides a very useful risk assessment. Atrial fibrillation is common in LVH and coronary disease.

In the *kidneys*, long-term damage to blood vessels can lead ultimately to kidney failure.

Although often associated in the minds of the public with headache, hypertension itself is largely asymptomatic and so is more often discovered only during a routine check. Isolated readings should be followed by accurate automated measurements over periods of time and under ambulatory conditions, preferably over 24-hour periods. Contributory factors (e.g. underlying endocrine disease) must be identified, as must other risk factors and complications such as kidney damage.

Management

The aim is to reduce both the systolic and diastolic pressures first by *lifestyle measures*, including correction of obesity, reduction of salt and alcohol intake, regular physical exercise, increased intake of fruit and vegetables and oily fish, reduced intake of saturated fats and cessation of smoking.

To these measures are added *antihypertensive drugs*, taking into account recommended target blood pressure levels, the threshold for which is set lower in diabetics who should always be regarded as at particularly high risk. A variety of types of antihypertensive drugs, with differing modes of action, is in current use in various combinations and the development of a suitable regimen depends on individual response, convenience, side effects, etc. Most people require combination therapy using two or three drugs in low doses to reduce unwanted side effects.

Adjuvant therapy with *low dose aspirin* aims to depress platelet activity, the benefits of which are regarded as outweighing the increased risk of cerebral haemorrhage if the blood pressure is well controlled. In the presence of raised blood cholesterol, *statins* are used to offset the consequent increased risk of developing coronary artery disease. These agents have now been shown to exert several additional beneficial actions on various cardiovascular risk factors.

Faults in posture and muscles

These may include any of the postural faults described in Chapter 3.

Good teaching practice

This would include:

- understanding that there may be underlying cardiovascular disease
- awareness that headaches or dizziness may be an indication for drug therapy review
- understanding that moving too quickly from supine to standing could result in postural hypotension (a side effect of antihypertensive agents) or that bruising could result from depression of platelet activity
- avoidance of overexertion and straining.

CORONARY HEART DISEASE

Coronary heart disease (CHD) is the most common form of heart disease and seems likely to become the major cause of death worldwide. Death rates in the UK are amongst the highest in Western Europe; however, they are falling. Atheroma is usually the basis of CHD, leading to impaired coronary blood supply with anginal pain and disorders of heart rhythm. There is the ever-present possibility of coronary thrombosis with myocardial infarction and sudden death.

Management

This comprises detailed advice on lifestyle, together with medication. Attention should be paid to cessation of smoking, attaining an ideal body weight, and taking exercise regularly, but not to a severe or unaccustomed degree, especially after a heavy meal or in very cold weather.

Sublingual nitrates should be carried for use before undertaking exertion that is known to induce angina.

Anxiety and misconceptions that may be contributing to disability should be dispelled. Some people avoid all forms of exertion because they fear that any anginal pain signifies permanent ischaemic myocardial damage.

Medication centres on *antiplatelet therapy* with low-dose aspirin or clopidogrel, and *antianginal therapy* with nitrates, beta-blockers and calcium channel blockers.

Invasive procedures in current use comprise coronary artery bypass grafting (CABG) and percutaneous coronary interventions (PCI) by balloon arterioplasty or coronary artery stent implantation.

Oxygen and full dose aspirin are the two most valuable first aid measures in acute myocardial infarction (heart attack) and may be given even in advance of the arrival of skilled assistance.

Faults in posture and muscles

These may include any of the postural faults described in Chapter 3.

Good teaching practice

This would include:

- ensuring that exercise occurs at least 1 hour after meals and that the venue is sufficiently warm
- being aware that exercise intensity should increase but must be monitored by a health professional
- ensuring the person always has their sublingual nitrates, etc., readily available
- avoiding overexertion or straining.

CEREBROVASCULAR DISEASE

Cerebrovascular accidents (CVAs) are the third most common cause of disability and death in the developed world after cancer and ischaemic heart disease, the mechanism being either brain ischaemia from occlusion of blood vessels or haemorrhage from their rupture causing physical damage to brain tissue.

The most likely CVA presentation is an *acute focal stroke*, although in the elderly there may be a more gradual decline in cerebral function into dementia. In acute focal stroke there is the sudden appearance of a specific deficit in function, usually a hemiplegia, with the possible addition of a higher functional deficit such as aphasia (speech deficit) or visual field loss.

A stroke deficit may be *transient,* with recovery within 24 hours, *evolving* beyond a period of 6 hours, or *complete* and not worsening. When a cerebral artery is occluded, an area of brain tissue is damaged from the loss of the oxygen supply to which it is acutely sensitive. This is commonly due to arteriosclerosis or following an embolism in which some insoluble thrombotic debris is carried into the cerebral arterial system from the heart, aortic arch or carotid arteries. The heart can become a source of embolism in atrial fibrillation if anticoagulants have not been used so that there is atrial thrombus from which fragments can become detached and enter the cerebral circulation. However, local compensatory changes in the cerebral vessels can offset the effect of the primary occlusion, in some cases to a remarkable degree.

The other possible cause of ischaemic brain tissue damage is an intracerebral haemorrhage where a blood vessel ruptures within the brain substance, or in an area already damaged by an embolism, or when a nearby subarachnoid haemorrhage has occurred with bleeding into the space surrounding the brain as might be more the case in younger age groups.

Risk factors for stroke include increasing age, heredity, a previous stroke, heart attack or other vascular event, hypertension, diabetes, hyperlipidaemia, smoking, alcohol excess and oral contraceptives.

Management

Management of a completed stroke centres on limiting the extent of brain damage, preventing complications, reducing disability, rehabilitation and preventing recurrences.

However, cases of subarachnoid, as opposed to intracerebral, haemorrhage require neurosurgical intervention to control bleeding from the blood vessel responsible, in which a small 'berry' aneurysm will have ruptured.

Thrombolytic and anticoagulant drugs may be used, but of these aspirin is the least controversial with a lower risk of haemorrhagic complications than with the other agents.

Rehabilitation starts at the earliest opportunity, initially in a specialized stroke unit if possible, with the then likelihood of accelerated functional recovery that for the subject is the most important aim.

Faults in posture and muscles

These may include any of the postural faults described in Chapter 3.

Good teaching practice

This would include:

- awareness of associated problems affecting sight, hearing, speech and balance
- consideration of general weaknesses due to enforced inactivity, as well as functional deficits due to the condition
- strengthening muscle groups that help to maintain independence during everyday activities
- allowing time for the individual to exercise effectively
- ensuring torso muscle control is adequate for safe spine mobilization
- using props, supports and specialized Pilates' equipment to increase exercise efficiency by reducing any unwanted gravitational effects on posture and balance
- avoiding overexertion and fatigue
- assisting a gradual return to normal everyday activities.

CHRONIC OBSTRUCTIVE PULMONARY DISEASE

Chronic obstructive pulmonary disease (COPD) is the term now used to cover chronic bronchitis and emphysema. It is a slow, progressive disorder with airflow obstruction leading to impaired lung function that, although to a large degree fixed, may still respond partially to bronchodilator therapy.

The term *chronic bronchitis* refers to the coughing up of sputum regularly over an extended period; *emphysema* refers to the permanent destructive enlargement of the distal airspaces. In the majority of cases, the two conditions overlap considerably.

Cigarette smoking is the most important single cause, by inducing persistent airway inflammation, but other irritants such as dust and air pollution may be involved, depending on occupation, etc. As the condition develops, there are episodes of cough and sputum, usually after winter colds, getting gradually worse over time until cough is present throughout the year. Subjects are then prone to repeated chest infections, breathlessness on exertion, coughing and wheezing with thick sputum and active use of accessory muscles of respiration, especially the scaleni and sternomastoids. A relative increase in thoracic anteroposterior diameter gives rise to the term 'barrel chest'.

Management

This centres first on complete and permanent cessation of smoking, ideally by joining a formal cessation programme, and elimination of environmental and occupational factors as far as possible. Chest infection that aggravates breathlessness and worsens lung function should receive prompt antibiotic treatment. Bronchodilators, both anticholinergic and beta sympathomimetic, should be used regularly and in combination. Inhaled anti-inflammatory corticosteroids may also be used but, like antibiotics, their use should be confined to exacerbations and not on a long-term basis. Exercise should be encouraged in order to improve performance and ultimately reduce breathlessness.

Faults in posture

These may include kyphosis/kypholordosis (see also Chapter 3).

Good teaching practice

This would include:

- ensuring that the venue is sufficiently warm
- ensuring medications such as inhaled anti-inflammatory corticosteroids, etc., are readily available
- being aware that the fear of breathlessness may hinder an individual's progress
- being aware that exercise intensity should increase but must be monitored by a health professional
- using upright positions to assist breathing efficiency
- avoiding the prone position with a support under the abdomen as this compromises breathing efficiency
- avoiding overexertion or straining.

ASTHMA

Bronchial asthma is a disorder in which chronic airway inflammation and increased airway responsiveness result in chest tightness and wheeze, cough and breathlessness. There is a variable degree of airflow obstruction, reversible with treatment. Whilst the condition may be severe and progressive in some cases, others are symptom- and sign-free between attacks.

Asthma is common and is increasing in prevalence, although for reasons that are not clear, but early exposure to aeroallergens and cigarette smoke may be factors in genetically susceptible persons. It is known to run in families and there are associations with other allergic phenomena, including rhinitis, urticaria and eczema.

Environmental sources of allergens may be indoor such as house mites, other insects and pets, spores, cigarettes, cooking and other sources of fumes. Outdoor allergens include grass and flower pollens, allergens from crops, and fumes from motor traffic and industrial sites.

Some drugs – including especially aspirin, as well as NSAIDs, beta-blockers by their specific pharmacological

2

effects on smooth muscle and a variety of drugs associated with histamine release – can cause bronchoconstriction in some people.

Other aggravating factors include respiratory tract infection, smoking, exercise, cold air and, in some cases, severe anxiety and stress.

Management

This involves education towards understanding the nature of the condition, avoidance of precipitating factors if known, and the correct choice and use of inhaled bronchodilators and anti-inflammatories, for which devices with more effective aerosols are now being developed.

Faults in posture

These may include kyphosis (see also Chapter 3).

Good teaching practice

This would include:

- awareness of precipitating factors such as the onset of a viral infection or stress
- ensuring that the venue is clean, warm, etc.
- ensuring that the person always has their inhaled anti-inflammatory corticosteroids, etc., readily available
- using upright positions to assist breathing efficiency as required
- avoiding the prone position with a support under the abdomen during active episodes of disease
- being aware that asthma sufferers may be fit and have a high limit of exercise tolerance.

GASTROINTESTINAL PROBLEMS

Gastro-oesophageal reflux

This condition, in which gastric contents reflux into the lower oesophagus to some extent, occurs occasionally in 30% of the population, causing the well-known symptoms of *heartburn* due to the strong acidity of gastric juice.

Occasional episodes of reflux are common in health, the reflux being cleared by oesophageal peristalsis and the residual acid being neutralized by alkaline saliva that is swallowed constantly so that actual symptoms do not occur.

However, prolonged exposure results in *gastro-oesophageal reflux disease*, with symptoms of heartburn from actual oesophagitis. Factors predisposing to prolonged exposure include a low oesophageal sphincter tone that permits reflux when intra-abdominal pressure

is raised, as in obesity, during pregnancy, when straining or from Pilates core strengthening exercises.

Hiatus hernia

This may be associated with reflux because the pressure gradient between abdominal and thoracic cavities that causes pinching of the oesophagus at the diaphragmatic hiatus is lost. However, the relationship between hiatus hernia and reflux is poor, some persons with large herniae having no reflux symptoms and vice versa.

The major symptoms of heartburn and regurgitation, even as far up as the pharynx, may be provoked by bending, straining and lying down. 'Waterbrash' may occur, with reflex secretion of alkaline saliva in response to acid entering the oesophagus.

Management

This includes lifestyle advice covering weight loss, avoidance of aggravating dietary factors and drugs to neutralize gastric acid or suppress its secretion. Ultimately, antireflux surgery may be required.

Inflammatory bowel disease

This term generally refers to ulcerative colitis (UC) and Crohn's disease (CD), both of which pursue a relapsing and remitting course and are largely indistinguishable, except that, whilst UC is confined to the colon, CD may occur anywhere in the entire gastrointestinal tract from the mouth to the anus, not only in the terminal ileum.

Management

Management of these lifelong conditions, with their psychosocial implications, requires counselling and educational support as a basis for long-term drug and nutritional therapy.

Up to 60% of those with UC require surgical removal of, possibly, the entire colon and rectum, thus effecting a cure.

Up to 80% of those with CD require surgery, but recurrences may follow in a previously healthy gastrointestinal tract. Surgical resection therefore aims to be conservative in extent to avoid ultimately extensive loss of functioning bowel, but in both forms of inflammatory bowel disease there is the likelihood of a colostomy that must be borne in mind when Pilates core strengthening exercises are being performed.

Both conditions can be associated with a so-called 'enteropathic' arthritis.

Arthritis and bowel disease

Patients with ulcerative colitis and with regional ileitis (Crohn's disease) are susceptible to inflammatory arthritis, so-called 'enteropathic' arthritis. Large lower limb joints are mostly involved and the arthritis coincides with exacerbations in the bowel disease. The arthritis is relieved when the ulcerative colitis is relieved by total colectomy but it may persist in Crohn's disease, which is less amenable to curative surgery. Although sacroiliitis and ankylosing spondylitis can both coexist with bowel disease, unlike enteropathic arthritis they pursue independent courses.

Irritable bowel syndrome

This is a form of functional bowel disorder in which abdominal pain is associated with bowel actions, or a change of bowel habit is associated with abdominal distension and irregular bowel actions. It is thought to occur in 20% of the population, although only half of these seek medical advice. The syndrome, which affects mostly young women, leads to absenteeism from work and impaired quality of life. There may be associated dyspepsia, chronic fatigue syndrome, dysmenorrhoea, dyspareunia, or a history of panic attacks or physical or sexual abuse.

The common symptoms of colicky abdominal pain, cramps and bloating, worsening during the day, are relieved by bowel actions that may alternate between constipation and diarrhoea, although one or the other predominates, but physical examination and investigations are generally normal.

Management

This is based on reassuring the person accordingly and dispelling common fears of cancer. Otherwise relapse can often be related to stressful life events and difficulties with interpersonal relationships.

Together with their frequently anxious and stressed demeanour, these persons may have difficulty in carrying out Pilates core strengthening exercises on account of abdominal pain, cramps and bloating, especially if there is a tendency to provoke incontinence. However, with perseverance the exercises may improve symptoms as well as generating improved self-esteem and well-being.

Faults in posture

These may include any of the faults described in Chapter 3.

Good teaching practice

This would include:

- awareness of possible psychological issues
- understanding that a colostomy is not in itself a contraindication for exercise but will need bearing

in mind when agreeing an appropriate schedule for exercising
- awareness that symptoms such as colicky abdominal pain, cramps and bloating may worsen during the day
- understanding that core strengthening exercises may initially be difficult due to abdominal symptoms
- an emphasis on breathing and relaxation to help reduce abdominal symptoms
- awareness that side lying, sitting or standing positions may be needed to avoid gastric reflux syndrome or general discomfort when exercising.

NECK, SHOULDER AND ARM PROBLEMS

The neck and shoulder are two of the most common sites of musculoskeletal pain associated not only with heavy manual workloads and increasing age, but also more insidiously with long-term faulty postural habits. *Depression* may also be an underlying psychological factor.

Although pain may follow injury to bony or soft tissue elements, it is always essential to exclude nerve root pain, bony pathology or underlying infection or malignancy.

Whilst the neck moves constantly when awake, the shoulder girdle, of which the shoulder joint is a major component, articulates with the ribcage, and the whole joint, comprising capsule, ligaments, tendons and bursae, is extremely mobile, as is the entire shoulder girdle. The stability of the glenohumeral or shoulder joint relies on the rotator cuff. Laxity of the cuff, with impairment of supporting muscle tone because of pain, leads to shoulder joint instability.

NECK PAIN

This may arise in the cervical vertebral column, particularly in *rheumatoid arthritis*, in which it can be associated with *atlantoaxial subluxation*, or in *ankylosing spondylitis* with osteophyte pressure. Cervical nerve root pain may arise because of a *prolapsed intervertebral disc*.

Neck and arm pain with muscle spasm may follow a rapid acceleration–deceleration or 'whiplash' injury.

Pain may arise solely in soft tissue, as *myofascial pain* that can be reproduced by pressure on so-called 'trigger points' that can often be located as small knots within muscles.

2

Acute torticollis, also termed 'wryneck'

This consists of sudden onset of muscle pain with stiffness and there is usually lateral neck flexion. It may follow intense activity or immobility in an awkward position, or minor muscle strain. Other causes include facet joint 'locking' intervertebral disc problems and upper respiratory or other viral infections; however, in some cases there is no obvious precipitating factor. There may be lateral muscle spasm with limitation of movement, but with usually no other abnormal findings provided cervical disc rupture, vertebral fracture or dislocation has been excluded.

Cervical strain

This is a muscle–tendon injury following overloading or excessive stretching of the muscles supporting the shoulder girdle: trapezius, sternocleidomastoid, scaleni, levator scapulae and the rhomboids. Mechanisms of injury include hyperextension, hyperflexion, rotation and lateral flexion. Pain and limitation of movement develop over hours or overnight.

Cervical sprain

This is an injury to ligamentous and capsular elements supporting the cervical facet joints following neck hyperextension or hyperflexion. Pain and limitation of movement develop more rapidly than with cervical strain. In both conditions the differential diagnoses include acute torticollis and cervical vertebral and disc injuries.

Faults in posture

These may include a mobile or fixed kyphotic posture with a forehead position; scoliosis or scoliosis/kyphosis; any postures involving persistent, awkward head and neck positions as might be seen in professional dancers or athletes (see Chapter 3).

Good teaching practice

This would include:

- awareness of warning signs and symptoms such as pain, paraesthesia and muscle weakness – refer for medical opinion
- initially correcting postural and shoulder girdle alignment and muscle function
- introducing isotonic neck muscle exercises and progressing to active exercise, including mobilization and stretching, only when advised by a health professional
- being aware that cervical spine mobilization may always be inappropriate in cases of ongoing

degenerative disease (*when the internal diameter of the cervical vertebral foramina is reduced during movement, nerve constriction within the narrowed foramina occurs, so producing neurological symptoms; this problem commonly resolves itself as the disease progresses and the affected discs fuse*)

- in such cases emphasis is placed on confining flexion and extension to the atlanto-occipital joint (with possibly a few degrees of flexion and extension occurring also in the atlantoaxial joint) and rotation to the atlantoaxial joint
- improving overall spine function, including lumbar and thoracic spine mobility, providing there are no contraindications such as pathology or pain
- addressing residual weakness in the upper limbs and hands
- gradually improving overall muscular strength, stamina and function.

SHOULDER PAIN AND INJURIES

Most shoulder pain is of soft tissue origin, most commonly from rotator cuff tendinitis and tears, osteophytes of the adjacent acromial process or from shoulder joint instability, especially in younger and more active people. A long-standing rotator cuff tear can lead eventually to shoulder joint arthritis. Pain may be felt over the whole shoulder area, worse when using the raised arm, or at night if lying on the affected side. Larger tears will be associated with muscle wasting and weakness. Calcifying tendinitis is a form of rotator cuff syndrome where calcific deposits form within the cuff. A dull ache may progress to acute pain with fever and systemic upset requiring analgesics, NSAIDs and supervised mobilization and stretching.

Chronic shoulder injuries

These are common in athletes from swimming, throwing or the use of racquets, and include *impingement syndrome* which occurs where soft tissues of the rotator cuff and subacromial bursae repeatedly impinge between the acromial process and the head of the humerus so that a rotator cuff tendinitis and acromial bursitis arise and become chronic, with the possible development of a rotator cuff tear, commonly in the supraspinatus tendon. Pain predominates, especially at night. In some cases, impingement syndrome is secondary to a series of shoulder joint subluxations.

Frozen shoulder, with capsular adhesions, occurs more often in middle age and is commoner in diabetics, although not usually as an isolated problem. It is a form of adhesive capsulitis, often precipitated by pain in or around the shoulder that has necessitated prolonged immobilization, as when fractures or dislocations have been rested in a sling. There may be an acute inflammation with synovitis, etc. Pain tends to be worse at night and there may be progressive restriction of movement with associated muscle wasting. Daily mobilization after injuries helps to avoid a frozen shoulder that can otherwise become chronic and difficult to resolve.

Shoulder pain may also be associated with shoulder joint arthritis, cartilage injuries, cervical nerve root or brachial plexus entrapment or neuritis, or thoracic outlet nerve compression.

Shoulder pain may also be purely localized to the *acromioclavicular joint* that may likewise be subject to arthritis or sprain.

Chronic, work-related upper limb pain

This has become a well-recognized syndrome involving a variety of possible causal factors. Pain is the main symptom that may initially have a local cause such as carpal tunnel syndrome at the wrist, flexor or extensor tenosynovitis of the hand, or lateral or medial epicondylitis at the elbow (tennis or golfer's elbow, respectively). Pain develops and spreads proximally to involve possibly the whole arm. The severity and extent of the pain may be disproportionate to the physical findings and can cause great distress. It is commonly associated with the use of keyboards, but also sudden or unwelcome changes in working practices or relationships, job insecurity or other disharmony at work. Because of the possible neurophysiological and psychosocial mechanisms involved, reference to a specialist pain relief unit may be advisable.

Fibromyalgic syndrome

This term describes the occurrence of widespread musculoskeletal pain and hyperanalgesic tender spots, frequently around the shoulder, with no recognizable cause. It presents frequently in general practice and in rheumatology clinics, constituting diagnostic and therapeutic challenges that unduly consume health care resources. Whilst physical examination excludes systemic illness, and clinical findings are unremarkable, there may also be stiffness, poor sleep patterns, depression and other psychological factors. Pressure on normally mildly tender spots produces acute pain and distress. Investigation of headaches, dizziness, paraesthesiae and possible systemic causes will have revealed nothing significant.

The constant feature is pain, exacerbated by emotional and physical stress. There may be associated chronic fatigue, migraine or other headaches, irritable bladder and bowel syndromes, as well as panic attacks, anxiety, depression and poor concentration that may have been fully investigated already.

While management now tends to centre on complementary and alternative medicine, superimposed upon education and relaxation, pacing of activities with graded exercise is important. Such pacing aims to break down everyday activities into realistic and achievable components. This generates a sense of accomplishment and a regain of control. Graded exercise aims to improve the patient's general physical fitness so as to increase strength, stamina and flexibility.

Faults in posture

These may include a mobile or fixed kyphotic posture with a forehead position, scoliosis or scoliosis/kyphosis (see Chapter 3).

Good teaching practice

This would include:

- awareness that pain could be related to neck pathology
- starting shoulder joint mobilization in accordance with medical treatment (see regimen for regular home exercises)
- increasing loads and ranges of joint motion as advised by a health professional
- improving postural and shoulder girdle alignment and stabilization, particularly before upper limb movements
- improving overall spine function, including lumbar and thoracic spine mobility if appropriate
- understanding that full recovery of shoulder function may take anything up to 2 years.

Note: Exercises for rehabilitation after surgery or injury are carefully graded as seen below.

- *Stage 1*: This would include exercises such as:
  - standing with the arms hanging by the sides of the body and shrugging the shoulders
  - swinging the affected arm – the body weight is transferred from one foot to the other and the arm follows the body's movement
  - when supine, using the unaffected arm to move the affected arm through increasing ranges of shoulder flexion.
- *Stage 2 – at up to 6 weeks after stage 1*: When supine, increasing ranges of shoulder flexion with assistance and then unassisted but with shortened

2

levers. Scapula depression at the end of shoulder flexion would be occurring towards the end of stage 2.

■ *Stage 3*: This aims to increase scapula and joint mobilization as well as stability. Exercises might include:
  – when facing a wall with the elbows bent, reaching the arms forwards to creep the fingers up the wall (depressing the scapulae) before opening the arms to the side to describe two circles on the wall
  – clasping the wrist of the affected arm with the hand of the other arm behind the back and, with the shoulders back and down, gently moving the hands up the back.

Specific shoulder girdle strengthening (as in traditional Pilates exercises) would occur after stages 1, 2 and 3.

BACK PROBLEMS

Chronic thoracic and lumbar back pain

Many individuals, both athletic and non-athletic, experience chronic back pain on a daily basis. Whilst not related to any significant acute episode, such pain could be due to long-standing poor posture, faulty lifting and handling procedures, intervertebral disc abnormalities or structural vertebral deformities.

Chronic muscle strain

This can be a common cause of pain in the lower back where repetitive muscle activity results in progressive and cumulative damage at the muscle fibre level. At the same time pain may arise in intervertebral discs or facet joints. Examination will show limitation of movement due to pain and there may be muscle spasm and localized tenderness.

In general, this is a self-limiting condition, resolving without formal medical attention within 3–4 weeks with the help of analgesics and lower back and abdominal stretching and strengthening exercises. Deterioration or failure to respond within 3–4 weeks is an indication for specialist referral.

Lumbar interspinous bursitis

Irritation and inflammation of these structures may cause backache in the lumbar region, exacerbated by hyperextension and relieved by flexion of the lumbar spine. One or more interspinous bursae may be involved and there may be adjacent muscle spasm that, together with pain, limits movement. Analgesia and a graded

resumption of activity are indicated while the bursitis is allowed to resolve.

Iliac apophysitis

This is an inflammation of the growth plate that will later form the iliac crest on the top of each iliac wing. It is a condition of adolescents not yet skeletally mature. There may be tenderness along the iliac crest and spasm of related muscles with limitation of movement. Like chronic muscle strain, this condition tends to be self-limiting and responds to the same measures.

Low back pain

This affects at least 70% of the population in developed countries and constitutes a major socioeconomic problem.

There are many causes, not only within the spine itself, but in association with malignancy, sepsis or systemic disease. Structural causes of low back pain may be of generalized mechanical origin or associated specifically with facet joint arthritis, annular tearing or collapse of an intervertebral disc, spondylosis or spondylolisthesis. In addition, there may be an inflammatory process – discitis, sacroiliitis or spondylitis – or, in older age groups, osteoporotic vertebral collapse. History taking should cover the type of onset, as well as occupational, athletic and general systemic factors. It is especially important to exclude underlying factors when the onset is in comparatively young, or in elderly, patients.

Low backache with leg pain

Leg pain is a feature of many spinal conditions in which backache may be absent. *Sciatica*, where leg pain radiates to the foot, is most commonly due to intervertebral disc prolapse compressing the adjacent lumbar nerve root in the intervertebral foramen. A fall in disc water content with age may contribute to annular tears that may occur acutely and allow the nucleus pulposus to prolapse through the tear, leading to further nerve compression. *Spinal stenosis* may be a factor in older patients and *facet joint arthritis* is common, especially in association with disc pathology.

Non-specific back pain comprises up to 85% of cases due to the effects of mechanical and postural stresses upon vertebral and paravertebral structures.

Localized back pain occurs more specifically in spondyloarthopathies affecting the spine and sacroiliac joints. There may be an associated more peripheral arthritis, as in ankylosing spondylitis and psoriatic arthritis, or in enteropathic arthritis, as in ulcerative colitis and Crohn's disease.

Spondylolysis and spondylolisthesis

These are not uncommon causes of backache, especially in athletes.

In spondylolysis there is a defect in the facet joint structure of a lumbar vertebral arch that, if bilateral, can permit a spondylolisthesis whereby the vertebra above becomes displaced anteriorly on the one below. Pain may range from minimal to severe, together with radiation to the legs signifying neurological involvement. There may be a localized tenderness and, in spondylolisthesis, there may be a palpable forward displacement of the spine of the slipped vertebra. A related factor may be a stress fracture in the vicinity of the facet joint following long-standing repeated hyperextension stresses. Specialist referral is indicated in both these conditions.

Sacroiliac joint pain

This may be felt in the lower back or thigh as well as in the buttock. The joint is synovial but bound by strong ligaments. Pain may be of mechanical origin or there may be a sacroiliitis.

Thoracic and lumbar disc disease

In the *thoracic region* the discs between T10 and T11, T11 and T12, and T12 and L1, and in the *lumbar* region between L4 and L5 and L5 and S1, are those most commonly involved. Compared with acute muscle and ligament strains, there may be no history of trauma at the time of onset of pain associated with thoracic disc herniation. If the disc has herniated laterally then there will be chest or abdominal wall pain at the relevant level due to spinal nerve irritation or compression. If the disc herniates centrally there may be no pain at all, but rather stiffness and weakness in the lower limbs due to cord compression. In this case, specialist referral is indicated. However, thoracic disc herniation is rare.

Lumbar disc herniation is associated with pain in the midline or paravertebral regions but as there may be no history of injury at the time of onset, the pain may seem to be of muscular origin and be felt in the lower back and buttock. However, pain radiating to the leg, ('sciatica') is always suggestive of disc herniation. With more severe compression, pain may give way to numbness and weakness. Local tenderness over the area of the disc concerned may be accompanied by flattening of the lumbar contour and limitation of movement secondary to muscle spasm. Backache due to disc degeneration rather than herniation is distinguished by neurological examination of the lower limbs during specialist referral, although a simple straight-leg raising sciatic nerve tension test is a very sensitive indicator of nerve root compression from disc herniation.

Initially bouts of back pain with sciatica may well respond to rest, analgesics and graded resumption of activity, but chronic pain and a neurological deficit require specialist assessment with a view to possible surgery.

Scoliosis and kyphosis

These chronic ongoing deformities of the spine are generally asymptomatic, being without pain or disability. Any associated chronic pain is an indication for further investigation.

Scoliosis is an abnormal lateral curvature of the spine that may be more obvious when viewed from behind, particularly when the subject bends forward to touch toes in which the characteristic rib hump is most obvious.

Kyphosis is an exaggeration of flexion of the normal curvature of the thoracic spine, seen most easily when viewed from the side.

Both scoliosis and kyphosis are associated with alterations in the normal range of movement of the thoracic and lumbar spine and may be associated with impaired lung function to a degree dependent on the anatomical distortion. In more severe cases surgical stabilization will usually be performed.

Ankylosing spondylitis

This is a chronic inflammatory arthritis with a predilection for the sacroiliac joints and spine with progressive stiffness and fusion of the axial skeleton. Commoner in males, onset is slow with recurring stiffness and back pain radiating to the buttocks that may be misdiagnosed as sciatica. Whilst the lumbosacral area is usually affected first, the disease process ascends slowly to involve possibly the entire vertebral column. Spinal rigidity and disuse lead to secondary osteoporosis and risk of spinal fracture. Nearly half of cases develop peripheral arthropathies, usually symmetrical with additional tendinitis, bony tenderness and general fatigue. There may be extra-articular inflammatory features involving the cardiovascular system, the eye and the prostate gland. Exercise regimens to combat stiffness and maintain mobility are important and regular swimming is an ideal form of exercise in these cases.

Arthritis and bowel disease

See page 68.

Lumbar facet syndrome

Like other synovial joints, the facet joints of the vertebral segments can become inflamed, with pain aggravated

2

by lumbar extension and rotation, and relieved by flexion. In the majority of cases there is also pre-existing disc disease.

Faults in posture

These may include, in particular, lordosis and scoliosis (see Chapter 3).

Good teaching practice

This would include:

- awareness of warning signs and symptoms such as pain, paraesthesia and muscle weakness that require onward referral
- understanding that regular exercise may relieve aching or throbbing pains and stiffness due to inflammatory processes such as arthritis
- recognizing that mechanical pain due to injury (e.g. intervertebral disc prolapse) presents as a sharp pain or dull ache that worsens as the day progresses and is relieved by rest
- understanding that such pain is a contraindication to exercise until assessed by a health professional; initial treatment would include rest and physiotherapy
- initially focusing on correcting spine alignment and stability
- assessing iliopsoas for weakness, tightness and performance during exercising
- performing spine mobilization only when regular home exercises are prescribed
- avoiding spine extension in people with spondylolysis, spondylolisthesis, lumbar facet syndrome and spinal stenosis
- avoiding lumbar flexion after lumbar disc prolapse until a health professional has confirmed its safety (after full recovery loaded lumbar flexion is always contraindicated unless there is normal thoracic and lumbar spine mobility well controlled by efficient core strength)
- addressing residual weaknesses in the back, posterior hip (especially the lower fibres of gluteus maximus) and lower limb muscles
- improving lumbar and thoracic spine mobility if appropriate, as well as overall posture, muscular strength and stamina.

HIP PROBLEMS

Pain from the hip joint tends to be felt in the groin or the front of the thigh and can often be referred to the knee, so masking its true origin. Pain felt posteriorly in the buttock is more likely to originate from the lumbar spine. Hip pain is a common cause of limping.

Hip pain and stiffness in adults is mostly due to osteoarthritis, but may also be due to rheumatoid, or possibly psoriatic arthritis or ankylosing spondylitis in which stiffness tends to predominate. Hip replacement arthroplasty is the ultimate and most effective measure. Osteoporotic hip fracture is particularly common in elderly women and requires surgical stabilization or femoral head hemiarthroplasty.

Other causes of hip pain may be avascular necrosis of the femoral head (Paget's disease) or malignancy involving the pelvis. Soft tissue sources of hip pain include trochanteric bursitis and tears of the acetabular labrum.

Hip disease in children may present more with limping than with hip pain. Alternatively, the pain may, misleadingly, be referred to the knee joint. *Congenital dislocation of the hip* usually presents before the age of 5, whilst *osteonecrosis of the femoral epiphysis (Perthes' disease)* usually occurs in boys between 5 and 10 years of age. *Slipped upper femoral epiphysis* is typically seen in overweight boys, although girls are not immune. Both hips may be affected and surgical stabilization is required. Knee pain is a common presentation but other causes of hip pain in children include septic arthritis, transient synovitis (*irritable hip*) and juvenile chronic arthritis.

Faults in posture

These may include, in particular, lordosis, scoliosis and sway back posture. There may be associated faults in leg and foot alignment (see Chapter 3).

Good teaching practice

This would include:

- understanding that pain due to inflammatory processes such as in arthritis can be relieved by mobilization, but that mechanical pain initially requires rest and physiotherapy
- understanding that limping (particularly in children) could be an indication of hip rather than knee pain
- addressing associated weakness and tightness in the lower back, posterior hip and lower limb muscles (gluteus maximus, the hamstring and quadriceps muscles being particularly vulnerable to wasting, tightness and loss of performance)
- exercising the lower fibres of gluteus maximus
- exercising the hamstring muscles concentrically and eccentrically and improving flexibility with caution
- addressing muscle imbalances within the quadriceps (vastus medialis is nearly always more

affected as it is only fully active during the last 10–20 degrees of knee extension)

- assessing iliopsoas for weakness, tightness and performance and exercise accordingly
- improving foot function and balance, particularly when standing on the affected leg (if appropriate)
- improving overall postural alignment, core strength and control.

KNEE PROBLEMS

Pain in the knee usually follows injury but may occur spontaneously and pain referred from the hip is a common pitfall. There is usually stiffness and evidence of effusion within the joint that fills out the depressions on either side of the kneecap and may be associated with a 'patellar tap' on clinical examination.

Knee pain in adults commonly follows sporting injuries such as a twisting force during football with a major tear of a meniscus or of a cruciate ligament producing a sudden swelling of the whole knee indicative of bleeding into the joint. A more slowly developing effusion suggests a smaller menisceal tear. Chronic pain and swelling usually indicate rheumatoid or osteoarthritis, but other causes include psoriatic arthritis and ankylosing spondylitis. Loose bodies may be produced in osteoarthritis causing instability and intermittent pain. *Osteochondritis dissecans*, with separation of articular cartilage from underlying femoral or tibial bone, can lead to pain, swelling and instability or 'giving way'. In *patellar maltracking*, the kneecap may be totally displaced (dislocated) or partially displaced (subluxated), either by a direct blow or by a strong muscular contraction. *Patellar subluxation*, seen more in girls with patellar maltracking, usually responds to exercise regimens.

Bursae that occur at several sites around the knee may also become inflamed and painful.

Common causes of *knee pain in children* include *chondromalacia patellae* with softening of the cartilage on the articular surfaces of the kneecap. Seen in adolescent girls, it tends to settle at maturity. *Osteochondritis of the tibial tubercle* (Osgood–Schlatter's disease) is seen in adolescent boys with localized pain, tenderness and swelling of the patellar tendon insertion. It is usually a self-limiting condition.

A similar condition involves the distal pole of the patella and the proximal attachment of the patellar tendon (Sinding–Larsen–Johansson's disease).

Lock knee

This phenomenon is associated with menisceal tears that, when extensive, can displace into the joint and cause a mechanical block that prevents full knee flexion or, more particularly, full extension. The so-called 'bucket-handle tear' is particularly associated with this phenomenon. The knee can often be unlocked by self-learned methods involving flexing, extending, then passively rotating the joint so that the displaced and trapped segment of meniscus is freed and mobility is restored.

Faults in posture

These may include any of the described postural faults but especially lordosis and sway back posture, lower limb malalignments such as medial or lateral hip rotation, tibial bowing or knock knees, and pronated or supinated feet (see Chapter 3 and address as appropriate).

Good teaching practice

This would include:

- encouraging avoidance of aggravating activities
- being aware that knee problems must be considered together with hip, ankle and foot function (if ankle joint mobility is compromised, the knee and hip as well as the small joints in the feet will be affected)
- understanding that liaison with health and other professionals (e.g. podiatrists) may be ongoing
- addressing associated weakness and tightness in the lower back, posterior hip and lower limb muscles (gluteus maximus, the hamstring and quadriceps muscles being particularly vulnerable to wasting, tightness and loss of performance)
- exercising the hamstring muscles concentrically and eccentrically and improving flexibility with caution
- addressing muscle imbalances within the quadriceps (vastus medialis is nearly always more affected as it is only fully active during the last 10–20 degrees of knee extension)
- assessing the patella for lateral tracking – this occurs when vastus medialis is weakened and tensor fasciae latae is tightened – and performing strengthening and stretching exercises as appropriate
- assessing iliopsoas for weakness, tightness and performance and exercise accordingly
- improving foot function and balance, particularly when standing on the affected leg (if appropriate).

LOWER LEG PROBLEMS

These may often occur as a result of overuse injury common in endurance sports such as long distance running, cycling and swimming. Common sites are around the knee, the Achilles tendon and the shin area ('shin splints'). In Achilles tendinitis there is inflammation around the tendon with inflammation and swelling of the tendon and sheath following repetitive overuse.

Shin splints refers to a chronic painful condition located in the shin area of the lower leg, medial, lateral or posterior to the tibia. Mechanisms involved may include tibial periostitis, stress fracture or chronic compartment syndrome.

In *tibial periostitis* there is pain on the side of the tibia, typically in the middle third, that is associated with the late landing and push off phases of running. It usually fades with warm-up but in severe cases it is present throughout running and jumping. This so-called traction periostitis is thought to arise where the muscles attached to the bone are overstressed, leading to irritation at the musculoperiosteal junction.

Stress fracture is an important differential diagnosis in lower leg pain where the mechanism is repeated stressful muscle contractions around the bone. Whilst the muscles gain in strength, bone strength does not respond at the same rate; if the stress continues, numerous microfractures occur which may develop into a full stress fracture. Symptoms start with a dull pain after exercise. Later, pain may increase to occur with every foot stride during walking, but is concentrated in the injured area compared with the more diffuse nature that occurs in other conditions such as traction periostitis.

Muscle strain in the lower limb

This is an injury to a muscle–tendon unit caused by overloading or excessive stretching around the knee or ankle as already explained with regard to neck or shoulder girdle muscles.

Muscle sprain in the lower limb

This follows an injury to ligamentous and capsular structures around the knee or ankle.

ANKLE AND FOOT PROBLEMS

In most cases these are associated with injuries. Over half of all sports injuries occur in the lower limb and, of these, one-third occur in the ankle and foot. The vast majority involve only soft tissue and may be acute or chronic, usually as a result of overuse. Damage may be associated with particular sports and activities, especially skiing, running, ballet, football and gymnastics.

Ankle and foot sprains may involve the medial and lateral ankle ligaments. Acute lateral ligament sprain usually results from excessive inversion or plantar/dorsiflexion of the foot and is best managed by strap support once fracture has been excluded. Unsuccessful treatment may lead to chronic strain and laxity of the ligament that may require surgical reconstruction rather than persevering with exercise regimens that can ultimately fail. Sprains of the much stronger medial ligament are rare. If there is pain and swelling of both sides of the ankle, there may be tarsal involvement with subtalar instability. In high ankle sprain there may be damage to the distal tibiofibular articulation with tenderness over the interosseous membrane.

Peroneal tendon injuries may occur in skiing and football, with tenosynovitis, tendinitis and tearing of these relatively weak structures.

Plantar calcaneonavicular (spring) ligament sprain follows a twisting injury of the mid-foot, with tenderness of the medial arch of the sole.

Achilles tendon injuries, comprising tendinitis and rupture, are common, difficult to treat and usually occur with overtraining. Complete or partial rupture may follow a violent contraction of the calf muscle complex during the push-off phase of running or racquet sports, or during balletic leaps (grands jetés). Whilst complete tears require surgical repair, partial tears that are more difficult to diagnose may require surgical excision of scar tissue. Associated tendinitis and bursitis respond to rest, NSAIDs, ultrasound and eccentric calf muscle exercise.

Stress fractures should be suspected when an athlete has bone pain with a normal radiograph. They may be a fatigue type, resulting from increased loading in normal bone, or from normal loading in bone weakened by osteoporosis as in female ballet dancers and gymnasts in whom anorexia has led to amenorrhoea. Sites involved may include lower tibia, calcaneum, navicular, etc. depending on the physical activity or sport that was involved. Treatment is based on rest, immobilization, analgesia and attention to training details.

Nerve entrapment around the foot and ankle may involve the tibial, sural, saphenous or peroneal nerves.

Morton's neuroma, with pain typically between the third and fourth metatarsal heads, feels like walking with a pebble under the ball of the foot. Treatment centres on orthotics with shoe modification, NSAIDs, stretching, corticosteroid injections, massage, surgical release, neuroma excision, etc., indicative of the difficulty that may arise with this condition.

Plantar fasciitis is a common cause of crippling heel pain with localized tenderness. Treatment with analgesics, stretching and corticosteroid injections may, if unsuccessful, require surgical fascial release.

Metatarsalgia, with forefoot pain between the metatarsal heads, is vague and related to impact sports. After excluding Morton's neuroma, treatment centres on stretching, analgesics, orthotics, etc.

Hallux valgus (bunions) occurs in members of the general public who persevere with fashionable but ill-fitting, unsuitable footwear. However, it arises especially in ballet dancers who incur a chronic repetitive injury. Treatment in these subjects aims to delay the prolonged debilitating effect of surgical intervention on their professional skills for as long as possible by means again of orthotics, analgesics, etc.

Hallux rigidus from a stiff and painful first metatarsophalangeal joint arises from microtrauma or osteoarthritis seen in push-off sports, especially in those with long, narrow feet. Strong, stiff-soled footwear may be required.

Ankle pain not related to trauma, sport, etc., may occur with synovitis, as in RA or OA, or gout.

Compartment syndromes

In *acute compartment syndrome* there is early severe pain due to increased pressure within a confined muscle compartment, leading to ischaemia and the possibility of tissue necrosis and a useless limb. Causes are soft tissue trauma, with or without fracture, crush injuries and extreme athletic exercising. The lower leg muscle compartments are most commonly involved, although the condition can occur in the forearm when the brachial artery is damaged following a supracondylar fracture of the radius, with fragment displacement, leading to the condition of *Volkmann's ischaemic contracture*.

Early recognition and prompt treatment are essential before pallor, pulselessess and paralysis supervene. Treatment may ultimately involve surgical release if rest, moderate elevation and analgesia have not brought early relief.

In *chronic compartment syndrome* the onset is more subtle, occurring after prolonged training. As with trauma, the situation is aggravated by exercise when increased blood flow further enlarges the muscle and obstructs its venous outflow. Further engorgement results eventually in slowing of the arterial inflow and ischaemic pain develops. Pain therefore comes on after exercise has begun, becoming so severe that rest is essential before running can be resumed. Chronic compartment syndrome occurs most commonly on the lateral side of the tibia, in the anterior muscle compartment, but other leg compartments can be involved. Tibial periostitis and stress fracture can be ruled out by the absence of tibial tenderness, although all three conditions can coexist. Treatment again involves rest, analgesia and attention to footwear, with the possibility of eventual release fasciotomy.

Faults in posture

These may include any of the described postural faults but especially lordosis and sway back posture, lower limb malalignments such as medial or lateral hip rotation, tibial bowing or knock knees, and pronated, supinated or flat feet (see Chapter 3).

Good teaching practice

This would include:

- encouraging avoidance of aggravating activities
- understanding that referral to a podiatrist may be appropriate
- understanding that only health professionals should perform the early mobilization required for injuries such as ligament sprains – this occurs even when swelling is still present
- improving thigh as well as lower limb and foot muscle function
- assessing and improving soleus muscle function and flexibility – exercises such as heel raises, and bending the knees slowly with the heels still lifted improve its eccentric contractibility (deceleration action), an important part of rehabilitation for Achilles tendon injuries and problems
- improving overall calf muscle strength and flexibility with plantarflexion and extension exercises, using a resistance band as exercise tolerance improves
- improving intrinsic foot muscle function including finer movement control (e.g. as required in picking up a tissue with the toes)
- being aware that recurrent, severe or poorly managed sprains can lead to permanent ankle instability
- improving proprioception and balance, particularly of the affected limb.

Chapter 3

Anatomy review – the torso, lower limbs and feet

THORACIC CAGE

BONES AND JOINTS

The *walls of the thoracic cage* comprise the thoracic vertebral column posteriorly and the sternum anteriorly, with the ribs and costal cartilages ranged between (Fig. 3.1).

The *sternum* comprises three distinct parts: the body with the manubrium attached superiorly and the xiphoid process attached inferiorly. It connects with the ribs through the flexible hyaline costal cartilages.

The *costal cartilages* of the first to the seventh ribs articulate with the sternum itself. The cartilages of the eighth, ninth and tenth ribs are inserted into the seventh costal cartilage so as to join the sternum. The cartilages of the eleventh and twelfth so-called 'floating ribs' are just caps on their anterior ends. These cartilages act to increase the flexibility of the anterior thoracic cage, particularly in the lower region where the cartilages of the eighth, ninth and tenth ribs merge and attach to the costal cartilage of the seventh rib, as described above.

MOVEMENTS OF THE RIBS, COSTAL CARTILAGES AND STERNUM

Main joints of the thoracic cage

The thoracic intervertebral joints and the articulations between the ribs and the vertebral column lie posteri-orly, whilst anteriorly are the manubriosternal and xiphisternal joints, the sternocostal joints between the costal cartilages of the first to the seventh ribs and the sternum, and the interchondral joints between the tips of the cartilages of the eighth to the tenth ribs and their successive proximal cartilages.

The *thoracic vertebral* articulations include secondary cartilaginous joints and synovial joints, and the articulations between the ribs and the bodies and transverse processes of the thoracic vertebrae at both the costovertebral and costotransverse joints.

The *costovertebral joints* are formed by the two facets on each side of the head of the rib articulating with the sides of two adjacent thoracic vertebral bodies, and the *costotransverse joints* are formed by the tubercle of the rib articulating with the transverse process of its adjacent vertebra.

Joint movement

A limited range of movement is possible at both the costovertebral and costotransverse joints, but they allow only small gliding and twisting motions during inspiration and expiration. However, because of the length of the ribs these small posterior joint movements are amplified into much greater excursions in the lateral and anterior areas of the chest wall during breathing.

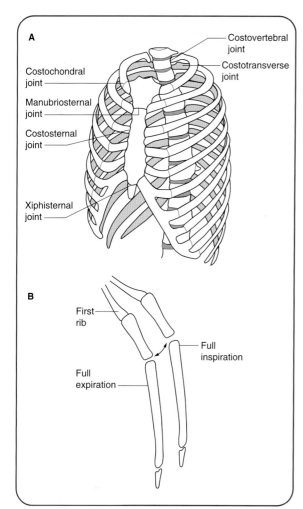

Figure 3.1 **A** Joints of the thorax. **B** Movements of the sternum during respiration (seen laterally). Reproduced with permission from Palastanga et al (2002).

The manubriosternal and xiphisternal joints are secondary cartilaginous joints between the body of the sternum, manubrium and xiphoid process. Both allow a small range of movement during breathing.

The sternocostal joints lie between the costal cartilages of the first to the seventh ribs and the sternum. The first sternocostal joint is a primary cartilaginous joint that prevents significant movement between the rib and the sternum. The other six joints are synovial joints that allow gliding motions between the articular surfaces of the costal cartilages and the sternum required during breathing.

The eighth and ninth interchondral joints are synovial and allow small gliding motions for increased rib mobility, while the tenth interchondral joint, being fibrous, is relatively fixed.

The movements of the ribs, sternum and diaphragm increase and decrease the volume of the thoracic cage to produce the breathing cycle.

During inspiration, the upper ribs move their anterior ends upwards, the manubriosternal joint bends slightly allowing the sternal body to move forwards and upwards with the upper ribs, the lower ribs move outwards and upwards and the diaphragm moves downwards. This increases the dimensions of the thoracic cage and its enclosed lungs. The subatmospheric pressure thereby created between the thoracic cavity and the atmosphere causes air to be drawn into the lungs.

During passive expiration the ribs and sternum descend, and the diaphragm relaxes and ascends, returning the thoracic cage and the lungs to their normal size. This revives the pressure gradient between the lungs and the outside environment and air is expelled from the lungs.

'Pump' and 'bucket handle' rib action

During breathing the second to the fifth ribs move up and down with almost no lateral displacement and their action is considered to be like a pump drawing water from a well, a so-called 'pump' action.

In contrast, the anterior ends of the eighth to the tenth ribs shift laterally as they move up and down towards the horizontal, and their action is considered to be more like raising a handle from the side of a bucket, a so-called 'bucket handle' action.

Whilst the intermediate ribs (the sixth and seventh) demonstrate both 'pump' and 'bucket handle' actions, the first, eleventh and twelfth ribs are not that involved in increasing the volume of the thoracic cage.

MUSCLES INVOLVED IN BREATHING

Inspiration	Expiration
Diaphragm	Transversus abdominis
Scalenes	Internal obliques
Intercostals	External obliques
Levatores costarum	Latissimus dorsi
Serratus posterior superior	Transversus thoracis
	Subcostals
	Serratus posterior inferior

3

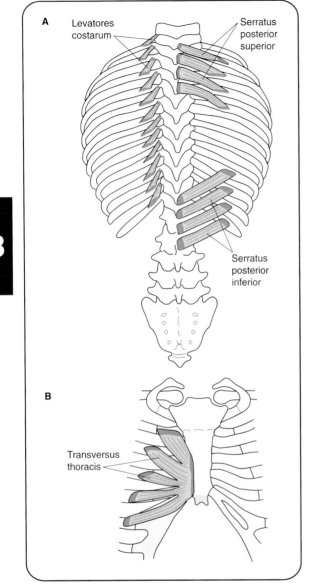

Figure 3.2   A The left levatores costarum, and the right serratus posterior superior and inferior muscles, posterior view. **B** The left transversus thoracis muscle on the inner surface of the thoracic cage. Reproduced with permission from Palastanga et al (2002).

Inspiration

The *diaphragm* is a dome-shaped musculotendinous leaf separating the thoracic and abdominal cavities (Fig. 3.2). It has several major points of origin around its circumference: the xiphoid process; the deep surfaces and cartilages of the seventh to the twelfth ribs; the lumbar vertebrae via the 'right crus' and 'left crus', ligaments

that arise from the bodies of the lumbar vertebrae L1–L3 and L1–L2, respectively; and the arcuate ligaments that attach to the lumbar vertebrae.

Its insertion is unlike that of any other muscle as it does not attach to bone but to its own central tendon, a strong, interlacing arrangement of fibrous tissue. The central tendon contains an opening to transmit the vena cava and there are other openings for the descending aorta and the oesophagus.

In normal breathing the dome-shaped diaphragm contracts and its central tendon descends to increase the capacity of the thoracic cage and produce inspiration. It then relaxes and controls the rate at which air is expelled from the recoiling lungs during expiration.

In forced expiration as occurs during coughing and sneezing, the abdominal muscles contract and increase intra-abdominal pressure as the diaphragm relaxes. This pushes the abdominal contents against the diaphragm, thereby increasing its upward displacement as it ascends. This increase in its upward motion further reduces lung volume and forces air from the lungs.

The *external, internal and innermost intercostal muscles* lie between adjacent ribs in three separate layers. Although there is controversy about the active role of these muscles during breathing (some of the external intercostal muscles possibly assist elevation of the rib below), together they help to maintain the tone and integrity of the intercostal spaces and chest wall during breathing.

Levatores costarum are short, strong muscles lying on each side of the spine between the seventh cervical and eleventh thoracic vertebrae. They attach superiorly to the transverse process of one vertebra and inferiorly to the upper border of a rib one or two levels below. They assist rib elevation during breathing and can also help to produce rotation and lateral flexion of the spine.

Serratus posterior superior lies deep to the rhomboids and the muscle fibres attach diagonally from the sides of the spinous processes of the seventh cervical, first, second and third thoracic vertebrae to the second, third, fourth and fifth ribs, respectively. It assists rib elevation during breathing.

Expiration

Transversus thoracis lies behind the sternum and ribs in the anterior thoracic wall. The muscle fibres originate from the posterior surface of the xiphoid process and lower region of the sternum and run superolaterally to attach to costal cartilages of the second to the sixth ribs. When transversus thoracis contracts, it pulls on the costal cartilages and lowers those ribs to assist expiration.

The subcostals are muscle slips found mainly in the thoracic region lying between the ribs across two intercostal spaces. They assist in lowering the ribs and producing expiration.

'Serratus posterior inferior lies deep to latissimus dorsi, arising from the spinous processes T11, T12, L1 and L2 and their supraspinous ligaments via the thoracolumbar fascia. It helps to pull the lower four ribs downwards and backwards' (Palastanga et al 2002, p. 483).

The muscles of the anterior abdominal wall are very important during breathing as they act with the diaphragm to alter the volume and internal pressures of the thoracic and abdominal cavities.

In normal breathing

- During inspiration the abdominal muscles relax and reduce intra-abdominal pressure, allowing the diaphragm to lower as it contracts.
- During expiration the abdominal muscles passively contract and increase intra-abdominal pressure, assisting the diaphragm's upwards motion as it relaxes.

In forced expiration

- The abdominal muscles actively contract and further increase intra-abdominal pressure as the diaphragm relaxes. This pushes the abdominal contents against the diaphragm, increasing its upward displacement as it ascends. This in turn increases intrathoracic pressure that forcefully compresses and deflates the lungs.
- Forced expiration, and breath holding that activates the abdominal muscles whilst anchoring the diaphragm, both have a stabilizing and protective effect on the spine, and these breathing patterns may be used unconsciously to prepare for or during heavy lifting or similar strenuous activities.

VERTEBRAL COLUMN

See anatomical body charts on page xii.

BONES AND JOINTS

The vertebral column comprises 24 mobile vertebrae: 7 cervical, 12 thoracic and 5 lumbar; and 9 fused vertebrae; 5 in the sacral region forming the sacrum and 4 in the coccygeal region forming the coccyx.

The intervertebral joints occur from between the first and second cervical vertebrae, called the atlas and axis, respectively, to the lumbosacral junction between the fifth lumbar and first sacral vertebrae, the latter forming the base of the triangular sacral bone. Finally, the sacrococcygeal joint links the fifth sacral vertebra at the apex of the sacral bone with the coccyx. The joint between the skull and the first cervical vertebra (the atlas) is called the atlanto-occipital joint and that between the atlas and the second cervical vertebra (the axis) is called the atlantoaxial joint. These two specialized cervical vertebral joints are designed to allow the head to nod and to turn from side to side.

The intervertebral discs separating the vertebrae account for approximately one-quarter of the length of the vertebral column and function as shock absorbers during everyday activities, particularly walking and running.

The adult vertebral column has four curvatures: anterior convexities in the cervical and lumbar regions called lordoses and anterior concavities in the thoracic and sacrococcygeal regions called kyphoses. These curves, together with the intervertebral discs, give the vertebral column its pliancy, and an ability to absorb axial compressive forces and thereby provide a flexible support for the trunk.

MOVEMENTS OF THE VERTEBRAL COLUMN AND THE MAIN MUSCLES INVOLVED

Cervical spine

Flexion and extension

The total range of movement in the lower cervical region is about 25 degrees of flexion and 85 degrees of extension, and the least mobile joint is between the last cervical and first thoracic vertebrae.

To control flexion from the upright position, the postvertebral neck muscles (trapezius, splenius capitis, longissimus capitis, semispinalis capitis) and most of the small suboccipital muscles act bilaterally against the weight of the head.

To flex the head from the supine position the sternocleido-mastoid, longus capitis and the short muscles between the atlas and occiput (the suboccipital muscles) contract bilaterally.

The atlanto-occipital joint between the occipital condyles of the skull and the first cervical vertebra allows a total range of approximately 20 degrees of movement. Flexion and extension, together with a slight rotational motion, occur as the occipital condyles slide on the lateral masses of the atlas; full rotation occurs at the atlantoaxial joint.

Lateral flexion, rotation and circumduction

Lateral flexion of the neck is initiated by muscle action on that side and is then limited by the opposing articular facets, intervertebral disc compression and the flexibility of the contralateral cervical facet joint capsules.

Lateral flexion at the atlanto-occipital joint is limited to some 8 degrees and occurs as the occipital condyles move against the atlas. The axis moves against the third cervical vertebra so that the atlantoaxial joint is not specifically involved in lateral flexion.

In the lower cervical region the total range of movement is about 40 degrees of lateral flexion to each side and this is accompanied by a slight degree of rotation towards the flexed side. This occurs as the shape and orientation of the cervical articular facets prevent pure lateral flexion.

In *rotation* the skull and first cervical vertebra move as one unit and, with the head beginning erect, approximately 15 degrees of movement to each side may be achieved. As the head turns, it nods slightly on top of the spine and the chin drops minimally. This adjustment occurs as a result of the oblique orientation of the lateral joint surfaces and the slight convexity of the facets on the axis. If the head is tilted slightly backwards and away from the motion as the head turns, the range of rotation may be increased. The suboccipital sterno-cleido-mastoid and trapezius muscles produce rotation.

Circumduction combines flexion, extension, lateral flexion and rotation, and involves the whole array of deep and superficial neck muscles.

Thoracic spine

Flexion and extension

In the thoracic spine the total range of movement is between 50 and 70 degrees. Overall the thoracic spine is more mobile in flexion, as extension is limited by the impact of the articular and spinous processes between adjacent vertebrae as well as the tension in the anterior longitudinal ligament. Also, flexion is much freer in the lower thoracic spine due to the length and comparative flexibility of the lower ribs.

The postvertebral muscles pay out bilaterally so as to control flexion from the upright position; from the supine position the muscles of the anterior abdominal wall – in particular, rectus abdominis and the obliques – bring about flexion.

The anterior abdominal wall muscles control extension from the upright position; from the supine position extension occurs through postvertebral muscle action.

Psoas major and the anterior abdominal wall muscles control extension from the upright position whilst the postvertebral muscles produce extension from the prone position.

Lumbar spine

Flexion and extension

The lumbar spine is relatively free in flexion, its total range of movement being approximately 55 degrees. In extension the range of movement is approximately 30 degrees.

Flexion from the upright position is controlled by the postvertebral muscles on both sides being limited by tension in the posterior part of the intervertebral disc, the posterior longitudinal ligament, the ligamenta flava, and the inter- and supraspinous ligaments.

From the supine position the concentric bilateral actions of psoas major and the muscles of the anterior abdominal wall – in particular, rectus abdominis and the obliques – produce flexion.

Psoas major and the anterior abdominal wall muscles control extension from the upright position; from the prone position the postvertebral muscles, assisted by quadratus lumborum contracting bilaterally, produce it. Quadratus lumborum also assists lateral stability as the lumbar spine extends (Palastanga et al 2002, p. 512).

Thoracic and lumbar spine

Lateral flexion and rotation

The ranges of motion in both the thoracic and lumbar spine, as in the cervical spine, vary greatly between individuals and change with age, the ranges of motion being greatest in childhood and adolescence and possibly reducing by as much as 50% by the time an adult reaches 30 years of age.

Lateral flexion is greatest when in the upright position and is reduced when the normal curves of the spine are diminished (as when sitting) or reversed (as in spine flexion and extension). In addition, spine mobility in rotation is compromised and possibly lost when the normal spinal curves are reversed as in spine extension.

Lateral flexion is initiated by the concentric muscle action of anterior abdominal wall muscles and the quadratus lumborum on the side of flexion, and then controlled by the eccentric muscle action of those same muscles on the opposite side. The eccentric muscle action of the opposing side begins at about 10 degrees of lateral flexion.

The spinal muscles can also produce lateral flexion, erector spinae contracting unilaterally to produce lateral flexion with rotation to the side of the contraction and multifidus producing lateral flexion as well as extension and rotation at all levels of the vertebral column. Additionally, intertransversarii found in the cervical and lumbar regions can contract unilaterally to produce lateral flexion on the side of the contraction; however, both intertransversarii and multifidus act more importantly as stabilizers of the vertebral column during lateral flexion.

Thoracic spine

The lower half of the thoracic spine is more mobile in lateral flexion than the upper half and the total range of movement is between 20 and 25 degrees to each side. As in the cervical spine, lateral flexion is associated with rotation and for each degree of lateral flexion there is approximately one degree of vertebral rotation away from the side flexion motion, i.e. the spinous processes turn towards the concavity of the curve. During lateral flexion the ribcage modifies accordingly as the movement increases, becoming expanded on the elevated side and contracted on the opposite side.

In the thoracic spine the shapes of the vertebral bodies and their alignment to form a gentle posterior thoracic curve allow rotation to occur. The ranges of rotational motion are reduced and possibly lost when the curve is increased as in an exaggerated thoracic kyphosis or reversed as in thoracic spine extension.

The thoracic spine has an approximate range of 35 degrees to each side, the movement being comparatively free between the sixth and ninth thoracic vertebrae and comparatively limited towards the pectoral and pelvic girdles.

The muscles of the anterior abdominal wall largely produce thoracic spine rotation, in particular the oblique abdominal muscles. When the left internal obliques and the right external obliques contract together, the trunk rotates to the left.

Semispinalis, along with the muscles of the anterior abdominal wall, produces trunk rotation; when one side contracts, the trunk rotates to the opposite side.

Multifidus and the rotators can also produce rotation in the thoracic region but their most important role is one of stabilizing the vertebral segments through their lengthening and shortening as required to stabilize adjacent vertebrae.

Lumbar spine

The total range of lateral flexion in the adult spine is between 20 and 30 degrees to each side, possibly half of that available in the spine of a prepubescent child. However, as lateral flexion and rotation occur concurrently, and rotation is restricted by the shape and orientation of the lumbar facet joints, lateral flexion in the lumbar spine is limited throughout the total age range and even more so at the lumbosacral joint where rotation is normally minimal. However, rotation may become freer with increasing lumbar flexion, and this can be a feature of spinal dysfunction that leads to lumbar vertebral disc prolapse.

Both side flexion and rotation in the lumbar spine are prevented in lumbar extension due to the closely packed orientation of lumbar facet joints.

PELVIC GIRDLE

BONES AND JOINTS

The *pelvic girdle*, like the pectoral girdle, comprises three bones: the ilium, ischium and pubis that together form an innominate bone on each side. The left and right innominate bones then articulate anteriorly at the symphysis pubis and posteriorly with the sacrum at the left and right sacroiliac joints, so completing the bony pelvis.

The *sacrum*, comprising the five fused sacral vertebrae, is roughly triangular in shape with the base, formed by the first sacral vertebra, articulating with the fifth lumbar vertebra at the lumbosacral junction. The coccyx, comprising four fused coccygeal vertebrae, articulates with the fifth sacral vertebra, the apex of the triangular sacrum, at the sacrococcygeal joint.

The *pelvis* supports and protects the pelvic viscera, supports and transfers the body weight through the vertebral column to the lower limbs, and provides joint movement that assists correct lower limb function, as well as providing attachments for muscles. In the female, it also provides support for the birth canal.

The *sacroiliac joints* between the ilium and sacrum are united and stabilized by powerful ligaments in and around the joints. The orientation of the joints' surfaces allows slight gliding and rotary movements during everyday activity.

In addition, the sacrum itself undergoes some 5 degrees of forward rotation independent of the ilium when the body moves from erect to supine. This sacral mobility is increased during pregnancy, and during childbirth there is a complex sacral movement that is analogous with nodding of the head.

The *lumbosacral junction* between the last lumbar vertebra and first sacral segment is part of the vertebral column and is potentially its weakest link. This is due to the incline of the superior sacral surface and the tendency for the fifth lumbar vertebra to slide on it and move downwards and forwards. However, this movement is prevented by the arrangement of the overlapping bony articular processes of the adjacent fifth lumbar and first sacral vertebrae, together with the strong ligamentous attachments that fix and stabilize the joint. Normal lumbosacral joint movements are flexion, extension and lateral flexion, and the degree of movement available varies from person to person and depends on age.

In children between the ages of 2 and 13 years the lumbosacral joint is very mobile and provides up to 75% of the total range of flexion and extension of the lumbar spine. However, this mobility reduces during puberty and adulthood so that by 35 years of age the average range of flexion and extension available is approximately 18 degrees and this reduces further as people age. Lumbosacral mobility in lateral flexion is considerably less than in flexion and extension, being approximately 7 degrees in children, 1 degree in mature adults and absent in the elderly.

The *sacrococcygeal joint* between the last sacral and first coccygeal segments allows passive flexion and extension during defecation and childbirth. This mobility is frequently lost by old age as degenerative changes fuse and eliminate the joint.

MUSCLES OF THE PELVIC FLOOR

These comprise the *levator ani* and *coccygeus*. Each levator ani muscle arises in a continuous manner from the inner surfaces of the bones of the pelvis and the obturator membrane. From this extensive origin each muscle slopes down to form a gutter-like diaphragm that separates the pelvic cavity from the perineum. The muscles join only at their anterior and posterior margins, between which they accommodate the anal canal posteriorly, the urethra in the male and both the vagina and urethra in the female.

The combined muscle tone of levator ani and coccygeus plays an important role in supporting the contents of the pelvic cavity, and when contracted actively the muscles affect the openings of the pelvic floor. This is of particular importance in the female during and following childbirth.

Abdominal muscles and their different roles

In producing expulsive actions

To expel the contents of the stomach, bladder, bowel and womb, the anterior abdominal wall muscles contract to flatten the abdominal wall and produce expulsive actions as the appropriate sphincter muscles relax.

For vomiting, micturition, defecation and parturition, as the abdominal muscles contract the diaphragm maintains its tone and resists an upward displacement, thereby further increasing intra-abdominal pressure and compressing the pelvic organs.

In coughing and sneezing, as the abdominal muscles contract and intra-abdominal pressure increases, the diaphragm relaxes and accepts an upward displacement, thus forcing air from the lungs.

In protecting and stabilizing

The abdominal muscles provide a corset-like structure to protect and maintain the contents of the pelvic and abdominal cavities whilst their muscle tone supports and cushions the spine during everyday activities.

This protective effect on the spine is of particular importance before and during strenuous lifting or handling when breath holding that simultaneously activates the abdominal muscles and anchors the diaphragm can occur instinctively. Also, when sitting up from the supine position the abdominal muscles act to stabilize the lumbar spine as the upper body moves forwards and upwards.

In trunk flexion

The rectus abdominis, the internal and external obliques and psoas major and minor are involved in trunk flexion. Bilateral, concentric contractions of the rectus abdominis and the obliques will draw the thoracic cage and pelvis towards each other and, when the ribs are fixed, their actions produce a posterior pelvic tilt, moving the anterior pelvis towards the lower ribs.

From the supine position, and acting with the abdominal muscles independently of iliacus, psoas major can produce vertebral column flexion by using its lower attachment as a fixed point.

The more poorly developed psoas minor can also produce weak lumbar spine flexion.

In trunk extension

Quadratus lumborum is a large, flat, quadrilateral muscle of the posterior abdominal wall running between the pelvis and the twelfth rib deep to erector spinae. It assists lumbar vertebral column lateral stability whilst helping erector spinae to produce lumbar vertebral column extension (Palastanga et al 2002, p. 473–474).

In trunk rotation

The internal and external oblique abdominal muscles and the postvertebral muscles (multifidus, rotatores and semispinalis) produce trunk rotation.

Rotation to the left is produced by the combined actions of the left internal and right external obliques, and rotation to the right is produced by the right internal and left external obliques acting together. Rotation may be passively or actively accompanied by trunk flexion, so drawing the thoracic cage towards the pelvis as it turns to one side.

In lateral trunk flexion

The right rectus abdominis, acting together with the right internal and external obliques and the right side of erector spinae, produces trunk movement to the right side; conversely, the muscles on the left side of the body produce trunk movement to the left.

The *transversus abdominis* arises from the inguinal ligament, the iliac crest, the thoracolumbar fascia and the inner surfaces of the costal cartilages of the lower six ribs interdigitating with the attachments of the diaphragm. It wraps horizontally around the abdominal cavity to form the innermost of the three sheets of muscle that comprise the anterior abdominal wall.

The *internal oblique muscle* is the middle sheet of the three layers. It also arises from the inguinal ligament, the iliac crest and the thoracolumbar fascia, but fans vertically, horizontally and obliquely to form a flat sheet of muscle between the ribcage and pelvis.

The *external oblique muscle* arises by fleshy slips from the outer borders of the lower eight ribs and costal cartilages; these interdigitate with the origins of serratus anterior above and the insertions of latissimus dorsi below. Being the most superficial of the three muscle layers, the external oblique fibres run downwards and medially from the ribs towards the inguinal ligament.

All three muscle layers have sheet-like tendinous insertions that converge towards the midline and join in an arrangement to form sheaths on the left and right sides that enclose each rectus abdominis muscle.

Whilst the transversus abdominis insertion forms the deep surface layer of the rectus sheath, and the external oblique the superficial surface layer, that of the internal oblique splits to unite with both the deep and the superficial layers of the rectus sheath. The sheaths then reunite and blend to form the linea alba which spans the midline between the xiphisternum and pubic crest.

The rectus abdominis arises via two tendons from the front of the symphysis pubis and pubic crest, extends the length of the anterior abdominal wall and inserts into the anterior surfaces of the xiphoid process and the costal cartilages of the fifth, sixth and seventh ribs in a horizontal line. The right and left sides of rectus abdominis are enclosed within tendinous intersections and these sheaths fuse together medially to blend into the linea alba.

FASCIAE OF THE TRUNK

- Superficial fascia
- Deep fascia
- Thoracolumbar fasciae.

The *superficial fascia* lies within the walls of the trunk where it provides a fatty protective covering for blood vessels, nerves and underlying organs, as well as a connection between the skin and deep fascia and between the complicated arrangements of membranous layers throughout the body and limbs.

The *deep fascia* covers the anterior, lateral and posterior aspects of the torso and varies in thickness and strength depending on the role it is required to perform. In both the thoracic and anterior abdominal walls it is comparatively thin and elastic to allow expansion, whilst in the neck and upper back regions it is dense and strong, providing protection for the neck and underlying cervical spine and a covering for the superficial muscles that attach the upper limbs to the trunk.

It attaches between the thoracic and lumbar vertebral spines, the spine and acromion process of the scapula, and the iliac crest and the back of the sacrum.

'Laterally it is continuous with the deep fascia of the axilla, the thorax and the abdomen: it also blends with the deep investing fascia of the arm. Deep to the superficial muscles of the back is found an extremely strong layer of the deep fascia, the thoracolumbar fascia' (Palastanga et al 2002, p. 483).

The *thoracolumbar fascia* comprises anterior, middle and posterior layers that enclose paraspinal muscles.

The anterior layer is the thinnest of the three layers. It covers the front of quadratus lumborum, separating its medial part from psoas major, and attaches medially to the fronts of the lumbar transverse processes. Laterally it blends with the middle layer to form a narrow band that extends from the last rib to the iliac crest.

The middle layer is continuous with the fascial coverings of sacrospinalis and the lateral borders of the posterior aponeurosis of transversus abdominis. It covers the posterior surface of quadratus lumborum, separating its medial part from sacrospinalis, and extends from its medial attachments to the tips of the lumbar transverse processes to blend superiorly with the lumbocostal ligament.

The posterior layer lies between erector spinae and the superficial back muscles, thereby forming a sheet that covers the posterior surface of the deep back muscles as it extends upwards from the sacrum and iliac crest to attach to the angles of the ribs lateral to the iliocosto-cervicalis and blend with the aponeurosis of serratus posterior superior.

In the sacral and lumbar regions it interweaves with the tendinous expansion of latissimus dorsi and serratus posterior inferior to form the strong posterior lumbar fascia. This becomes continuous with the deep fascia above the loin.

HIP JOINT

BONES, MOVEMENTS AND THE MUSCLES INVOLVED

The hip joint comprises the acetabulum (to which all three elements of the innominate bone contribute) and the head of the femur, the ball and socket arrangement of which permits freedom of movement around three axes in accordance with a broad range of physical activities.

The shapes of the bones, the strength and proximity of the muscles crossing the joint and the strong surrounding joint capsule all make for joint stability. Muscles contributing to keeping the femoral head in firm contact with the acetabulum have fibres that run more parallel with the femoral neck and include iliopsoas, pectineus, gluteus minimus and medius, the obturators, the gemelli, quadratus femoris and piriformis.

Conversely, the actions of muscles whose fibres run along the femoral shaft (e.g. the adductors) have a tendency to destabilize the hip joint. Although the healthy hip is able to withstand this tendency, joints already compromised by impairments in bones and muscles may be adversely affected. In extreme cases this may lead to joint dislocation, either superiorly or anteromedially, the latter being a result of attempting to adduct an extended, laterally rotated joint (Palastanga et al 2002, p. 325).

Movements of the hip and the main muscles involved

The hip joint allows flexion, extension, adduction, abduction, medial and lateral rotation, as well as circumduction, and, because the femoral head is set at an angle to the femoral shaft, all these movements involve associated rotation of the femoral head within the acetabulum.

Hip flexion

- Iliopsoas
- Rectus femoris
- Pectineus
- Sartorius.

Iliopsoas comprises iliacus, psoas major and psoas minor. *Iliacus* originates from the inner surface of the ilium. *Psoas major and minor* originate from the body and the sides and lower borders of the transverse processes of the twelfth thoracic vertebra, from the five lumbar vertebrae and the lower borders of their transverse processes, from the sacrum, and from all the intervening lumbar intervertebral discs.

Iliacus and psoas major are inserted just below the lesser trochanter of the femur and psoas minor inserts into the iliopubic eminence and fascia iliaca. Iliacus and psoas major act together to flex the hip and are involved in activities that pull the lower limb up in front of the trunk as in walking, running, etc., and when raising the legs from the floor in the supine position.

In sitting up from the supine position they pull the body weight away from the floor as the abdominal muscles flex the trunk. Here, lifting the head early to curl the upper body forwards assists the iliopsoas to control the lumbar spine as it pulls the body up from the floor. Iliopsoas is thought by some authorities to be a lateral hip rotator but this remains unconfirmed.

Rectus femoris originates from the anterior inferior iliac spine and the roughened groove immediately above the acetabulum. It attaches via a thick tendon to the upper border of the patella, with some fibres passing around the patella to help form the patellar tendon which carries on into the tibial tuberosity. Although part of the quadriceps group of muscles, it works independently with iliopsoas to flex the hip.

Pectineus originates from an area approximately 2.5 cm wide on the front of the pubis, just below the crest. It inserts along a roughened line from the lesser trochanter to the linea aspera.

Pectineus flexes and adducts the hip and works with iliopsoas to raise the legs from the floor in the supine position.

As with many muscles, pectineus may perform different actions when the body position reverses the relative positions of its origin and insertion as, for example, when sitting as opposed to standing. With the hip joint flexed at a right angle, the muscle fibres pass forwards and upwards, thus still permitting adduction but now with extension and lateral rotation added. Pectineus is possibly a medial hip rotator but this is not confirmed.

Sartorius originates from the anterior superior iliac spine and the area just below. It is inserted into the medial condyle of the tibia. The 'tailor's muscle' – so-called as it produces cross-legged sitting – flexes, laterally rotates and abducts the hip. It is engaged in activities that involve simultaneous hip and knee flexion with hip lateral rotation – for example, lower limb action during breaststroke swimming.

Hip extension

- Gluteus maximus
- Hamstrings
- Semitendinosus
- Semimembranosus
- Biceps femoris.

Gluteus maximus is the largest posterior hip muscle, originating from the ilium, sacrum and coccyx, and passing in two layers to its two insertions, one more posteriorly into the gluteal tuberosity of the femur and one more laterally between the two layers of fasciae latae, helping to form the iliotibial band.

When gluteus maximus acts from above, its upper attachment towards the back of the thigh allows it to pull the femur backwards to extend the flexed hip. This occurs powerfully during stepping upwards, climbing and running. Its lower attachment, being more towards the lateral aspect of the thigh, tends to encourage hip lateral rotation during hip extension.

Gluteus maximus also plays important roles in maintaining upright postures. In standing it acts to balance the pelvis on the femoral head and helps to raise the medial longitudinal arch of the foot. In sitting it relieves pressure on the ischial tuberosities by regular static, dynamic, unilateral or bilateral contractions so as to lift the body weight from or change its distribution over its supporting surfaces.

In forward bending from the upright position it acts eccentrically with the hamstrings and erector spinae to control the body's motion during hip and spine flexion. During returning from flexion gluteus maximus and the hamstrings extend the hip as erector spine extends the spine.

Gluteus maximus is much less involved during normal walking and this can contribute to its loss of tone and shape in people who live sedentary lives or who, due to age, illness or injury, are unable to perform more energetic walking or similar activities.

The *hamstrings* cross the hip and knee joints posteriorly and so are involved both in hip extension and knee flexion. When standing or in the prone position with the knees extended the hamstrings and gluteus maximus act together to extend the hip.

During hip extension when returning the body from forward flexion to the upright position they act maximally, and they also act strongly when sustaining the body in a leaning forward position as, for example, when preparing to race from a starting block.

The hamstrings, together with the abdominal muscles anteriorly and gluteus maximus posteriorly, control the tilt of the pelvis and help to maintain the normal lumbar lordosis.

They also have a role during walking by acting eccentrically to slow down the forward swing of the tibia and prevent the knee snapping back into extension.

Semitendinosus is on the medial aspect of the femur. It originates from the femoral ischial tuberosity and is inserted via a long tendon into the medial condyle of the tibia.

When acting from above, semitendinosus flexes the extended knee and when the knee is partially flexed it medially rotates the knee. If the foot is fixed, it acts to laterally rotate the femur and pelvis on the tibia.

When acting from below, semitendinosus is involved in hip extension and, with its lower attachment being more towards the lateral aspect of the thigh, it tends to encourage hip lateral rotation as the hip extends.

Semimembranosus originates from the upper lateral aspect of the ischial tuberosity and travels down the posteromedial aspect of the thigh deep to semitendinosus to insert via a tendon into the posteromedial surface of the medial tibial condyle. Here its tendinous fibres fan in every direction but laterally they come together to form the oblique popliteal ligament. Semimembranosus acts synergistically with semitendinosus to extend the hip.

Biceps femoris originates from a long head that arises with the tendon of semitendinosus from the lower medial facet on the ischial tuberosity and a short head from the linea aspera on the lower half of the posterior thigh. The long head forms a muscle that runs downwards on the posterolateral aspect of the thigh, and in the lower third of the thigh its narrowing tendon blends with the muscle fibres of the short head to travel conjointly towards the posterolateral aspect of the knee where it joins the head of the fibula by two separate attachments. Biceps femoris acts synergistically with semitendinosus and semimembranosus as a hip extensor and knee flexor.

When the knee is partially flexed, biceps femoris rotates the knee laterally on the thigh; when the lower limb is fixed, it medially rotates the femur and pelvis on the tibia.

Hip abduction

- Gluteus medius
- Gluteus minimus
- Tensor fasciae latae.

Gluteus medius lies on the lateral upper portion of the posterior surface of the hip with its broad upper fascial attachment spreading between the iliac crest above and the sciatic notch below. This strong layer of fascia travels to enclose gluteus medius laterally and gluteus maximus posteriorly before its fibres run both forwards and backwards then downwards to merge into a flattened tendon that is inserted into the upper outer surface of the greater trochanter of the femur.

When the pelvis is fixed, gluteus medius will abduct the hip joint and its anterior fibres will assist medial hip rotation. When the lower limb is fixed, gluteus medius will tilt the hip of the same side downwards whilst raising the hip on the opposite side, and its anterior fibres will tend to rotate the opposite side of the pelvis forwards.

Gluteus maximus and gluteus medius are close companions and the upper fibres of gluteus maximus may be involved during hip abduction. Also, when sitting, piriformis is well positioned for hip abduction and plays an important role in this particular situation.

Gluteus medius is important during walking and running as it controls the position of the pelvis during weight bearing on one leg. In the single leg stance phase of walking it acts strongly on the supporting side to maintain the pelvis level and prevent the opposite hip dropping, thus allowing the raised leg to swing through and forwards for the next step. A malfunctioning gluteus medius allows the pelvis to drop on the side of the raised leg as it swings through. This easily recognized motion is termed the 'Trendelenburg sign'.

Gluteus minimus is the smallest and deepest of the gluteal muscles, originating from a broad base covering the upper gluteal surface of the ilium to be inserted via a tendon into the anterior superior aspect of the greater trochanter of the femur. With its upper attachment fixed, its anterior fibres medially rotate the hip; when its lower attachment is fixed, it acts to keep the pelvis level and prevent the opposite hip dropping.

Tensor fasciae latae is a small dense muscle that lies on the superior anterolateral portion of the hip. Its upper fascial attachment is into the outer upper iliac crest and its insertion via a long strong band of fascia is into the iliotibial band between its two layers, just below the level of the greater trochanter. It works with the glutei to abduct and medially rotate the hip and may also assist hip flexion.

Acting with gluteus maximus it will tighten the iliotibial band and its posterior fibres may assist lateral hip rotation.

As tensor fasciae latae is a link between the pelvis and lower limb during weight bearing, it assists the control of the pelvis and femur on the tibia.

Hip adduction

- Adductor magnus
- Adductor longus
- Adductor brevis
- Gracilis
- Pectineus.

Adductor magnus originates from the edge of the inferior ramus of the pubis, the ischium and ischial tuberosity, and is inserted along the whole length of the linea aspera, the inner condyloid ridge and the adductor tubercle of the femur. It is the largest and most posterior muscle of the adductor group and comprises two sec-

tions: a hamstring part and an adductor part that, when working together, adduct the hip. The hamstring part of the muscle assists hip extension and possibly hip lateral rotation during adduction.

Adductor longus originates from the anterior surface of the body of the pubis just below its crest and is inserted into the middle third of the linea aspera. It is a long, slim, triangular muscle lying partially over adductor magnus towards the middle of the thigh. Adductor longus adducts the thigh and assists both in flexing the extended hip and extending the flexed hip. Its role as a hip rotator is still unconfirmed.

Adductor brevis originates from just below adductor longus at the front of the body of the pubis and is inserted in front of adductor magnus into the upper half of the linea aspera. Its upper and lower parts lie posterior to pectineus and adductor longus, respectively. Adductor brevis adducts the hip but its role as a hip rotator is still unconfirmed.

Gracilis originates from the front and the descending medial edge of the inferior ramus of the pubis. It runs down the medial aspect of the thigh, past the knee joint, and inserts just below the tibial condyle on the anteromedial surface of the tibia.

Although gracilis assists hip adduction, it acts mainly to bring about and control knee flexion – for example, it helps the hamstrings to flex the knee during the early swing phase of walking; it aids strong knee flexion for pulling the body forwards on a sliding seat during rowing; it controls and helps to maintain the flexed knee when riding a horse. In addition, when the knee is already flexed, it assists hip medial rotation.

Pectineus originates from an area approximately 2.5 cm wide on the front of the pubis, just below the crest. It inserts along a roughened line from the lesser trochanter to the linea aspera.

Pectineus flexes and adducts the hip (see hip flexion).

Hip rotation – lateral

- Piriformis
- Obturator internus and externus
- Gemellus superior and inferior
- Quadratus femoris.

The actions of these muscles must first be considered in the anatomical position where they act together to help to control the movements of the hip and pelvis and to bring about external rotation of the femur. During the one legged stance of walking they act to keep the pelvis level and during the swing-through phase of walking they produce lateral rotation of the supporting limb. Also, when being supported on one leg, they contract strongly to turn the body forcefully away from the leg.

This action occurs when swinging a cricket bat or throwing a ball.

However, these muscles take on completely different roles when the hips are flexed as in sitting, crawling and rolling over when lying down. Here they act as hip abductors and control the movements of the pelvis over the flexed hip and thigh.

Piriformis is a triangular muscle lying behind the hip joint with both its base and apex in the gluteal region. It originates from the second to the fourth sacral segments, the ilium and the pelvic surface of the sacrotuberous ligament – the sacrum and ischial tuberosity – and is inserted into the medial surface of the greater trochanter of the femur. In the anatomical position piriformis laterally rotates the hip but in the sitting position it abducts the hip.

Obturator internus is also a triangular muscle that originates from the inner surface of the obturator membrane, the surrounding bony margins of the obturator foramen and the pelvic surface of the ilium.

Some fibres run laterally but most run backwards and downwards where they merge to pass as a narrow tendinous band through the lesser sciatic foramen. The tendon then changes direction to travel forwards and laterally to be inserted into the medial surface of the greater trochanter of the femur. In the anatomical position obturator internus laterally rotates the hip but in the sitting position it tends to abduct the hip.

Gemellus superior and *gemellus inferior* originate from the gluteal surface of the iliac spine and the upper part of the ischial tuberosity, respectively, and run laterally to merge and blend with the tendon of the obturator internus. The gemelli act to assist obturator internus.

Obturator externus, another triangular-shaped muscle, originates from the outer surface of the obturator membrane and the surrounding margins of the obturator foramen. The fibres mostly run backwards and downwards where they merge to form a tendon that runs across the back of the neck of the femur to be inserted into the trochanteric fossa of the femur. In the anatomical position obturator externus laterally rotates the hip but in the sitting position it tends to abduct it.

Quadratus femoris originates from the anterior surface of the sacrum, the posterior portions of the sacrum and the obturator membrane. It is inserted into the superior and posterior aspects of the greater trochanter. In the anatomical position quadratus femoris laterally rotates the hip but when the hip is flexed it abducts it.

Hip rotation – medial

- Anterior part of gluteus medius
- Anterior part of gluteus minimus
- Tensor fasciae latae
- Pectineus.

Gluteus medius and *gluteus minimus* act strongly to abduct the hip and maintain the pelvis level during walking and running (see hip abduction).

When the pelvis is fixed, the anterior fibres of both gluteus medius and gluteus minimus assist hip medial rotation.

Tensor fasciae latae acts with the glutei to abduct the hip (see hip abduction) and assists hip medial rotation.

Pectineus flexes and adducts the hip (see hip flexion) and is thought by some authorities to play a role in medial hip rotation, although this is unconfirmed.

KNEE JOINT

BONES, MOVEMENTS AND THE MUSCLES INVOLVED

3

The long bones of the lower limb are the femur, tibia and fibula.

The knee joint comprises the articulating surfaces of the enlarged condyles at the distal end of the femur and the proximal end of the tibia, together with the patella, developed from a floating sesamoid bone embedded in the quadriceps group of muscles. The posterior surface of the patella has facets that fit over the condyles of the femur and when standing it is held loosely by its tendons at the front of the knee.

The fibula is the small, laterally situated lower leg bone and is not actually part of the knee joint. However, it provides attachments for important knee structures and therefore contributes to knee function.

Movements of the knee and the main muscles involved

The knee joint is a large, complex joint but its movements are principally knee flexion and extension. However, when the knee is bent the tibia can swing medially and laterally and can rotate. The patella shifts laterally as the knee bends.

Knee flexion

- Hamstrings
- Semitendinosus
- Semimembranosus
- Biceps femoris
- Popliteus.

Although the role of the *hamstring muscles* in hip extension is important, they are primarily involved in knee flexion. Also, knee rotation when the knee is flexed is brought about by hamstring muscle activity.

3

Semitendinosus is on the posteromedial aspect of the thigh. It originates from the ischial tuberosity of the femur and is inserted via a long tendon into the medial condyle of the tibia. When acting from above, semitendinosus flexes the extended knee; when the knee is partially flexed, it medially rotates it.

Semimembranosus originates from the upper lateral aspect of the ischial tuberosity and travels down the posteromedial aspect of the thigh deep to semitendinosus to insert via a tendon into the posteromedial surface of the medial tibial condyle. Here its tendinous fibres fan in every direction but laterally they come together to form the oblique popliteal ligament. Semimembranosus acts with semitendinosus to flex the knee.

Biceps femoris originates from a long head that arises with the tendon of semitendinosus from the lower medial facet on the ischial tuberosity and a short head from the linea aspera on the lower half of the posterior thigh. The long head forms a muscle that runs downwards on the posterolateral aspect of the thigh, and in the lower third of the thigh its narrowing tendon blends with the muscle fibres of the short head to travel conjointly towards the posterolateral aspect of the knee where it joins the head of the fibula by two separate attachments. Biceps femoris acts together with semitendinosus and semimembranosus to flex the knee. When the knee is partially flexed, biceps femoris rotates the knee laterally on the thigh.

The *popliteus* originates from the posterior surface of the lateral condyle of the femur and is inserted into the upper posteromedial surface of the tibia. It is the only true flexor of the knee and, with the hamstrings, it can bring about medial rotation of the knee.

Knee extension

- Quadriceps femoris
- Rectus femoris
- Vastus lateralis
- Vastus intermedius
- Vastus medialis
- Tensor fasciae latae.

The *quadriceps muscles* act collectively to extend the knee. They are attached to the patella and their attachments also cross the front of the knee as part of the patellar tendon to be inserted into the tibial tuberosity.

The patella and its tendon provide a pulley effect for the quadriceps that gives it a mechanical advantage during knee extension.

Rectus femoris originates from the anterior inferior iliac spine and the roughened groove immediately above the acetabulum. It is attached via a thick tendon to the upper border of the patella, with some fibres passing around the patella to help form the patellar

tendon between it and the tibial tuberosity. It acts with the other quadriceps muscles to extend the knee.

The three vasti muscles are mainly concerned with knee extension when the hip is already flexed, or as it moves into flexion, and during such activities as kicking a football or extending the knees to come out of a squat, which they achieve with little rectus femoris involvement. However, they do act together with the rectus femoris to extend the knee during walking, running, jumping, etc.

Vastus lateralis has an extensive origin comprising the intertrochanteric line, the inferior and superior borders of the greater trochanter, the gluteal tuberosity, the upper half of the linea aspera, the fasciae latae and the lateral intermuscular septum. It is inserted into the lateral border of the patella and, via the patellar tendon, into the tibial tuberosity. It acts with the other quadriceps muscles to extend the knee.

Vastus intermedius originates from the upper anterior aspect of the femur and is inserted into the upper border of the patella and via the patellar tendon into the tibial tuberosity. It acts with the other quadriceps muscles to extend the knee.

Vastus medialis originates from the length of the linea aspera and the medial condyloid ridge and inserts into the medial, upper aspect of the patella and via the patellar tendon into the tibial tuberosity. It acts with the other quadriceps muscles to extend the knee.

Tensor fasciae latae originates from the outer, upper iliac crest and is inserted via a strong band of fibrous tissue called the iliotibial band into the lateral condyle of the tibia and the head of the fibula. Although it acts mainly to flex, abduct and rotate the hip, it also plays a minor role in knee extension and rotation of the flexed knee.

ANKLE JOINT AND FOOT

BONES, MOVEMENTS AND THE MUSCLES INVOLVED

The ankle joint is a synovial hinge joint formed by the articular surfaces of the distal ends of the tibia and fibula and the body of the talus.

Bony structure of the foot (including tarsus and phalanges)

The *tarsus* comprises the calcaneum and talus, the cuboid and navicular, and the three cuneiform bones.

The *talus* lies posteriorly between the lower limb bones above, the calcaneum below and the other tarsal bones in front. It has no muscle attachments but is important for transmitting the body weight from the tibia down to the calcaneum and forwards to the navicular and other tarsal bones.

The *calcaneum* is a large, oblong-shaped bone with a pronounced backwards prominence that forms the heel. It articulates with the talus superiorly and the cuboid anteriorly. The calcaneum provides attachments for ligaments that bind it to the other tarsal bones as well as for the plantar aponeurosis: a thick fibrous band of connective tissue running along the plantar surface of the foot.

The *navicular* articulates with the head of the talus behind and with the three cuneiform bones in front.

The next row, comprising the cuboid laterally and three cuneiforms medially, articulates with the next row, comprising the metatarsals.

The five *metatarsals*, lying distal to the tarsus, articulate with the row of proximal phalanges in the toes, and so on.

Movements of the ankle and foot and the main muscles involved

The ankle joint is purely a hinge joint and allows flexion and extension. However, ankle joint movements normally have associated subtalar and midtarsal joint motions that allow inversion and eversion of the forefoot.

The posterior muscles of the leg comprise the tibialis posterior, the gastrocnemius and soleus which plantarflex and invert the forefoot.

Muscles plantarflexing the ankle joint

- Gastrocnemius
- Soleus
- Plantaris
- Peroneus
- Tibialis posterior.

The *gastrocnemius* is an easily palpable muscle at the upper posterior aspect of the calf. It has two origins, its medial and lateral heads arising from the posterior surfaces of the medial and lateral femoral condyles, respectively. It is inserted as a part of the Achilles tendon into the posterior surface of the calcaneum. Gastrocnemius is an effective plantarflexor when the knee is extended but its efficacy is reduced when the muscle is shortened as during plantarflexion with the knee flexed.

The *soleus* lies deep to gastrocnemius and originates from the posterior surfaces of the tibia and fibula. It extends the length of the calf to also be inserted as part of the Achilles tendon into the posterior surface of the calcaneum. The soleus is important, as it is always active during plantarflexion at the ankle. When the knee is extended, it works efficiently; however, when the knee is flexed and the action of gastrocnemius is reduced, soleus is required to work correspondingly harder.

Although both gastrocnemius and soleus work during movements that propel the body upwards (hopping, skipping, jumping, etc.), these and other activities such as classical ballet dancing on point depend heavily upon soleus. Therefore, gastrocnemius is exercised most effectively when plantarflexing with the knee extended (heel raising with straight legs) and soleus when the knee is flexed (heel raising with the knee slightly bent, ankle mobilization against resistance with the knee bent, as well as hopping, jumping, etc.).

Plantaris is a long slender muscle running down the back of the leg. It originates from the lateral supracondylar ridge of the femur, the popliteal surface of the femur and the capsular structures of the knee, and is inserted into the calcaneum or the adjacent tendinous attachments. It acts with gastrocnemius and soleus to bring about plantarflexion at the ankle.

The anterior muscles of the leg include the tibialis anterior and the peroneus longus and brevis which dorsiflex and evert the foot, respectively.

Muscles dorsiflexing the ankle joint

- Tibialis anterior
- Extensor digitorum longus
- Extensor hallucis longus
- Peroneus tertius.

Tibialis anterior is a long muscle at the front of the leg, originating from the upper two-thirds of the anterior–lateral surface of the tibia and passing downwards and medially to be inserted into the inner aspect of the medial cuneiform bone and the base of the first metatarsal bone. Tibialis anterior dorsiflexes the ankle joint and acts with tibialis posterior to turn the foot to face medially so as to invert it. Tibialis anterior plays an important role in helping to maintain the balance of the body over the feet in standing and during changes in posture; it also assists with control over the placement and use of the foot during walking, running, etc.

Extensor digitorum longus is also at the front of the leg and originates from the lateral condyle of the tibia and the head and upper two-thirds of the anterior surface of the fibula. It passes down the leg, its tendon passing over the front of the ankle to merge with the complicated arrangement of membranous attachments between and surrounding the bones of the forefoot. Tendinous slips from this arrangement attach extensor digitorum

3

longus to the dorsal aspects of the middle and distal phalanges of the four lesser toes. Extensor digitorum longus assists ankle dorsiflexion. It extends the four lesser toes, assists extension of the interphalangeal joints and during walking and running helps to keep the toes clear of the ground until the heel strike of the action has been accomplished.

Extensor hallucis longus is again found running down the front of the leg but lies deep to and between tibialis anterior and extensor digitorum longus. It originates from the middle two-thirds of the anterior aspect of the fibula and inserts into the base of the distal phalanx of the great toe.

This muscle is able to powerfully dorsiflex the foot at the ankle joint and it acts to extend all the joints of the great toe. This is particularly important during running as the toes must be flexed during ankle plantarflexion to assist the powerful thrusting foot action necessary for the foot to leave the ground. The toes must then extend during ankle dorsiflexion to prepare for the next heel strike.

Peroneus tertius is a small muscle originating from the distal third of the anterior aspect of the fibula and is inserted into the base of the fifth metatarsal. It is a weak dorsiflexor of the ankle.

Muscles everting the foot

- Peroneus longus
- Peroneus brevis
- Peroneus tertius.

Peroneus longus originates from the head and superior lateral aspect of the fibula. It lies along the lateral aspect of the leg and its long tendon follows an intricate route around the bony and reticular structures of the ankle and foot to insert finally into the undersurfaces of the medial cuneiform and first metatarsal bones. This complicated arrangement allows it to be part of the supportive sling under the middle of the foot and to contribute to the strength and integrity of the lateral weight-bearing arch of the foot. This is particularly important for ankle stability when standing on one leg and raising the heel to stand on tiptoe, and during walking or running over uneven ground.

Peroneus longus acts with peroneus brevis and peroneus tertius to evert the foot. It also acts with peroneus brevis to assist gastrocnemius and soleus during plantarflexion.

Peroneus brevis originates from the lower two-thirds of the lateral aspect of the fibula and is inserted into the plantar surface of the fifth metatarsal bone. With peroneus longus and tertius it everts the foot and also assists in maintaining the strength and integrity of the supporting arches of the foot.

Peroneus tertius is a small muscle originating from the distal third of the anterior aspect of the fibula and is inserted into the base of the fifth metatarsal. It is both a weak ankle dorsiflexor and evertor of the foot.

Muscles inverting the foot

- Tibialis posterior
- Tibialis anterior.

Tibialis posterior, the deepest of the posterior leg muscles, originates from the posterior surface of the upper half of the interosseous membrane and the adjacent surfaces of the tibia and fibula, and is attached to the lower inner surfaces of the navicular and cuneiform bones, as well as to the bases of the second, third, fourth and fifth metatarsal bones.

It is the main invertor of the foot and, like all the muscles that enter the foot behind the malleoli, is able to produce ankle plantarflexion. Tibialis posterior action increases support for the underside of the foot and particularly helps to maintain the longitudinal arch. It is exercised through performing heel raises and inversion exercises against resistance.

Tibialis anterior dorsiflexes the ankle joint and assists tibialis posterior to turn the foot to face medially and bring about foot inversion (Thompson & Floyd 1998).

Intrinsic muscles of the foot

The intrinsic muscles of the foot include, on the dorsal surface of the foot, extensor digitorum longus which acts to dorsiflex the four lesser toes, and on the plantar side of the foot several layers of small muscles that plantarflex, abduct and adduct the toes, independently or simultaneously. These muscles are important for maintaining the intricate relationships between the bony structures of the feet during standing and walking. In addition, their development and strength are needed to prevent weak foot conditions that lead to ongoing and possibly permanently disabling problems.

Summary of intrinsic muscles

Extension of the toes

- *Extensor hallucis longus* extends the great toe and dorsiflexes the foot at the ankle joint.
- *Extensor digitorum longus* extends the four lesser toes, assists the lumbricals to produce extension at the interphalangeal joints and assists ankle dorsiflexion.
- *Extensor digitorum brevis* assists extensor hallucis longus in extending the great toe and extensor digitorum longus the lesser toes.
- The *lumbricals* flex the toes at the metatarsophalangeal joints whilst extending them at the interphalangeal joints.

Flexion of the toes

- *Flexor digitorum longus* flexes the four lesser toes, their distal and proximal interphalangeal joints and metatarsophalangeal joints. It also assists foot plantarflexion at the ankle.
- *Flexor accessorius* assists flexion of all the joints of the lesser toes.
- *Flexor digitorum brevis* initially flexes the proximal interphalangeal joints and then the metatarsophalangeal joints of the lesser toes.
- *Flexor hallucis longus* flexes all the joints of the great toe and assists plantarflexion of the foot.
- *Flexor hallucis brevis* flexes the metatarsophalangeal joint of the great toe.
- *Flexor digiti minimi brevis* flexes the metatarsophalangeal joints and assists the maintenance of the longitudinal arch.
- The *dorsal interossei* act with the plantar interossei to produce flexion of the metatarsophalangeal joints.
- The *lumbricals* flex the toes at the metatarsophalangeal joints whilst extending them at the interphalangeal joints. They play an important role during walking, as they help to keep the toes separated and prevent so-called 'clawing' during the propulsive phase of gait.

Abduction of the toes

- *Abductor hallucis* abducts and helps to flex the great toe at the metatarsophalangeal joint.
- *Abductor digiti minimi* abducts the smallest of the lesser toes at the metatarsophalangeal joint and helps to flex this joint.

Adduction of the toes

- *Adductor hallucis* adducts the great toe and flexes the first metatarsophalangeal joint.
- The *plantar interossei* adduct the third, fourth and fifth toes towards the second and flex the metatarsophalangeal joints of the three lesser toes.

References

Palastanga N, Field D, Soames R 2002 Anatomy and human movement, 4th edn. Butterworth-Heinemann, Oxford

Thompson CW, Floyd RT (eds) 1998 Movements of the ankle and foot. In: Manual of structural kinesiology, 13th edn. McGraw-Hill Education, New York

3

Chapter **4**

Exercises for core stabilization and efficient movement

CORRECT RESTING BODY POSITIONS

HEAD AND CERVICAL SPINE ALIGNMENT

Head and cervical spine alignment in standing and sitting

Viewed from side

- The normal cervical and thoracic spinal curves are intact with the head balancing on top of the spine (Fig. 4.1).
- A plumb line falls through the middle of the mastoid process, just in front of the glenohumeral joint.
- The back of the neck is lengthened and the eyes look directly ahead.

Viewed from front and back

- The head and cervical spine are aligned with the thoracic and lumbar spine to achieve whole body symmetry.

Head and cervical spine alignment in supine

Viewed from side

- The head may rest on the floor or suitable supports to maintain the normal cervical and thoracic curves (Fig. 4.2).
- Supports are commonly used to prevent cervical spine extension (recognized by the chin poking forwards) in those people with an exaggerated thoracic kyphosis.

Viewed from head to feet

- The head and cervical spine are aligned with the thoracic and lumbar spine to achieve whole body symmetry.

General points

The position should feel comfortable with the neck muscles appearing relaxed. It may be necessary to try a variety of supports (e.g. neck or small pillow, rolled

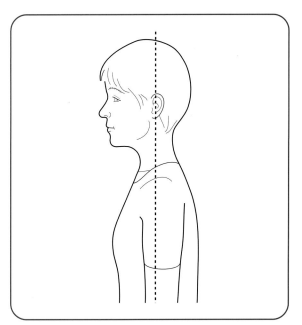

Figure 4.1 Ideal neck posture. Redrawn with permission from Oliver (1999).

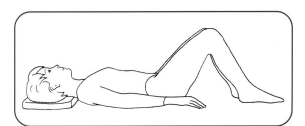

Figure 4.2 Correct head and neck position in supine.

towel) to achieve correct resting alignment. These may need adjusting as exercises progress – for example, head supports can restrict spine movement when progressing from small pelvic tilts to full pelvic curls. The use of head supports for an individual should be continuously reviewed as spine mobility and overall posture improve.

PECTORAL GIRDLE AND SCAPULAR ALIGNMENT IN STANDING AND SITTING

Viewed from side

■ The normal thoracic curve is intact so that the ribcage is balanced over the pelvis and lower limbs (Fig. 4.3).
■ The line of gravity falls in front of the glenohumeral joint approximately through the centre of the acromion process.
■ The glenohumeral joint is neutral in rotation, the proximal and distal ends of the humerus aligned in

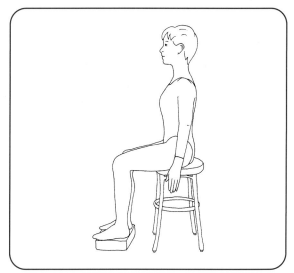

Figure 4.3 Correct pectoral girdle alignment in sitting.

the same vertical plane with the palms of the hands facing the body and the thumbs facing forwards.

Viewed from front

■ The ribcage should be centred over the pelvis and lower limbs with the shoulders facing directly forwards.

Viewed from back

■ The scapulae lie flat against the ribcage between the second and seventh thoracic vertebrae with their vertebral borders parallel to and approximately 7.5 cm from the midline of the spine.
■ They are rotated approximately 30 degrees anterior to the frontal plane to follow the curve of the ribcage (Sahrmann 2002).

NEUTRAL SPINE IN STANDING, SITTING AND SUPINE

The pelvis is in neutral and the normal spinal curves are intact but not exaggerated (Figs 4.4 & 4.5).

Neutral spine in standing

Viewed from side

■ The cervical, thoracic and lumbar curves are intact.

Neutral spine in sitting

Viewed from side

■ The cervical and thoracic curves are intact but the lumbar curve appears slightly less than in standing.
■ The body weight balances over the ischial tuberosities.

4

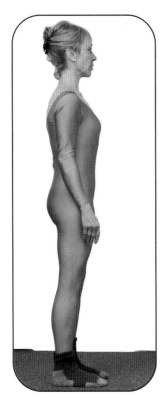

Figure 4.4 Neutral pelvis in standing.

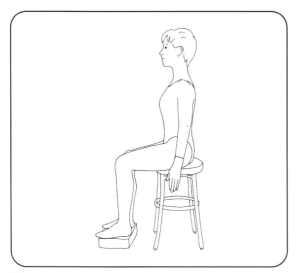

Figure 4.5 Neutral pelvis in sitting.

Neutral spine in supine

Viewed from side

- The normal cervical and thoracic curves are apparent but the lumbar spinal curve may appear less than when viewed in standing (Fig. 4.6).

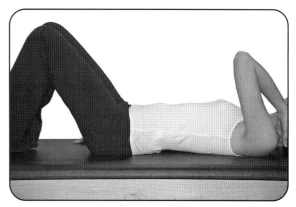

Figure 4.6

- The spine's true alignment may be obscured by the effects of gravity on soft structures surrounding the lumbar spine and pelvis.

NEUTRAL PELVIS

When the body is supine the pelvis lies in the transverse plane. Using the anterior superior iliac spine (ASIS) and pubis as landmarks, a triangle traced with the fingers between these points lies parallel with the floor.

IMPRINTED SPINE (RELAXED BACK POSITION)

When the body is supine the pelvis is positioned with a posterior tilt to eliminate the normal lumbar curve. Using the ASIS and pubis as landmarks, the pubis is positioned at a higher level than the ASIS (Fig. 4.7).

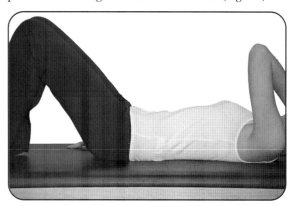

Figure 4.7

SUPINE POSITION: NEUTRAL LUMBAR SPINE AND PELVIS

Body position

Lying on the back with the hips and knees flexed approximately 90 degrees and the hips neutral in rotation. The heels are aligned with the axes of the hip joints. The normal spinal curves are intact (Fig. 4.8).

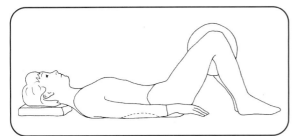

Figure 4.8 Neutral lumbar spine and pelvis.

General points

The position should be stable and comfortable. To achieve the best possible alignment and comfort, use supports with discretion under the head, back, hips, shoulders or feet. If the arms are not comfortable with the palms to the floor, allow them to turn to face the palms to the ceiling. To assist pectoral girdle alignment and stability, cue to press the little fingers lightly into the floor. To correct lower limb alignment, place a chi ball or cushion between the thighs or instruct the student to gently activate the short leg adductor muscles (brevis and magnus). To maintain lumbar spine alignment, cue to reach the 'sitting bones' and crown of the head in opposite directions and relax the lower back muscles.

Equipment

Neck pillow, pillow, rolled towels, chi ball; yoga blocks or a small box may be used to raise the feet.

Observable features

Viewed from side

- An elongated upper spine with intact cervical and thoracic curves.
- The chin is slightly dropped to relax the superficial neck muscles.
- The eyes look directly ahead.
- Correct pectoral girdle alignment allowing the shoulders to open and drop back to the floor.
- The arms lying beside the body with the elbows softly rounded.
- The glenohumeral joints are in slight medial rotation so that the palms of the hands face towards the floor with the fingers following the line of the arms.
- An elongated lumbar spine with the lumbar curve intact (the pubic bone is in same transverse plane as the ASIS).

Viewed from head to feet

- The head, upper torso, pelvis and lower limbs align to achieve whole body symmetry (Fig. 4.9).
- The chin is slightly dropped to relax the superficial neck muscles.

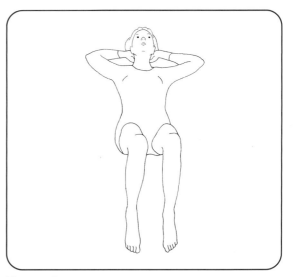

Figure 4.9

- The eyes look directly ahead.
- The lower limbs and feet are placed so that a line can be taken from the axis of each hip joint (a point slightly medial to the ASIS) through the middle of the knee joint to between the second and third toes.
- The feet make contact with the floor so that the weight is distributed over the tripod of weight bearing.

Common problems

- Rounding the shoulders: Use tactile cues to encourage breadth across the collarbones.
- Tensing the back, extending the spine and pushing the ribcage away from the floor: Use the breath to improve relaxation of the spinal muscles so that the breastbone can drop back towards the spine and the ribs can align correctly with the pelvis; this allows the abdominal muscles to achieve their optimum length and tone.
- Tightening the hip flexors: Cue to relax the toes, feet, thighs and posterior hip muscles; cue to release and lengthen through the groins.

See Table 4.1 for Teaching points.

SUPINE POSITION: IMPRINTED LUMBAR SPINE

This position is used during exercising when abdominal muscle strength is insufficient to stabilize the lumbar spine, or when first attempting more challenging exercises.

Body position

Lying on the back with the hips and knees flexed approximately 90 degrees and the hips neutral in rotation (Fig. 4.10). The heels are aligned with the axes of

Table 4.1   Teaching points – Supine position: neutral lumbar spine and pelvis

Focus on	Examples of verbal/visual cues
Creating a correctly aligned and relaxed, comfortable position	Centre yourself on the mat Use sufficient head support to achieve relaxed neck muscles and comfort Align the heels with the sitting bones Reach the sitting bones for the heels Lengthen from the crown of the head through to the sitting bones On breathing out, relax the tongue in the throat and imagine your body and limbs sinking into warm sand
Achieving a neutral spine and pelvis	Trace your fingers along a triangle formed between the pubic bones and the hip bones. The triangle is to lie parallel with the floor Imagine a small space under the lower back – just enough to allow a glimmer of light to shine through Imagine the pelvis as a bowl of water and the surface of the water is absolutely level and still

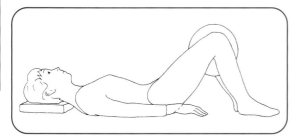

Figure 4.10   Imprinted spine.

the hip joints. The pelvis is in a slight posterior tilt with the lumbar spine flattened.

General points

The position should be stable and comfortable. To achieve the best possible alignment and comfort, use supports with discretion under the head, back, hips, shoulders or feet. If the arms are not comfortable with the palms to the floor, allow them to turn to face the palms to the ceiling. To assist pectoral girdle alignment and stability, cue to press the little fingers lightly into the floor. To correct lower limb alignment, place a chi ball or cushion between the thighs or instruct the student to gently activate the short leg adductor muscles (brevis and magnus). To create and maintain a flattened lumbar spine, cue to gently activate the pelvic floor and lower abdominal muscles.

Equipment

Neck pillow, pillow, rolled towels, chi ball; yoga blocks or a small box may be used to raise the feet.

Observable features

Viewed from side

- An elongated upper spine with intact cervical and thoracic curves.
- The chin is slightly dropped to relax the superficial neck muscles.
- The eyes look directly ahead.
- Correct pectoral girdle alignment allowing the shoulders to open and drop back to the floor.
- The arms lying beside the body with the elbows softly rounded.
- The glenohumeral joints are in slight medial rotation so that the palms of the hands face towards the floor with the fingers following the line of the arms.
- An elongated lumbar spine with a flattened lumbar curve (the pubic bone is higher than the ASIS).

Viewed from head to feet

- The head, upper torso, pelvis and lower limbs align to achieve whole body symmetry.
- The chin is slightly dropped to relax the superficial neck muscles.
- The eyes look directly ahead.
- The lower limbs and feet are placed so that a line can be taken from the axis of each hip joint (a point slightly medial to the ASIS) through the middle of the knee joint to between the second and third toes.
- The feet make contact with the floor so that the weight is distributed over the tripod of weight bearing.

Table 4.2   Teaching points – Supine position: imprinted spine

Focus on	Examples of verbal/visual cues
Creating a correctly aligned and relaxed, comfortable position	Centre yourself on the mat Use sufficient head support to achieve relaxed neck muscles and comfort Align the heels with the sitting bones Reach the sitting bones for the heels Imagine the groins as deep valleys On breathing out, relax the tongue in the throat and imagine your body and limbs sinking into warm sand
Using abdominal muscle activation and relaxation of the lower back muscles to create the posterior pelvic tilt	Imagine the pelvis as bowl of water. Using the pelvic floor muscles and lower abdominal muscles, tilt the bowl to spill one drop of water towards your navel Keep the lower back muscles relaxed and the abdominal muscles gently working to maintain this position Trace your fingers around the edges of the triangle to see if the pubic bone is higher than the hip bones Use your fingers to see if your normal lower back curve has flattened to the floor

Common problems

- Using the legs to push the back to the floor: Cue to maintain relaxed hamstring and gluteal muscles.
- Tightening the hip flexors to create or maintain the 'imprinted' position: Cue to relax the toe, thigh and posterior hip muscles; cue to think of making deep valleys in the groins.
- Poor relationship between the ribcage and pelvis due to thoracic spine extension and/or lumbar spine lordosis: Consider using a pillow behind the upper body to curl it forwards to facilitate abdominal control.

See Table 4.2 for Teaching points.

PRONE POSITION

Body position

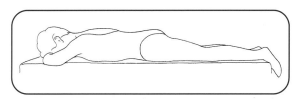

Figure 4.11

Lying prone, preferably on a mat or a raised bed that enables the ankles to relax as the feet drop over the edge (Fig. 4.11). The arms are bent with the elbows pointing to the side, and the hands resting one on top of the other to make a support for the forehead. The spine is lengthened and the limbs are symmetrically aligned. The abdominal muscles are drawn gently towards the spine, supporting the natural lumbar curve and the groins are soft and lengthened.

General points

The position should feel comfortable and be stable so that correct body and limb alignment may be maintained during exercising. Supports may be placed in the axillae for upper body comfort. A small pillow may be placed under the body to reduce an exaggerated lumbar lordosis. A rolled towel may be place between the thighs to maintain leg alignment.

Initially, it may be necessary to allow a student with tight hip flexors to slightly abduct the hips to achieve a comfortable, stable position. Where possible, maintain the hips neutral in rotation unless otherwise stated.

Equipment

Neck pillows, small pillows, rolled towel. *Note*: Large pillows should not be used between the lower ribs and the pelvis as this may affect the breathing effort, particularly in those individuals with pathology that compromises breathing such as asthma, respiratory disease, etc.

Observable features

Viewed from side

- An elongated upper spine with intact cervical and thoracic curves.
- The chin is slightly dropped to relax the superficial neck muscles.
- An elongated lumbar spinal curve.

Viewed from head to feet

- The head, upper torso, pelvis and lower limbs align to achieve whole body symmetry.
- The hips are neutral in rotation and lie parallel to one another.
- The feet are placed so that a line can be taken from the axis of each hip joint – a point slightly medial to the posterior superior iliac spine (PSIS) – through the middle of the heels to between the second and third toes.

Common problems

- An exaggerated lumbar lordosis: For students with poor abdominal muscle control or tight hip flexors it may be helpful to place a small pillow under the body to support and lengthen the lumbar spine.
- For students with neck problems, position on a stack of mats at least 8–10 cm high so that the elbows fall lower than the chest and the head can drop forwards onto the hands; this allows the cervical spine to lengthen.
- For students with shoulder problems, supports may be placed in the axillae whilst the head rests on the hands, or a small support may be placed under the forehead whilst the arms remain at the sides of the body.

See Table 4.3 for Teaching points.

SIDE LYING POSITION FOR EXERCISING THE UPPER LEG

Body position

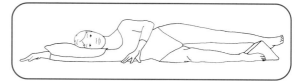

Figure 4.12

Side lying with the lower leg flexed approximately 90 degrees at the hip and knee (Fig. 4.12). The upper leg extends in line with the body or slightly in front of the hips (with no more than 10 degrees of flexion) and rests on the floor or a support at about hip height. The lower arm reaches along the floor in line with the shoulder and the upper hand is placed on the floor in front of the body or on the upper hip to help keep the side of the body lengthened. (Alternatively, the upper arm may be supported by placing it on yoga blocks, a pillow or small soft ball, or magic circle.) The head rests on the extended lower arm or on a suitable support to establish correct head, neck and thoracic spine alignment.

General points

The position should feel comfortable and be stable so that correct body and limb alignment may be maintained during exercising. For beginners and those with limited core control it may be necessary to flex the thoracic spine just enough to allow the sternum to drop down and back towards the spine. This can improve abdominal muscle control during exercising.

Table 4.3   Teaching points – Prone position

Focus on	Examples of verbal/visual cues
Correct spine alignment	Centre yourself on the mat
Creating a comfortable rest position for the student	Use supports appropriately
Lengthening through the groins	Lift the right leg slightly, stretch through the groin and reach the right leg out of the hip then return it to the mat Repeat with the left leg Think of lengthening through the groins and lower back
Sufficient abdominal muscle engagement to support the lumbar spine	Imagine creating a space under the navel large enough for small piece of chocolate Maintain sufficient abdominal muscle work to prevent squashing or melting the chocolate

Equipment

Neck pillow, pillow, rolled towel, triangle, yoga blocks, chi ball, magic circle.

Observable features

Viewed from front

- The head and cervical spine are aligned with the thoracic and lumbar spine to achieve whole body symmetry.
- The superficial neck muscles should appear relaxed.
- The pectoral girdle should be well aligned, with the shoulder blades drawing down the back.
- The head is neutral in rotation and the eyes look directly forwards.
- The upper hip lies directly above the lower hip with the natural waist curve intact.

Viewed from above

- The spinal curves are intact but not exaggerated.
- The front and back of the torso should appear to be equally lengthened.
- The upper shoulder lies directly above the lower shoulder and the upper hip stacks directly above the lower hip.
- The lower arm aligns with the body.
- The upper leg aligns with the axes of the hips.

Common problems

- Extension of the cervical, thoracic or lumbar spine and subsequent loss of the correct relationship between the ribs and the pelvis: Place the student against a wall or other back support; cue for stronger abdominal muscle control.
- Rounding of the upper shoulder: Cue to broaden across the collarbones and slide the shoulder blades down the back.
- Twisting from the waist and rotating the pelvis forwards or backwards: Place the student against a wall or other back support; support the upper arm with a stack of blocks.
- Flexing the spine laterally such that the waist drops to the floor: Instruct the student to place a hand on the upper hip together with contracting the lower abdominal muscles more strongly; consider placing a support such as a small rolled towel under the waist.
- Placing the upper leg in a position of hip extension with lumbar spine extension: Cue for stronger abdominal muscle control; instruct the student to be aware that the upper foot should be lying within their range of peripheral vision when looking straight ahead; consider stretching the gluteal and lower back muscles.

See Table 4.4 for Teaching points.

SIDE LYING POSITION FOR EXERCISING THE LOWER LEG

Body position

Side lying with the upper leg in approximately 90 degrees of hip and knee flexion, the knee resting on a support at about hip height (Fig. 4.13). The lower leg is extended in line with the body or slightly in front of the

Table 4.4 Teaching points – Side lying position for exercising the upper leg

Focus on	Examples of verbal/visual cues
Comfort	Lie along a mat, lining the body up with the edge of the mat, or place your back against a wall Use neck supports and waist supports as required – a pillow between the head and arm, a small towel under the waist
Good pectoral girdle alignment and stability	Imagine the shoulder blades sliding down the back into rear hip pockets on the opposite sides
Alignment and length of the spine and lower limbs	Imagine the sitting bones and the crown of the head reaching in opposite directions Reach the upper leg out of the hip joint Feel that a hand could slide between the waist and the floor
The optimum position for torso stability and effective upper limb movement	Imagine the body stretched between two panes of glass that might shatter if the body leans forwards or backwards Imagine you are lying with your back against a wall

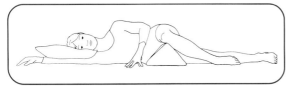

Figure 4.13   Side lying position for exercising the lower leg.

hips (with no more than 10 degrees of hip flexion). Both knees face directly forward. The lower arm reaches along the floor in line with the shoulder and the upper hand is placed on the floor in front of the body or on the upper hip to help keep the side of the body lengthened. (Alternatively, the upper arm may be supported by placing it on yoga blocks, a pillow or small soft ball, or magic circle.) The head rests on the extended lower arm or on a suitable support to establish correct head, neck and thoracic spine alignment.

General points

The position should feel comfortable and be stable so that correct body and limb alignment may be maintained during exercising. For beginners and those with limited core control it may be necessary to flex the thoracic spine just enough to allow the sternum to drop down and back towards the spine. This can improve abdominal muscle control during exercising.

Equipment

Neck pillow, pillow, rolled towel, triangle, yoga blocks, chi ball, magic circle.

Observable features

Viewed from front

- The head and cervical spine are aligned with the thoracic and lumbar spine to achieve whole body symmetry.
- The superficial neck muscles should appear relaxed.
- The pectoral girdle should be well aligned, with the shoulder blades drawing down the back.
- The head is neutral in rotation and the eyes look directly forwards.
- The upper hip lies directly above the lower hip with the natural waist curve intact.

Viewed from above

- The spinal curves are intact but not exaggerated.
- The front and back of the torso should appear to be equally lengthened.
- The upper shoulder lies directly above the lower shoulder and the upper hip stacks directly above the lower hip.

- The lower arm aligns with the body.
- The lower leg aligns with the axes of the hips.

Common problems

- Extension of the cervical, thoracic or lumbar spine and subsequent loss of the correct relationship between the ribs and the pelvis: Place the student against a wall or other back support; cue for stronger abdominal muscle control.
- Rounding of the upper shoulder: Cue to broaden across the collarbones and slide the shoulder blade down the back.
- Twisting from the waist and rotating the pelvis forwards or backwards: Place the student against a wall or other back support; support the upper arm with a stack of blocks.
- Flexing the spine laterally such that the waist drops to the floor: Instruct the student to place a hand on the upper hip together with contracting the lower abdominal muscles more strongly; consider placing a support such as a small rolled towel under the waist.
- Placing the lower leg in a position of hip extension with lumbar spine extension: Cue for stronger abdominal muscle control; instruct the student to flex the lower hip to about 20 degrees.

See Table 4.5 for Teaching points.

QUADRIPED POSITION

Body position

Four-point kneeling with the hips and knees flexed 90 degrees and the knees approximately hip distance apart (Fig. 4.14). The hips are neutral in rotation and the limbs are parallel and aligned so that the top of the feet face to the floor. The hands are in line with or just in front of the glenohumeral joints (if the arms are comparatively long). The glenohumeral joints are in slight lateral rotation and the arms are extended with the elbows softened to prevent hyperextension of the elbow joint. The little

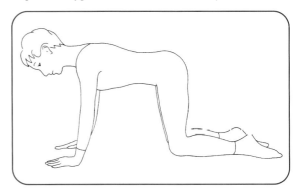

Figure 4.14   Quadriped position.

Table 4.5   Teaching points – Side lying position for exercising the lower leg

Focus on	Examples of visual/verbal cues
Comfort	Lie along a mat, lining the body up with the edge of the mat, or place your back against a wall Use neck supports and waist supports as required – a pillow between the head and arm, a small towel under the waist
Good pectoral girdle alignment and stability	Imagine the shoulder blades sliding down the back into rear hip pockets on the opposite sides
Alignment and length of the spine and lower limbs	Imagine the sitting bones and the crown of the head reaching in opposite directions Reach the lower leg out of the hip joint Feel that a hand could slide between the waist and the floor
The optimum position for torso stability and effective lower limb movement	Imagine the body stretched between two panes of glass that might shatter if the body leans forwards or backwards Imagine you are lying with your back against a wall

fingers press lightly into the floor to assist engagement of the pectoral girdle stabilizing muscles. The normal spinal curves are intact, with the back of the neck lengthened and the crown of the head reaching forward. The gaze is between the thumbs.

General points

The position should feel comfortable and be stable so that correct body and limb alignment may be maintained during exercising.

Equipment

Exercise mat or firm bed.

Observable features

Viewed from side

- The spine is elongated with the normal curves of the spine intact.
- The pectoral girdle is well aligned and stable with the shoulder blades flat on the ribcage.
- The back of the neck is lengthened with the superficial neck muscles appearing comparatively relaxed.
- The abdominal muscles are drawn up towards the spine.

Viewed from front

- The hands are placed under the shoulders and the knees are placed approximately under the axes of the hip joints, just medial to the ASIS.

Common problems

- Extension of the cervical, thoracic or lumbar spine and subsequent loss of the correct relationship between the head, neck, ribs and pelvis: Cue to lengthen through the back of the neck and to imagine holding a soft peach between the chin and the sternum; use the hands to direct the ribs to 'funnel down towards the pelvis'; cue to reach the crown of the head and the 'sitting bones' in opposite directions; trace the fingers along the spine to promote space between each vertebra.
- Hanging head: Cue to lift or float the head towards the ceiling whilst thinking of dropping the chin.
- Wrist pain: Decrease wrist extension by placing supports under the heels of the hands.
- Thoracic spine sagging down between the scapulae: Use the fingers to direct the sternum upwards towards the spine to establish the normal thoracic curve and allow the scapulae to flatten on the ribs; cue to slide the shoulder blades down and across the back.
- An exaggerated lumbar lordosis with poor abdominal muscle control over the lumbar spine: Cue to increase pelvic floor and lower abdominal muscle activation and to reach the 'sitting bones' and the crown of the head in opposite directions.
- Poor proprioception of body alignment in space: Initially consider the use of props such as a mirror, or by using a stick placed along the spine to feel where the normal spinal curves would lie; use visual imagery to cue the neutral pelvis alignment – for example, imagine the hip bones as lights shining directly to the floor below or the sitting bones as lights shining directly backwards.
- Should the contour of the paraspinal muscles be asymmetric, there could be a postural rotation of the lumbar vertebrae or uneven rotation in the hip joints. The latter is confirmed by asking the

Table 4.6 Teaching points – Quadriped position

Focus on	Examples of visual/verbal cues
Achieving a well-balanced position with the body weight distributed between the hands and the lower limbs	Kneel down and sit your bottom on your heels Keep the bottom in contact with the heels and curl the body, reaching the arms as far forward as possible along the floor Spread the fingers, push the hands into the floor and simultaneously slide the shoulder blades down the back Maintain shoulder girdle stability to draw the crown of the head forwards until you are supported over your hands and knees Adjust your position so that the shoulders are directly over the hands and the knees are over the hips
Good pectoral girdle alignment and stability	Draw the breastbone up towards the spine Imagine the shoulder blades sliding down the back into rear hip pockets on the opposite sides
Alignment and length of the spine and lower limbs	Imagine the sitting bones and the crown of the head reaching in opposite directions Reach the knees towards the floor

subject to rock back onto the heels. If lumbar spine rotation increases further as the subject reaches their end range of hip flexion motion, asymmetry of hip joint mobility is likely.

See Table 4.6 for Teaching points.

The classic Pilates repertoire

The Hundred, Roll-Up, Roll-Over, Leg Circles, Rolling Back, Single Leg Stretch, Double Leg Stretch, Spine Stretch, Open Leg Rocker, Corkscrew, See-Saw, Swan Dive, Single Leg Kick, Double Leg Kick, Neck Pull, Scissors, Bicycle, Shoulder Bridge, Spine Twist, Jackknife, Side Kick, Teaser, Hip twist with outstretched legs, Swimming, Leg Pull Front Support, Leg Pull Back Support, Side Kick Kneeling, Side Bend, Boomerang, Seal, Crab, Rocking, Control balance, Push-Up.

PREREQUISITE PREPARATORY EXERCISES

This covers basic sequences to achieve correct posture and efficient movement, thus providing the fundamental elements of the Pilates' mat and equipment repertoires.

In the following exercises and stretches these principles are implied and may be easily identified within each specific exercise 'aim'.

CONTROLLED BREATHING

Aim

To improve the efficiency of lung function and blood oxygenation.

To increase mental focus.
To improve the ability to relax so as to release unnecessary skeletal muscles tension.
To increase overall ribcage mobility.
To increase the vertical, lateral and anteroposterior dimensions of the ribcage during inspiration.
To encourage efficient exhalation.
To improve the performance of the pelvic floor and respiratory muscles throughout the breathing cycle.
To assist posture, musculoskeletal function and movement patterns.

Equipment

Exercise mat, gym ball, chair, dynaband; head supports to correct head/neck alignment and prevent neck and upper back tension.

Target muscles

Inspiration	Expiration
Diaphragm	Transversus thoracis
Intercostals	Subcostals
Levatores costarum	Serratus posterior inferior
Serratus posterior superior	External obliques
	Internal obliques
	Transversus abdominis
	Latissimus dorsi

Principles derived from Joseph Pilates' original tenets

1. *Efficient breathing* implies both efficient pulmonary ventilation and cardiovascular function. Controlled breathing patterns before and during exercise assist mental concentration and physical relaxation and may improve spine stability or mobility.
2. *Mental concentration* and control imply the exclusion of unrelated thinking so as to concentrate on and be fully aware of what one is feeling and doing.
3. *Relaxation* implies the simultaneous release of bodywide muscle tensions. Alternatively, it can refer to the relative relaxation of specific muscles of which their opposing muscles can then function efficiently.
4. *Correct spine elongation and alignment* are intrinsically linked to correct spinal stabilization, mobilization and underlying musculoskeletal function, so as to achieve ideal static and dynamic postures.
5. *Correct abdominal muscle control over spine stability and mobility* implies correct lumbar spine function through appropriate abdominal muscle activity.
6. *Correct function of each upper limb* requires a combination of correct pectoral girdle alignment and stability upon an underlying correctly aligned and stabilized spine.
7. *Correct function of each lower limb* requires a combination of correct pelvic girdle alignment and stability upon an underlying correctly aligned and stabilized spine.
8. *Precision* implies the ability to sense and identify the basic components of an action and then perfect the way they are performed.
9. *Flowing integrated movement.* Having achieved precision this implies an ability to perform the components correctly in sequence.
10. *Achieving muscular strength and stamina* requires adherence to all the above principles so as to eliminate any superfluous activity.

Sequence 1 – Relaxed breathing

Body position

Supine with 90 degrees of hip and knee flexion. The pelvis is slightly tilted posteriorly so as to flatten the lumbar spine and allow the back muscles to relax. The head is supported sufficiently to allow the superficial neck muscles to relax. The eyes are closed or the gaze is unfocused with the eyes looking directly forwards (Fig. 4.15A).

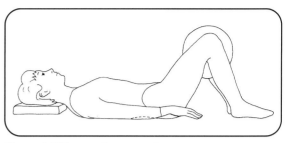

Figure 4.15A Breathing normally.

Action

Breathing normally for several minutes – encourage self-awareness to sense the movements of the sternum and ribs, the rate and pattern of the breathing cycle, and the relaxation and tightening of the muscles of the abdominal wall.

Following this (Fig. 4.15B–D):

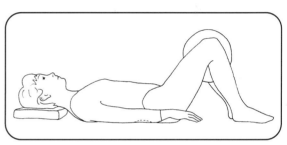

Figure 4.15B Breathing in.

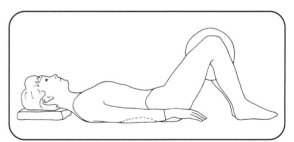

Figure 4.15C Breathing out.

Breathing actively

Breathing in – gently activate the pelvic floor and increase lung expansion, directing the breath more into the lower lobes of the lungs with increased mobilization of the lateral and posterior aspects of the thoracic cage. Simultaneously allow the anterior abdominal wall muscles to further relax to increase the descent of the diaphragm.

Breathing out – increase pelvic floor activation and tighten the lower fibres of transversus abdominis as exhalation begins. Maintain this gentle contraction to assist the ascent of the diaphragm as the lungs

4

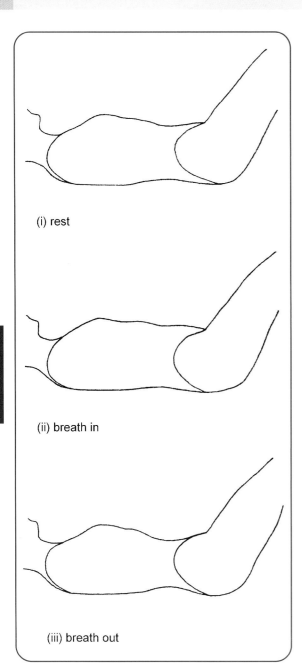

(i) rest

(ii) breath in

(iii) breath out

Figure 4.15D

continue to recoil and achieve a full deep exhalation. At the end of the breathing cycle the back muscles are fully relaxed so the sternum can drop down and back towards the spine to achieve the correct relationship between the upper and lower torso. This then allows each of the trunk muscles to achieve their optimum length.

Modification

To *assist breathing out* – place a dynaband or towel around the lower third of the thoracic cage and cross the ends in front of the chest. Gently pull the ends across the body so as to squeeze air out of the chest during exhalation. Release the tension during the next inhalation and repeat the sequence 5–10 times.

Progression

Directing the breath more into one side of the chest – prepare as in the Modification and focus on expanding first the right side and then the left side of the chest.

Common problems

- Breathing more into the upper lobes of the lungs: If the breathing patterns demonstrate a pronounced displacement of the sternum rather than the lower ribs, the lungs are not fully expanding. On *breathing in*, place the hands lightly over or a tie a dynaband around the chest approximately at the level of the seventh to twelfth ribs and encourage the student to direct the breath more into the lower lobes. On *breathing out*, use the hands or a dynaband to slightly compress the ribs so as to squeeze air from the lungs.
- An inadequate breathing effort overall: Modify the working position to focus more on mobilizing the posterior or lateral aspects of the ribcage – for example, as in lying prone or sideways over a gym ball; side lying with the legs and hips flexed and the upper leg supported on a pillow; sitting with the upper body resting forwards over a table; supported child pose with the upper limbs and head comfortably positioned. Use visual imagery to direct the breath as required.
- Overbreathing or 'trying too hard': Use visual imagery, the voice and/or music to create a calm atmosphere; focus more on fully *breathing out* and allow *breathing in* to occur passively.
- Initial difficulties with locating or feeling pelvic floor muscle tightening: Experiment with different visual imagery cues or body positions – for example, imagine urinating and then stopping the flow of urine midstream; perform side lying with the upper leg supported, lying prone or sitting on a gym ball.

Sequence 2 – Increasing posterolateral ribcage expansion

Prepare as for Sequence 1.

Breathing actively maintaining abdominal muscle control

Perform Sequence 1 whilst maintaining the pelvic floor and abdominal muscles more deeply contracted. Sense the support of the pelvic floor and abdominal wall assisting the expansion of the posterior and lateral aspects of the thoracic cage.

Sequence 3 – Forced expiration

Prepare as for Sequence 1.

Breathing more actively

Breathing in – breathe in deeply.

Breathing out – cough to stimulate pelvic floor and abdominal muscle activation as the exhalation begins. This pushes the abdominal contents up against the diaphragm, forcing it upwards, thus increasing its upward displacement as the exhalation progresses. As a result, the capacity of the chest is further decreased and air is forced from the lungs. The pelvic floor and abdominal muscle action can be controlled to assist the progression and depth of the exhalation.

Sequence 4 – Controlled breathing to assist spine stabilization and mobilization as required

During the breathing cycle there is normally slight spine extension on inhalation and passive flexion on exhalation. These unconscious motions can be harnessed to help elongate, stiffen and stabilize the spine during hip and shoulder joint mobilization (particularly the lumbar spine during hip flexion) or to assist segmental vertebral column mobilization during spine extension as well as flexion.

Active breathing can be used to assist control over spine stability during hip and shoulder joint mobilization (e.g. in the basic core stability exercises BCS4 and BCS5 the 'in breath' helps control lumbar spine stability during hip joint flexion), or it can be used to improve spine elongation and mobilization (e.g. as in the spine mobilization exercises). These exercises can be selected as required.

See Table 4.7 for Teaching points.

4

Table 4.7 Teaching points – Controlled breathing

Focus on	Examples of verbal/visual cues
Correct head and spine alignment without neck tension	Ensure the head is sufficiently supported to allow the neck and upper back to relax Allow the tongue to loll in the mouth and imagine the muscles of the face melting away
Correct pectoral girdle and lower limb alignment	Spread the collarbones apart and imagine the shoulder blades as skis sliding diagonally down and across the back Imagine the knees are suspended from the ceiling with strings
Relaxing the body throughout	Imagine the head, arms, back and feet sinking into warm sand Sense the weight of the whole body and allow it to drop into the floor
An efficient breathing cycle: inspiration	On 'breathing in': – imagine the shoulder blades as wings unfurling and preparing for flight – imagine the diaphragm as a dome-shaped leaf floating down into the pelvis – imagine the back and side ribs opening as louvre blinds that allow light into the lungs – sense the weight of the body spreading across the floor
An efficient breathing cycle: expiration	On 'breathing out', imagine: – the breastbone as a stone falling into the chest – the diaphragm as a hot air balloon floating gently up into the chest – the ribs closing together as louvre blinds – the shoulder blades sliding down across the back and sense the weight of the body dropping into the floor – the ribs as a concertina squeezing air from the lungs
An efficient breathing cycle: more active expiration	On 'breathing out', draw the lower abdominal muscles further back towards the spine

BASIC CORE STRENGTHENING EXERCISES

EXERCISE LIST

Supine lower abdominal muscle strengthening
  (Exercises BCS1–5)
  BCS1   Pelvic floor muscle toning
  BCS2   Lower abdominal muscle activation
  BCS3   Hip rolls
  BCS4   Leg slides
  BCS5   Thigh arcs

Prone posterior hip muscle strengthening
  (Exercises BCS6–8)
  BCS6   Gluteal squeezes
  BCS7   Gluteal strengthener with flexed
              knee
  BCS8   Hamstring curls

Side lying posterior hip muscle strengthening
  (Exercises BCS9–12)
  BCS9   The oyster
  BCS10   Upper leg lifts
  BCS11   Lower leg lifts
  BCS12   Body lengthening

Spine, hip and shoulder stabilization and mobilization –
  quadriped series (Exercises BCS13–19)
  BCS13   Head nodding
  BCS14   Head turning
  BCS15   Rocking
  BCS16   Arm lifts
  BCS17   Leg lifts
  BCS18   Arm and leg lifts
  BCS19   Cat

Supine spine mobilization (Exercises SSM20–22)
  SSM20   Pelvic tilt
  SSM21   Pelvic curls
  SSM22   Pelvic curls with arm lifts

Supine upper abdominal muscle strengthening
  (Progression from lower abdominal muscle
  strengthening) (Exercises SAS23–24)
  SAS23   Sit ups series
  SAS24   Sit ups with twist series

Prone spine mobilization (Exercises PSM25–26)
  PSM25   Cobra
  PSM26   Arrow

Side lying spine mobilization (Exercise SLM27)
  SLM27   Chest opener with spine twist

Knee strengthening (Exercise KS28)
  KS28   Quadriceps strengthening

SUPINE LOWER ABDOMINAL MUSCLE STRENGTHENING (EXERCISES BCS1–5)

Exercise BCS1 – Pelvic floor muscle toning

Aim

To enhance pelvic floor muscle tone and control.

Equipment

Exercise mat, box, bolster for between thighs, gym
  ball; head supports to correct head/neck alignment
  and prevent neck tension.

Target muscles

Levator ani and coccygeus acting together.

Body position

Supine with 90 degrees of hip and knee flexion –
  perform with a slight posterior pelvic tilt (the lumbar
  spine is flattened and the back muscles are relaxed).

Action 1

Breathing in – tighten the pelvic floor muscles.

Breathing out – lift the pelvic floor muscles without
  tensing the rest of the body. Hold this position
  while breathing normally for two or three breaths
  before allowing the muscles to gradually and
  completely release.

Repeat up to 10 times.

As stamina improves, the contraction can be held
  longer (up to 10 seconds whilst breathing normally)
  and the repetitions increased.

Note: This improves the performance of the slow
  twitch muscle fibres involved in pelvic and core
  stabilization.

Action 2

Perform the sequence faster in a rhythmical way,
  making sure that each contraction moves through
  its full range of movement, tightening and relaxing
  completely before each repetition.

Note: This improves the performance of the fast twitch
muscle fibres involved in micturition, defecation, childbirth and sexual intercourse. The pelvic floor muscles,
like other muscles, need regular exercise to maintain
health and performance. Encourage regular pelvic
floor exercising of the fast and slow twitch muscle
fibres throughout the day – for example, when cooking,
washing-up, etc., or even sitting waiting for traffic lights
to change! Also encourage their activation in preparation for changing position – when moving from sitting
to standing, getting in and out of bed, the car, etc. After
childbirth, the pelvic floor muscles should be strong
enough to sustain a contraction for at least 15 seconds
before they are challenged by activities such as jogging,
running, aerobics, etc.

Progression 1

Practise in conjunction with transversus abdominis activation in preparation for more strenuous exercise.

Progression 2

Perform as in Action 1 and hold for at least 10 seconds. Repeat up to 10 times.

Common problems

- Breathing patterns and pelvic floor muscle work not coordinated: Allow the student to find their own breathing rhythm.
- Breathing effort inadequate: Modify the working position to focus more on lateral breathing – for example, lying prone or sideways over a gym ball.
- Initial difficulties with locating or feeling pelvic floor muscle tightening: Experiment with different visual imagery cues or body positions – for example, imagine urinating and then stopping the flow of urine midstream; perform side lying with the upper leg supported; lying prone or sitting on a gym ball; lying on a slight slope with the head down (pelvis higher than the head) so that the action is gravity assisted.

See Table 4.8 for Teaching points.

Tactile cue suggestions

1. To increase breadth across the front of the chest – use the hands to stroke the collarbones from the sternum to their lateral aspects.
2. To establish the correct relationship between the upper and lower torso – on exhaling use the hands on the lower ribs to assist funnelling them down towards the pelvis.

Exercise BCS2 – Lower abdominal muscle activation (transversus abdominis activation)

Aim

To activate transversus abdominis with minimal recruitment of other anterior abdominal wall muscles.
To improve deep abdominal muscle control over spine stability.

Equipment

Exercise mat, box, bolster for between thighs, therapy ball; head supports to correct head/neck alignment and prevent neck tension.

4

Table 4.8 Teaching points – Pelvic floor muscle toning

Focus on	Examples of visual/verbal cues
Correct head and neck alignment without neck tension	Relax the tongue in the throat and imagine the muscles of the face melting away
Vertebral column length	Reach the crown of the head and the sitting bones in opposite directions
Correct pectoral girdle alignment and stability	Spread the collarbones apart and glide the shoulder blades diagonally down towards the centre of the back
Relaxing the body throughout	Imagine the head, arms, back and feet sinking into warm sand
Lower limb/feet placement	Imagine the knees are suspended from the ceiling with strings
Controlling activation of the pelvic floor muscles	Imagine urinating and then stopping the flow mid-stream Tighten the muscles around the vagina as if squeezing something (women only) Tighten the back passage as if to prevent passing wind Think of drawing the genitals up into the body (men only)
Total relaxation of the pelvic floor muscles after each contraction	Allow the muscles to release as if they were 'sighing' Allow the whole body to sink into the floor

Target muscles
Transversus abdominis.

Body position
Semi-supine – neutral pelvis (Fig. 4.16).

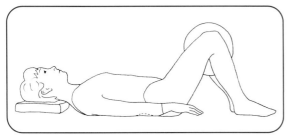

Figure 4.16 Breathing in.

Action

Breathing in – relax the abdominal muscles and fill the back and sides of the ribcage with air.

Breathing out – allow the back and chest muscles to relax and draw the abdomen just above the pubic bone (below the navel and approximately the lower third of the anterior abdominal wall) up and in towards the spine – this hollows just the lower abdominal area (Fig. 4.17).

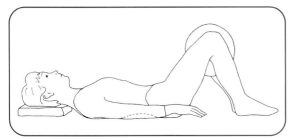

Figure 4.17 Breathing out.

Hold for 10 seconds.
Release slowly and relax completely at the end of the motion.
Repeat the sequence up to 10 times.

Modification 1

During *breathing in*, begin tightening the pelvic floor muscles. Then to assist transversus abdominis activation, lift the pelvic floor without tensing the rest of the body during *breathing out*.

Modification 2

Perform with a slight posterior pelvic tilt (the lumbar spine is flattened and the lower back muscles are relaxed).

Modification 3

Perform in four-point kneeling. Initiate the action with a pelvic floor muscle contraction and the teacher may lightly palpate multifidus to assist transversus abdominis muscle engagement.

Common problems

- Breathing and abdominal work not coordinated: Allow the student to find their own breathing rhythm.
- Core stability insufficient: Raise the feet onto a box or half barrel, or, if appropriate, lying supine on a roller assists firing the pelvic floor and lower abdominal muscles.
- Student unable to activate transversus abdominis without other muscle recruitment (indicated by spine or ribcage movement or lateral flaring/ tightening of the waist): Attempt the exercise in different body positions – for example, side lying with the upper body slightly rounded, supported prone position, lying over a gym ball, quadruped position to help fire transversus abdominis muscle action; cue to initiate the motion with a pelvic floor muscle contraction and lightly palpate multifidus.

See Table 4.9 for Teaching points.

(!) Precautions
- Individuals complaining of ongoing lower back, pelvic or abdominal pain should be referred for a physiotherapy or medical assessment.

(+) Contraindications
- Recent abdominal or pelvic surgery – seek medical advice.

Tactile cue suggestions

1. To increase breadth across the front of the chest – use the hands to stroke the collarbones from the sternum to their lateral aspects.
2. To establish the correct relationship between the upper and lower torso – on exhaling, use the hands on the lower ribs to assist funnelling them down towards the pelvis.
3. To assist transversus abdominis engagement – before exercising, instruct the student to place two fingers of each hand on the top of the hip and trace a line towards the centre of body until the fingers are still approximately 10 cm apart. Then instruct to press slightly inwards

and upwards and encourage the student to draw the abdominal wall away from the fingers.

4. To palpate multifidus – perform in the quadriped position. Locate the prominence of soft bulk in the lumbar paraspinal region and use the hands to lightly palpate this area as the cue is given to activate the pelvic floor muscles.

5. To test for transversus abdominis muscle action with minimal oblique abdominal muscle action – instruct the student to place the thumbs at the front of the hips and the fingers around to the back of the hips over the sacroiliac joints to feel for a change in muscle tone as the transversus abdominis contracts (initially this may be difficult to identify but improves with practice). Then instruct the student to place the hands higher around the waist to monitor oblique abdominal muscle activity. This area should remain comparatively relaxed throughout.

Exercise BCS3 – Hip rolls (independent bilateral hip abduction and adduction)

Aim

To maintain lumbar spine stability through abdominal muscle performance during independent, bilateral hip joint movement.

To improve oblique abdominal muscle performance.

Equipment

Mat, firm bed, half barrel, box or gym ball.

Target muscles

For maintaining a correct stable relationship between the upper torso and the pelvis – the isometric action of the pelvic floor, transversus abdominis and the obliques.

For pectoral girdle stability – latissimus dorsi, teres major and the middle and lower fibres of trapezius acting together.

Body position

Supine with 90 degrees of hip and knee flexion with the pelvis in neutral and the legs hip width apart. The arms lie beside the body, palms to the floor (Fig. 4.18A) or flexed with both hands behind the head.

Action

Breathing in – tighten the pelvic floor muscles.

Breathing out – lift the pelvic floor muscles and activate the transversus abdominis, drawing the lower portion of the abdominal wall upwards and inwards. Relax the upper back and allow passive thoracic spine flexion to drop the sternum down and back towards the spine (this action brings the lower ribs nearer to the pelvis and assists the torso muscles to achieve their optimum length).

Breathing in – maintain abdominal muscle control over the lumbar spine and move both legs towards the left until the back of the right hip feels as if it could lift away from the floor (this indicates the end of independent hip motion). The head moves

4

Table 4.9   Teaching points – Lower abdominal muscle activation

Focus on	Examples of visual/verbal cues
Correct head and neck alignment without neck tension	Relax the tongue in the throat and imagine the muscles of the face melting away
Vertebral column length	Reach the crown of the head and the sitting bones in opposite directions
Torso stability and the correct relationship between the upper torso and pelvis	On breathing in, imagine the back and front of the chest broadening On breathing out, soften the breastbone and allow it to drop down towards the spine Imagine the ribs sliding down the front of the ribcage
Lower limb/feet placement	Imagine the knees are suspended from strings
Activating just the lower anterior abdominal wall muscles	Draw the tummy from just above the pubic bone in and up Tighten and gently lift the pelvic floor muscles before drawing the tummy muscles in and up
Releasing tension in the back and the limbs during abdominal muscle activation	Imagine the head, arms, back and feet creating imprints in warm sand

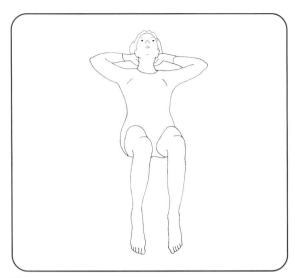

Figure 4.18A Body position for hip rolls.

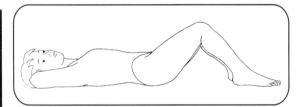

Figure 4.18B Hip roll to the left side.

gently away from the leg motion to help counterbalance it (Fig. 4.18B).

Breathing out – increase abdominal muscle activation, drawing the navel further towards the spine before drawing both legs back to their starting position (the lumbar spine and pelvis remain neutral and stable throughout).

Repeat 5–10 times each side.

Modification 1

Perform the basic exercise, abducting and adducting one leg at a time.

Body position

Supine with 90 degrees of hip and knee flexion with the lumbar spine flattened and the legs hip width apart.

Action

Breathing in – tighten the pelvic floor muscles.

Breathing out – lift the pelvic floor muscles and activate the transversus abdominis, then abduct the left hip to its end range of independent hip joint motion (the pelvis and lumbar spine remain stable).

Breathing in – adduct the left hip, drawing the leg back to its starting position.

Breathing out – maintain lower abdominal muscle activation.

Breathing in – adduct the left hip further towards the centre line of the body to stretch the lateral aspect of the left hip.

Breathing out – return the leg to its starting position.

Note: As lower abdominal muscle control improves, perform with a neutral lumbar spine/pelvic position.

Modification 2

Perform the basic exercise with an imprinted spine.

Modification 3

Perform the basic exercise with the feet raised on a half barrel or small box.

Modification 4

Perform the basic exercise with the legs hip width or wider than hip width apart (Figs 4.19A&B).

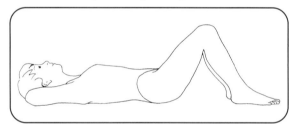

Figure 4.19A

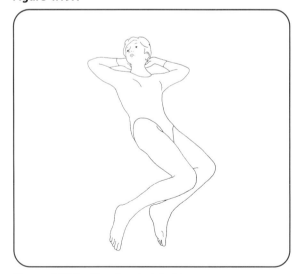

Figure 4.19B Hip roll to the left side.

As the knees move to one side, maintain abdominal muscle control over the lumbar spine and allow the pelvis to rotate. Increase abdominal muscle activation to draw the legs and pelvis back to the starting position (Fig. 4.20).

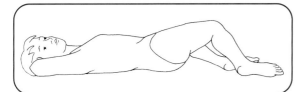

Figure 4.20   Hip rolls with legs wider than hip width apart.

Progression 1

Body position

Perform with the legs resting over a gym ball approximately hip distance apart with 90 degrees of hip/knee flexion (Figs 4.21A&B).

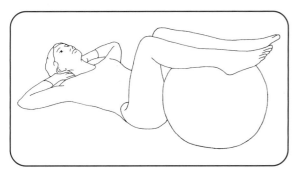

Figure 4.21A   Progression 1 – body position.

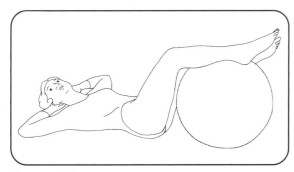

Figure 4.21B   Progression 1 – action.

Note: The arms can lie beside the body with the palms of the hands to the floor or be bent with the hands behind the head.

Action

Perform the sequence as for basic hip rolls, maintaining the lumbar spine and the pelvis in neutral throughout.

Progression 2

Body position

Perform with the legs extended and resting on a gym ball. Maintain the lumbar spine and pelvis in neutral throughout (Figs 4.22A&B).

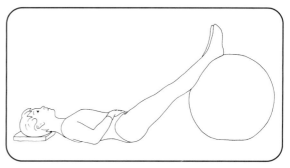

Figure 4.22A   Progression 2 – body position.

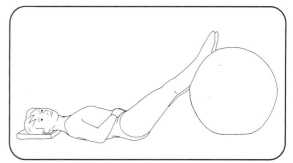

Figure 4.22B   Progression 2 – action.

Action

Breathing in – maintain abdominal muscle control over the lumbar spine and move both legs towards the left until the back of the right hip feels as if it could lift away from the floor (this indicates the end of independent hip motion). Stabilize the pectoral girdle, keeping both scapulae in contact with the floor and allow the head to turn in the opposite direction from the leg motion.

Breathing out – increase abdominal muscle activation, drawing the navel further towards the spine before allowing the spine to rotate so that the right hip lifts away from the floor towards the midline of the body and reach the legs away from the body. Maintain strong abdominal muscle control over the relationship between the lower ribs and the pelvis. The front and back of the body are equally lengthened and the lumbar curve is intact but not exaggerated. To increase the stretch, think of making space between the lower ribs and the pelvis.

Breathing in – maintain abdominal muscle activation.

Breathing out – increase the abdominal contraction to reverse the spine rotation, returning the pelvis and legs to their starting position.

Repeat on the left side.

Repeat up to five times on each side.

Progression 3

Perform with 90 degrees of hip/knee flexion without any leg support (Figs 4.23A&B).

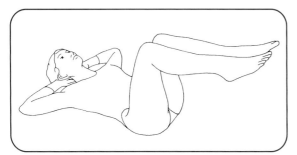

Figure 4.23A   Progression 3 – body position.

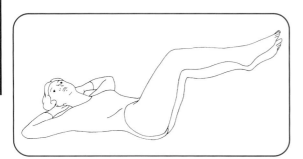

Figure 4.23B   Progression 3 – action.

Common problems

■ Initial problems with body position/pelvic alignment: Take time with exercise preparation, use appropriate body supports and monitor breathing patterns.

■ Neck/shoulder tension: Ensure correct head/cervical spine alignment with the use of appropriate supports and monitor breathing patterns.

■ Insufficient abdominal control over lumbar spine stability (identified by lumbar extension as the legs move away and lumbar flexion as the legs return to their starting position): Reduce hip range of movement; perform with the lumbar spine flattened throughout; raise the feet a little and perform with the lumbar spine flattened throughout. For uncoordinated lower limb movement, place a chi ball or other soft support between the knees.

See Table 4.10 for Teaching points.

Tactile cue suggestions

1. To increase breadth across the front of the chest – use the hands to stroke the collarbones from the sternum to their lateral aspects.
2. To increase awareness of and assist pelvic stability – instruct the student to rest their hands over the hip bones to assist pelvic control and feel any pelvic movement.
3. To assist transversus abdominis engagement – before exercising, instruct the student to place two fingers of each hand on the top of the hip and trace a line towards the centre of body until the fingers are still approximately 10 cm apart. Then instruct to press slightly inwards and upwards and encourage the student to draw the abdominal wall away from the fingers.
4. To assist oblique abdominal muscle engagement – instruct the student to place their hands on the anterolateral aspect of the abdominal wall (just below and to the side of the navel) to feel the muscle action as the legs move away from and then towards the body. Should further abdominal muscle control be required for pelvic stability, cue for the student to pull the abdominal wall away from the hands just before the legs move.

Exercise BCS4 – Leg slides (independent hip extension/flexion)

Aim

To improve abdominal muscle strength and control over lumbar spine stability during independent hip movement.

To mobilize the hip.

To improve the performance of the iliopsoas muscle during hip mobilization.

Equipment

Mat, firm bed, gym ball.

Target muscles

For core control – the pelvic floor, transversus abdominis and oblique abdominals acting together isometrically.

For pectoral girdle stability – latissimus dorsi, teres major and the middle and lower fibres of trapezius acting together.

For hip extension – the gluteus maximus and hamstring muscles acting concentrically to initiate hip extension.

Table 4.10 Teaching points – Hip rolls

Focus on	Examples of visual/verbal cues
Correct head and neck alignment without neck tension	Relax the tongue in the throat and imagine the muscles of the face melting away
Vertebral column length	Reach the crown of the head and the sitting bones in opposite directions
Breadth across the front and back of the torso	Broaden across the collarbones: on breathing in, visualize the back and sides of the chest filling with air
Maintaining a neutral and stable lumbar spine and the correct relationship between the lower ribs and the pelvis	On breathing out, allow the upper back muscles to release to sink the breastbone down and back towards the spine Imagine the ribs funnelling down into the pelvis Draw up the pelvic floor muscles and hollow the lower abdominal area just above the pubic bone towards the spine
Correct pectoral girdle alignment and stability	Imagine the shoulder blades as snowboards sliding diagonally down towards the centre of the back
Pelvic stability throughout	Imagine the head, arms, back and feet creating imprints in warm sand As the legs move to the right, feel the weight of the left hip dropping back to the bed and reach the knees to the right Feel the weight of both buttocks equally on the mat throughout

4

For hip flexion – iliopsoas and rectus femoris acting synergistically.

Body position
Supine with 90 degrees of hip and knee flexion with the pelvis in neutral, the legs approximately hip distance apart. The arms lie beside the body with the elbows slightly bent, palms turned to the floor (Fig. 4.24A).

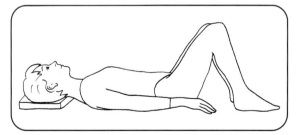

Figure 4.24A Leg slides – body position.

Action
Breathing in – tighten the pelvic floor muscles.
Breathing out – lift the pelvic floor muscles and activate the transversus abdominis.

Keeping the right hip neutral in rotation, slowly slide the right heel along the floor until the leg is fully extended (Fig. 4.24B).

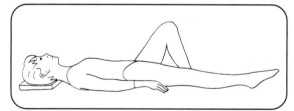

Figure 4.24B Leg slides – action.

Breathing in – maintain abdominal muscle engagement and simultaneously flex the right hip and knee to slide the leg to the starting position.
Note: The lumbar spine/pelvis should remain neutral and stable throughout. Inhaling as the hip flexes enhances lumbar spine stability.
Breathing out – repeat with the left leg.
Repeat 5–10 times with each leg

Modification 1
Perform the basic exercise with the lumbar spine imprinted and the upper body curled slightly forwards, supported from behind with a pillow or triangle (Fig. 4.25).

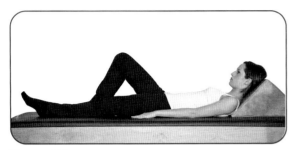

Figure 4.25   Leg slides – modification 1.

Modification 2

Body position

Supine with 90 degrees of hip and knee flexion with the lumbar spine imprinted (this position is maintained throughout). The left foot rests on a gym ball with the left knee and left hip flexed approximately 70 degrees. The right leg is bent with approximately 90 degrees of hip/knee flexion (Fig. 4.26).

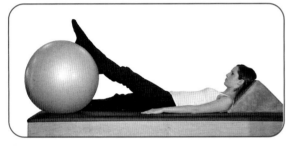

Figure 4.26   Leg slides – modification 2.

Action

Breathing in – to prepare.

Breathing out – activate the pelvic floor and lower abdominal muscles and extend the left hip. Continue hip/knee extension, rolling the ball away from the body until the left leg is fully extended.

Breathing in – maintain abdominal muscle engagement to flex the left hip, drawing the ball back towards the body. Flex the hip as much as possible, still maintaining the pelvis and lumbar spine stable (this may be more than 70 degrees).

Breathing out – repeat the leg extension and continue the sequence.

Perform five times with each leg.

Modification 3

Perform the basic exercise in the semi supine position with an imprinted lumbar spine.

Progression 1

Perform the basic exercise with the breathing reversed – *breathing out* as the hip flexes and *breathing in* as the hip extends, maintaining a neutral pelvis and lumbar spine throughout.

Progression 2

Body position

Perform the basic exercise with the lumbar spine and pelvis in neutral and add upper limb movement (Figs 4.27A&B).

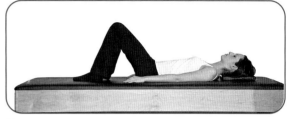

Figure 4.27A   Leg slides progression 2 – body position.

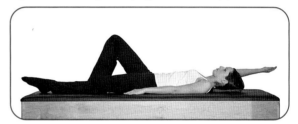

Figure 4.27B   Leg slides progression 2 – action.

Action

Breathing in – to prepare.

Breathing out – extend the left leg and flex the right shoulder, moving the right arm through a 180-degree arc to rest on the floor beside the head.

Breathing in – simultaneously return the left leg and right arm through the same ranges of motion to their starting positions.

Repeat on the other side.

Progression 3

Perform Progression 2 with the left leg and left arm moving simultaneously.

Common problems

■ Initial problems with body position/pelvic alignment: Take time with exercise preparation and use appropriate body supports.

■ Inadequate abdominal muscle control for lumbar spine stability: Consider curling the upper body forward with pillows (hospital bed pillow arrangement) or place a triangle behind the upper back; reduce hip range of movement; perform with the lumbar spine imprinted (see modifications).

■ Neck/shoulder tension: Use supports as required to correct head/neck alignment and cue for improved upper body relaxation.

■ Poor dynamic lower limb alignment: Cue to direct the heel of the active leg to align with the ischial tuberosity on the same side: if the knee falls in during the motion, perform the exercise with the hip of the active leg in slight lateral rotation; if the knee falls out during the motion, cue to activate the short adductor muscles (brevis and magnus). Ensure that the knee tracks along a line taken from the axis of each hip joint (a point slightly medial to the ASIS) through the middle of the knee joint to between the second and third toes.

■ Rectus femoris dominance during hip mobilization: Imagine the thigh floating towards the body in a current of water as the hip bends and floating away as the leg straightens; cue to maintain the toes and hamstrings as relaxed as possible.

See Table 4.11 for Teaching points.

⊘ Precautions

■ Neck and shoulder problems – provide sufficient support for comfort.
■ Lower back pathology – ensure efficient abdominal muscle control over lumbar spine stability and reduce the range of hip movement; increase the range of movement gradually as abdominal muscle control improves; consider modifications.
■ Hip and knee pathology – monitor the range of hip/knee motion and alignment.

➕ Contraindications

■ Advanced stages of pregnancy.
■ Back, hip or knee pain.
■ Symphysis pubis dysfunction – seek obstetric physiotherapy advice.

Tactile cue suggestions

1. To assist transversus abdominis engagement – before exercising, instruct the student to place two fingers of each hand on the top of the hip and trace a line towards the centre of body until the fingers are still approximately 10 cm apart. Then instruct to press slightly inwards and upwards and encourage the student to draw the abdominal wall away from the fingers.

2. To assist lumbar spine stability and maintain the correct relationship between the upper and lower torso – instruct the student to place their hands on the lateral aspect of the abdominal wall between the lower ribs and the pelvis to feel the space that is to be maintained throughout.

4

Table 4.11 Teaching points – Leg slides

Focus on	Examples of visual/verbal cues
Correct head and neck alignment without neck tension	Relax the tongue in the throat and imagine the muscles of the face melting away
Vertebral column length	Reach the crown of the head and the sitting bones in opposite directions
Breadth across the front and back of the torso	Broaden across the collarbones
Maintaining a neutral and stable lumbar spine and the correct relationship between the lower ribs and the pelvis	On breathing in, visualize the back and sides of the chest filling with air On breathing out, allow the upper back muscles to release to sink the breastbone down and back towards the spine
Pelvic stability throughout	Imagine the pelvis as a bowel filled with water. Keep the pelvis still so not a drop of water can be tipped out in any direction
Releasing tension in the groin of the exercising leg	Imagine the groin as a deep valley as the hip bends
Lumbar spine stability	Maintain gentle abdominal muscle engagement Visualize the sitting bones reaching towards the heels

Exercise BCS5 – Thigh arcs
(exercising the iliopsoas muscle)

Aim

To improve lower abdominal muscle tone.

To improve abdominal muscle control over lumbar spine stability during independent hip joint movement.

To improve iliopsoas muscle performance during hip mobilization.

Equipment

Mat, raised firm bed, half barrel, two small sensory balls, small head support.

Target muscles

For lumbar spine stability – erector spinae, the pelvic floor and transversus abdominis.

For hip mobilization – iliopsoas acting synergistically with rectus femoris (concentrically during hip flexion and eccentrically to control the return from flexion).

For pectoral girdle stability – latissimus dorsi and teres major acting together with the middle and lower fibres of trapezius.

Body position

Supine with approximately 90 degrees of hip and knee flexion, pelvis in neutral, feet hip distance apart. The arms lie beside the body with the palms turned to the floor (Fig. 4.28A).

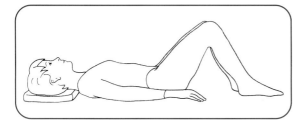

Figure 4.28A   Thigh arcs – body position.

Action

Breathing in – tighten the pelvic floor muscles.

Breathing out – lift the pelvic floor muscles and activate transversus abdominis.

Breathing in – flex the left hip and move the thigh in an arc until it is perpendicular to the floor (approximately 90 degrees of hip/knee flexion) (Fig. 4.28B).

Breathing out – the abdominal contraction may be increased to control lumbar spine stability as the leg returns to its starting position.

Repeat to each side up to five times.

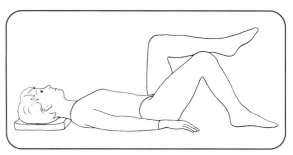

Figure 4.28B   Thigh arcs – action.

Modification 1

Perform with an imprinted lumbar spine throughout.

Modification 2

Perform with a reduced range of hip motion (begin with the feet resting on a half barrel or small box).

Modification 3

Perform with a small ball under each buttock to tilt the pelvis posteriorly (position these at approximately the level of the ischial tuberosities or a little higher).

Progression 1

Perform without conscious activation of the pelvic floor and abdominal muscles, allowing these to be comparatively relaxed throughout. Achieve pelvic stability through the use of visual imagery (see Teaching points).

Progression 2

Begin as in the basic exercise.

Body position

Semi-supine as for basic exercise, the lumbar spine imprinted or in a neutral position (Figs 4.29A–E).

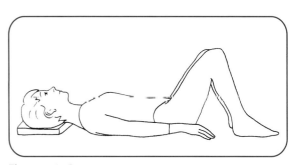

Figure 4.29A   Thigh arcs progression 2 – body position.

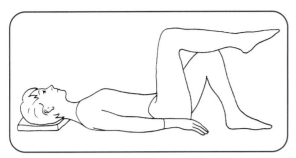

Figure 4.29B   Thigh arcs progression 2 – breathing in.

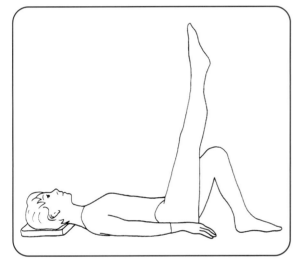

Figure 4.29C   Still breathing in.

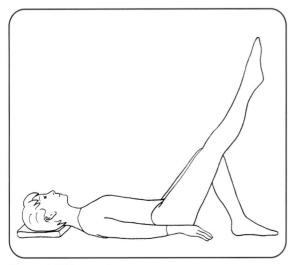

Figure 4.29D   Breathing out.

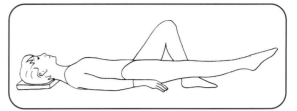

Figure 4.29E   Still breathing out.

Action
Begin as in the basic exercise.

Breathing in – flex the right hip and move the thigh in an arc until it is perpendicular to the floor (approximately 90 degrees of hip/knee flexion). Extend the knee and softly plantarflex the foot, pointing the toes to the ceiling.

Breathing out – increase abdominal muscle action as required to maintain lumbar spine stability; extend the hip, reaching the leg out of the hip joint as it lowers almost to the floor.

Breathing in – initiate knee flexion, drawing the foot towards the body, as if the toes are caressing the floor. Continue the motion by moving into hip flexion followed by knee extension and pointing the toes to the ceiling.

Breathing out – continue this smooth circular motion.

Repeat 5–10 times.

Progression 3
Toe dipping – bilateral hip flexion/extension.

Body position
Perform with a neutral pelvis and lumbar spine. The legs are hip distance apart with the hips and knees flexed 90 degrees and the feet softly plantarflexed. The arms lie beside the body with the palms turned to the floor (Figs 4.30A&B).

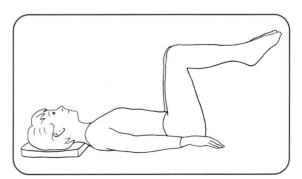

Figure 4.30A   Progression 3 toe dipping – body position.

4

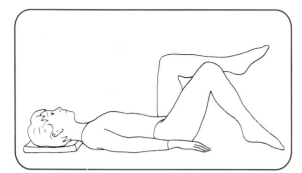

Figure 4.30B   Progression 3 – action.

Alternatively, place a small firm ball under each buttock to tilt the pelvis posteriorly and to imprint the lumbar spine (position the balls at approximately the level of the ischial tuberosities or a little higher). The legs are hip distance apart with the hips and knees flexed to maximum and the feet softly plantarflexed. The arms lie beside the body with the palms turned to the floor.

Action

Breathing normally – gently activate the pelvic floor and lower abdominal muscles to assist lumbar spine stability. Maintain this abdominal control as required.

Breathing in – to prepare.

Breathing out – keeping the left leg still, extend the right hip (maintain the same degree of right knee flexion), moving the thigh in an arc until the toes lightly touch the floor.

Breathing in – continue by flexing the right hip to maximum and simultaneously extending the left hip until the toes of the left foot touch the floor. The legs pass midway during the motion.

Breathing out – continue the motion.

Perform with easy flowing movements, integrating the breathing patterns with the leg action (breathe in cycles of two or four, depending on the speed of motion).

Progression 4

Toe dipping with diagonal alignment.

Body position

Flex both hips as in Progression 3.

Action

Keeping the lumbar spine and hips stable, move the lower legs towards to the right. Perform the sequence. Repeat on the other side.

Progression 5

Repeat as in Progression 1 without conscious abdominal muscle activation.

Common problems

- Rectus abdominis strongly activated: Cue for stronger pelvic floor and lower abdominal muscle activation and consider reducing hip range of motion (e.g. place the feet on a small box or half barrel).
- Inadequate abdominal muscle control for lumbar spine stability: Consider reducing hip range of motion or performing with the lumbar spine flattened throughout; cue for spine elongation (see Table 4.12 for Teaching points).
- Rectus femoris dominance over iliopsoas muscle action by a protruding band appearing on the anterolateral aspect of the groin prior to/during hip flexion: Consider the following: reduce hip range of motion (see Modifications); place the feet on an unstable surface such as a wobble cushion; ensure that the hip is not rotating laterally during the motion; cue for more effective iliopsoas action (see Table 4.12).
- Neck/shoulder tension: Use supports as required to correct head/neck alignment and cue for improved upper body relaxation.

! Precautions

- Lower back pathology – ensure efficient abdominal muscle control over lumbar spine stability (see Modifications); seek medical advice if unsure.
- Hip and knee pathology – monitor the range of hip/knee motion.

+ Contraindications

- Advanced stages of pregnancy.
- Back, hip or knee pain.
- Symphysis pubis dysfunction – seek obstetric physiotherapy advice.

Tactile cue suggestions

1. To increase awareness of and assist pelvic stability – instruct the student to rest their hands over the hip bones to assist pelvic control and feel any pelvic movement.
2. To assist transversus abdominis engagement – before exercising, instruct the student to place two fingers of each hand on the top of the hip and trace a line towards the centre of body

until the fingers are still approximately 10 cm apart. Then instruct to press slightly inwards and upwards and encourage the student to draw the abdominal wall away from the fingers.

3. Self-monitoring for rectus femoris dominance over the iliopsoas muscle – instruct the student to place their fingers in the anterolateral aspect of the groin during the motion.

PRONE POSTERIOR HIP MUSCLE STRENGTHENING (EXERCISES BCS6–8)

Exercise BCS6 – Gluteal squeezes (strengthening the lower fibres of gluteus maximus)

Aim
To exercise the lower portion of gluteus maximus.

Equipment
Mat, raised firm bed, trapeze table, a slim pillow, bolster or towel.

Target muscles
For lumbar spine stability – erector spinae, the pelvic floor and transversus abdominis muscles; the lower fibres of gluteus maximus contracting concentrically.

For pectoral girdle stability – gentle activation of the middle and lower fibres of trapezius, latissimus dorsi and teres major.

Body position
Lying face down, preferably on a mat or a raised bed that enables the ankles to relax as the feet drop over the edge. The arms are bent with the elbows pointing to the side, and the hands resting one on top of the other to make a support for the forehead. A slim pillow may be used under the body to help support and lengthen the lumbar spine as required (Figs 4.31A&B).

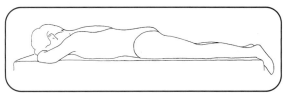

Figure 4.31A Prone position.

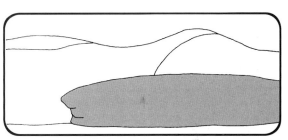

Figure 4.31B Pillow-supported prone position.

4

Table 4.12 Teaching points – Thigh arcs

Focus on	Examples of visual/verbal cues
Correct head and neck alignment without neck tension	Relax the tongue in the throat and imagine the muscles of the face melting away
Breadth across the front and back of the torso	Broaden across the collarbones
Correct pectoral girdle alignment and stability	Reach the little fingers for the heels Slide the shoulder blades down across the back
Releasing tension in the groin of the exercising leg	Imagine the groin as a deep valley as the hip bends Keep the ankles relaxed and imagine the toes dipping into and out of a pool of water
Exercising the psoas and rectus femoris synergistically	Imagine the iliopsoas muscle as a warm current of air flowing towards the body as the hip flexes, then flowing away as the hip extends Feel the weight of the leg as it lifts away from the floor
Correct dynamic leg alignment	Imagine the knee painting an arc as it moves through space

4

Action

Breathing in – tighten the pelvic floor muscles.

Breathing out – gently and simultaneously lift the pelvic floor muscles, hollow the lower abdominal area just above the pubic bone and begin squeezing the lower portion of the buttocks towards the midline. Continue this action until the lower fibres of gluteus maximus are firmly contracted (Fig. 4.31C).

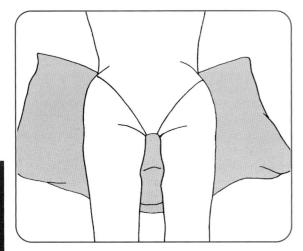

Figure 4.31C Gluteal squeezes – action.

Breathing in – slowly and simultaneously release the gluteal and abdominal muscle contractions.

Breathing out – to repeat.

Repeat up to 10 times.

Progression 1

The gluteal muscle contraction can be sustained for two or three breaths.

Progression 2

One side of the buttocks can be exercised whilst the other side remains relaxed.

Common problems

- Tension in the neck and upper trapezius muscles: Encourage lengthening through the back of the neck and light engagement of the scapulae stabilizing muscles.
- Tightening the lower back and creating a posterior pelvic tilt as the gluteal muscles engage: Encourage more gentle pelvic floor, abdominal muscle and gluteal muscle action together with more spine elongation.
- Asymmetrical gluteal muscle activity: Encourage the student to focus on the weaker side as the muscles engage; practise Progression 2 on the weaker side.
- Marked lateral hip rotation as the muscles contract: Encourage the student to focus on exercising just the lower portion of the buttocks and cue for more gentle muscle engagement.
- Inability to locate the specific muscles: Imagine turning the legs out to initiate the muscle contraction.

See Table 4.13 for Teaching points.

 Precautions and contraindications
- Advanced stages of pregnancy.
- Lower back problems made worse by lying in the prone position – perform the exercise lying over a gym ball or standing and leaning against a wall.

Table 4.13 Teaching points – Gluteal squeezes

Focus on	Examples of visual/verbal cues
Spinal elongation throughout	Lengthen through the back of the neck Reach the sitting bones towards the heels
Length in the groins	Lengthen the legs out of the hips before beginning the action
Sufficient pelvic floor and abdominal muscle activation to lengthen the lumbar spine	Imagine the sling of pelvic floor muscles as an elevator moving to the top of a high building Imagine a small piece of chocolate is lying under the body just below the navel; so as not to melt it, hollow the abdominal muscles towards the spine
Locating and activating the lower fibres of gluteus maximus with minimal rotation of the femurs	Imagine strings attached to the sitting bones being tied in a bow and drawing the sitting bones together

Tactile cue suggestions

1. To improve pectoral girdle alignment – place the hands firmly over the scapulae to direct them down and across the back (Fig. 4.32).
2. To assist lengthening through the groins before beginning the sequence – use the hands to gently lengthen one leg at a time. Do this by lifting the thigh just off the bed with the hip neutral in rotation, drawing it out of its hip joint and then lying it back on the bed.
3. To stimulate gluteus maximus muscle action – use the hands to gently tap the area or direct the gluteal creases to move towards each other.

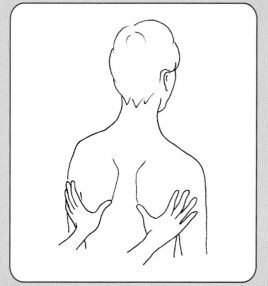

Figure 4.32   Directing the scapulae down and across the back.

Exercise BCS7 – Gluteal strengthener with flexed knee (gluteus maximus strengthener with hip extension)

Aim
To improve pelvic stability during hip extension through abdominal muscle control.
To enhance gluteus maximus performance.
To stretch the iliopsoas and rectus femoris muscles.

Equipment
Mat, raised firm bed, pillow, bolster or towel.

Target muscles
For lumbar spine stability and core control – erector spinae, and the pelvic floor and transversus abdominis acting together.

For hip extension – gluteus maximus.
For pectoral girdle stability – gentle activation of the middle and lower fibres of trapezius, latissimus dorsi and teres major.
For hip stability – the posterior muscles of the hip acting together. These muscles include gluteus medius and minimus, obturator internus, gemellus superior and inferior.

Body position
Prone with working knee flexed to maximum. The hamstring muscles are comparatively relaxed (Fig. 4.33A).

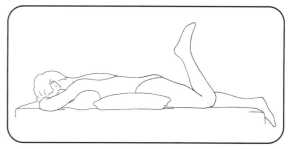

Figure 4.33A   Gluteal strengthener – body position.

Action
Breathing in – tighten the pelvic floor muscles.
Breathing out – contract the pectoral girdle stabilizing muscles, together with the pelvic floor and abdominal muscles, activate gluteus maximus on the working side and lift the thigh no more than 10 degrees away from the mat (abdominal muscle control should be sufficient to maintain a neutral and stable lumbar spine) (Fig. 4.33B).

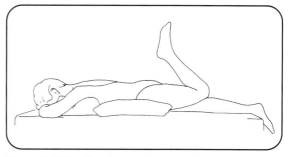

Figure 4.33B   Gluteal strengthener – action.

Breathing normally – hold this position initially for 3 seconds. As strength and stamina improve, the lift can be held for up to 10 seconds.
Breathing in – to prepare for lowering the leg.
Breathing out – to deepen the abdominal muscle contraction and lower the thigh to the mat.
Repeat up to five times.

Progression

Extend the knee before lowering the leg. Flex the knee to repeat (Figs 4.34A&B).

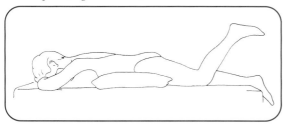

Figure 4.34A   Gluteal strengthener – progression.

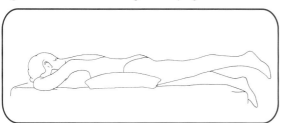

Figure 4.34B   Gluteal strengthener – progression.

Common problems

■ Neck tension: Encourage lengthening through the back of the neck and engagement of the scapulae stabilizing muscles.
■ Pelvic instability: Encourage stronger pelvic floor and abdominal muscle activation.
■ Lifting the thigh too high: Cue for reaching the knee away from the hip joint.

■ Overinvolvement of the hamstrings: Ensure the knee is able to flex more than 90 degrees.

See Table 4.14 for Teaching points.

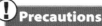

Precautions
■ Lower back pathology.

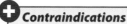

Contraindications
■ Knee pain during exercise – consider onward referral (there are a numerous possible causes, including muscle imbalance, faulty knee mechanics or other underlying pathology).

Tactile cue suggestions

1. To improve pectoral girdle alignment – place the hands firmly over the scapulae to direct them down and across the back.
2. To assist lengthening through the groins before beginning the sequence – use the hands to gently lengthen one leg at a time. Do this by lifting the thigh just off the bed with the hip neutral in rotation, drawing it out of its hip joint and then lying it back on the bed.
3. To stimulate gluteus maximus muscle action – use the hands to gently tap the area or direct the gluteal creases to move towards each other.

Table 4.14   Teaching points – Gluteal strengthener with flexed knee

Focus on	Examples of visual/verbal cues
Maintaining a neutral pelvis with a lengthened, correctly aligned spine	Lengthen from the crown of the head to the sitting bones
Efficient abdominal control throughout	Hollow the lower abdominal area, just above the pubic bone, to the spine
Length through the front of the hip throughout the exercise	Release the muscles at the front of the hip and reach the working thigh away Keep the groin of the working leg in contact with the floor throughout
Pectoral girdle and torso stability	Imagine the shoulder blades sliding down across the back
Correct working leg alignment	Keep the knee facing the floor as the leg lifts and lowers
Maintaining knee flexion with released hamstrings as the hip extends and returns from extension	Allow the knee to flex as much as possible so that the foot can drop towards the thigh
Maintaining pelvic stability, particularly during hip extension	Imagine lights on the pubic bones shining directly downwards as the hip extends
Relaxed feet and calf muscles throughout	Imagine the lower leg melting like warmed butter

Exercise BCS8 – Hamstring curls (hamstring muscle strengthener)

Aim
To collectively activate and equally strengthen the hamstring muscles.

To improve pelvic stability through abdominal muscle performance.

To stretch and improve flexibility of tensor fasciae latae and the quadriceps muscles.

Equipment
Mat, raised firm bed, slim pillow, bolsters or towels.

Target muscles
For lumbar spine stability – erector spinae, the pelvic floor and transversus abdominis (if required, assisted by a gentle contraction of the lower fibres of gluteus maximus).

For knee flexion – semitendinosus, semimembranosus and biceps femoris contracting concentrically; for knee extension these muscles contract eccentrically.

For pectoral girdle stability – gentle activation of the middle and lower fibres of trapezius, latissimus dorsi and teres major.

For hip stability – the posterior hip muscles acting together.

Body position
Prone (Figs 4.35A–D).

Action
Breathing in – activate the pelvic floor muscles.

Breathing out – lift the pelvic floor muscles and activate transversus abdominis (some lower gluteus maximus activation may also be required to assist pelvic stability but this should be omitted as core control improves).

Breathing in – lengthen the thigh out of the hip and flex the right knee, drawing the right heel towards the right ischial tuberosity. The knee should flex approximately 90 degrees.

Breathing out – extend the knee to slowly lower the leg to the floor.

Imagine the heel drawing through water during the action to increase exercise intensity.

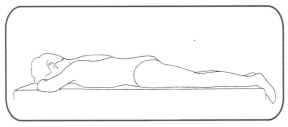

Figure 4.35A Hamstring curls – body position.

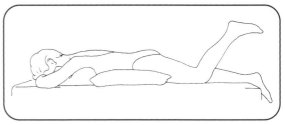

Figure 4.35B Hamstring curls – knee flexion.

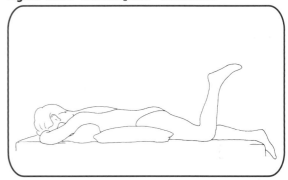

Figure 4.35C Hamstring curls – 90 degree knee flexion.

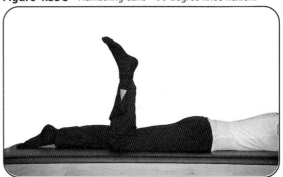

Figure 4.35D Hamstring curls – 90 degree knee flexion.

Repeat knee flexion and extension up to 10 times on each leg.

Progression
Perform the basic exercise 10 times on each leg, then perform the following sequence.

To prepare, flex the right knee to 90 degrees.

Breathing in – medially rotate the femur as far as possible without losing pelvic stability (Fig. 4.36A).

Breathing out – return the limb to the starting position.

Breathing in – laterally rotate the femur as far as possible without losing pelvic stability.

Breathing out – return the limb to the starting position (Fig. 4.36B).

Repeat two to three times on the right side, then two to three times on the left.

Note: This exercise stretches the hip's lateral and medial (including tensor fasciae latae) rotators.

4

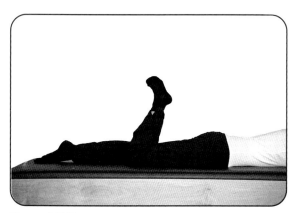

Figure 4.36A

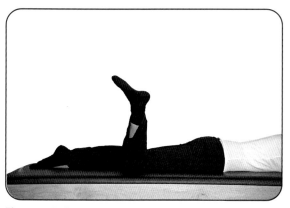

Figure 4.36B

Supports may be used in the axillae or under the torso for comfort or to correct alignment as illustrated (Fig. 4.37).

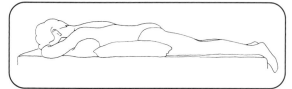

Figure 4.37   Supported prone position.

Common problems
- Neck tension: Encourage lengthening through the back of the neck and engagement of the scapulae stabilizing muscles.
- Lower back tension: Encourage more gentle pelvic floor and abdominal muscle activation, together with reaching the sitting bones towards the heels; consider placing a slim pillow under the lower torso to support the lumbar spine.
- Anterior pelvic tilt during flexion: Encourage stronger pelvic floor and abdominal muscle activation, together with gentle activation of the lower portion of gluteus maximus; instruct the

student to gently press the groin of the working leg into the mat throughout.
- Incorrect dynamic leg alignment: Imagine a pulley between the sitting bone and the heel drawing the heel towards and then lowering it away from the sitting bone.
- Malfunction of one or more of the hamstrings (this can be felt on palpation as uneven muscular activity at the back of the thigh): Palpate inactive muscles.

See Table 4.15 for Teaching points.

① Precautions
- Knee discomfort during exercise – supporting the knee on a small towel or bolster and reducing the range of knee flexion may eliminate discomfort. Alternatively, the range of motion can be reduced by placing a pillow or similar support under the shin (Fig. 4.38).

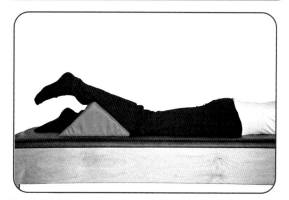

Figure 4.38

➕ Contraindications
- Knee pain during exercise – consider onward referral (there are a numerous possible causes including muscle imbalance, faulty knee mechanics or other underlying pathology).

Tactile cue suggestions

1. To improve pectoral girdle alignment – place the hands firmly over the scapulae to direct them down and across the back.
2. To assist lengthening through the groins before beginning the sequence – use the hands to gently lengthen one leg at a time. Do this by lifting the thigh just off the bed with the hip neutral in rotation, drawing it out of its hip joint and then lying it back on the bed.

3. To encourage hamstring muscle action – gently tap the muscles at the back of the thigh.
4. To assist dynamic alignment – align the heel with the ischial tuberosity of the same side.

SIDE LYING POSTERIOR HIP MUSCLE STRENGTHENING (EXERCISES BCS9–12)

Exercise BCS9 – The oyster (side lying strengthening for the lateral hip rotators and hip abductors)

Aim
To strengthen the lateral hip joint rotators and improve hip joint stability.

To improve lumbar spine stability through abdominal muscle control.

To improve oblique abdominal muscle performance during independent hip abduction and rotation.

Equipment
Mat, neck support, a small rolled towel for underneath the waist, a small pillow or towel to support the upper knee or ankle.

Target muscles
For lumbar spine stability and core control – pelvic floor and transversus abdominis acting together with erector spinae and the oblique abdominals.

For pectoral girdle stabilization – gentle activation of latissimus dorsi, teres major and the middle and lower fibres of trapezius.

For hip lateral rotation with flexed hip/knee – s[...] tensor fasciae latae, gluteus maximus (s[...] fibres) and biceps femoris.

For hip lateral rotation and abduction – piriformis, the obturators, the gemelli and quadratus femoris.

For hip medial rotation and adduction – the gluteals, tensor fasciae latae, piriformis, obturators, gemelli and quadratus femoris acting eccentrically to counteract the effects of gravity.

For hip abduction – gluteus medius and minimus.

For hip extension and lateral rotation – gluteus maximus and piriformis.

Body position
Side lying position (lying on right side) for exercising the left leg. Flex both hips and knees approximately 45 degrees. A pillow may be placed between the knees for comfort (Fig. 4.39A).

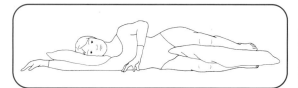

Figure 4.39A   The oyster – body position.

Action
Breathing in – activate the pelvic floor muscles.

Breathing out – stabilize the pectoral girdle, lift the pelvic floor muscles and activate transversus abdominis to stabilize the pelvis, then laterally rotate the left hip to its full range of movement, turning the left knee to face more towards the ceiling (Fig. 4.39B).

4

Table 4.15   Teaching points – Hamstring curls

Focus on	Examples of visual/verbal cues
Maintaining a lengthened, correctly aligned spine	Lengthen from the crown of the head to the sitting bones
Efficient abdominal control throughout	Hollow the lower abdominal area, just above the pubic bone, towards the spine
Length through the front of the hip throughout the exercise	Release the front of the hip and reach the working leg away
Shoulder alignment and girdle stability	Imagine the shoulder blades sliding down across the back
Correct dynamic lower leg alignment	Imagine a pulley between the sitting bone and the heel, drawing the heel towards and then lowering it away from the sitting bone
Relaxed feet and ankles as the calves should remain soft as the hamstrings contract	Imagine the lower leg melting like warmed butter
The collective, even muscular activity of the hamstring muscles	Imagine the lower leg is moving through water to create resistance

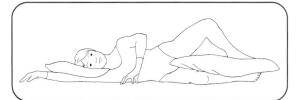

Figure 4.39B The oyster – action.

Breathing in – maintaining good abdominal muscle control and a stable lumbar spine, medially rotate the left hip to return the leg to its starting position.

Breathing out – to begin the next repetition.

Repeat up to 10 times.

Repeat on the other side.

Progression 1

Perform with the torso rotated slightly forwards – this is more challenging for the lateral hip rotators (Fig. 4.40).

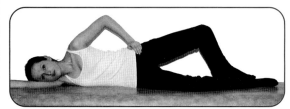

Figure 4.40

Progression 2

Hip extension, abduction and lateral hip rotation.

Body position

Side lying position (lying on right side) for exercising the left leg.

Action

Flex both hips and knees approximately 45 degrees, positioning the back approximately 15–30 cm away from a wall. The torso rotates forwards a little (just enough to face the pelvis slightly towards the floor). The upper hand may lie on the floor in front of the body or rest lightly on the upper hip. Maintaining pelvic alignment and knee flexion, extend the left hip until the left heel touches the wall, and then laterally rotate the left hip, turning the left knee to face more towards the ceiling (Fig. 4.41).

Breathing in – activate the pelvic floor muscles.

Breathing out – stabilize the pectoral girdle, lift the pelvic floor muscles and activate transversus abdominis to stabilize the pelvis, then slide the left

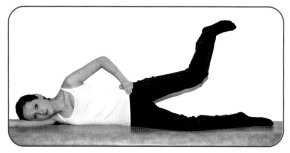

Figure 4.41

heel up the wall as far as possible without disturbing torso alignment.

Breathing in – maintain the lateral rotation and slide the left heel down to rest on the floor.

Breathing out – to repeat.

Repeat 5–10 times.

Repeat on the other side.

Progression 3

Perform at a faster speed, still moving through the full range of motion.

Common problems

■ Twisting from the waist and rotating the pelvis forwards or backwards: Place the student against a wall or other back support.

■ Flexing the spine laterally such that the waist drops to the floor: Instruct the student to place a hand on the upper hip together with contracting the lower abdominal muscles more strongly.

■ Moving the pelvis rather than the hip joint: Cue for lumbar spine stabilization with emphasis on lower abdominal muscle control.

See Table 4.16 for Teaching points.

⚠ Precautions

■ **Neck and shoulder pathology – modify rest position with appropriate supports.**

■ **Knee pathology – seek medical advice if unsure.**

■ **Hip pathology and/or surgery – monitor for pain-free action, seek medical advice if unsure.**

■ **Lower back problems – monitor for pain-free action, ensure adequate abdominal muscle control over lumbar spine stability.**

■ **Rheumatoid arthritis – monitor carefully for pain-free activity; ensure adequate abdominal muscle control over lumbar spine stability; consider shortening the lever length of the active leg and a reduced range of adduction motion.**

✚ Contraindications

- Knee pain during exercise – tight hip abductors together with weak hip adductors and/or tight hamstrings will alter patella tracking and knee mechanics; for onward referral.
- Adolescent knee pain – for onward referral.
- Acute spine, lower back, hip and knee pathology.

Tactile cue suggestions

1. To increase breadth across the front of the chest – use the hands to stroke the collarbones from the sternum to their lateral aspects.
2. To self-monitor gluteus medius activity – instruct the student to place a hand to the side and slightly to the back of the pelvis between the hips and the thigh.
3. To monitor spine stability and prevent pelvic rotation – instruct the student to place a hand on the upper hip.
4. To provide feedback on spine alignment and stability – instruct the student to perform the exercise lying with their back against a wall.

Exercise BCS10 – Upper leg lifts (hip abductor strengthening and stretching)

Aim
To strengthen and stretch the hip abductor muscles.
To improve lumbar spine stability through abdominal muscle performance.
To stabilize the lumbar spine during independent hip joint movement.

Equipment
Mat, neck support, a small rolled towel for underneath the waist, triangle or yoga blocks to support the upper leg.

Target muscles
For lumbar spine stability and core control – pelvic floor and transversus abdominis acting together with erector spinae and the oblique abdominals.
For pectoral girdle stabilization – gentle activation of latissimus dorsi, teres major and middle and lower fibres of trapezius.
For hip abduction – tensor fasciae latae, gluteus medius and minimus acting together concentrically.
For hip extension and lateral rotation – gluteus maximus and piriformis.

Body position
Side lying position (lying on right side) with the left leg resting on a support (Figs 4.42A&B).

4

Table 4.16 Teaching points – the oyster

Focus on	Examples of visual/verbal cues
Correct side lying alignment with the spinal curves intact	Reach the crown of the head and the sitting bones in opposite directions and allow the breastbone to soften on breathing out
The pelvis and trunk remaining perpendicular to the supporting surface so that the upper hip is aligned directly above to the lower hip	Hollow the lower abdominals towards the spin Stack the upper hip directly above the lower hip and maintain a small space under the waist
Stabilization of the pectoral girdle and the correct relationship between the upper torso and the pelvis	Slide the shoulder blades down the back and funnel the ribs down towards the pelvis On breathing out imagine putting on a corset or fixing a seatbelt across the hips
Stabilizing the pelvis and moving only in the hip joint to rotate the leg	Imagine a light on the kneecap beaming forwards up a wall and then towards the ceiling Place a hand to the side and slightly to the back of the pelvis between the hips and the thigh to feel the muscles contracting as the thigh moves
Rotating the active leg so the knee faces more towards the ceiling	Reach the knee away from the body as the leg rotates

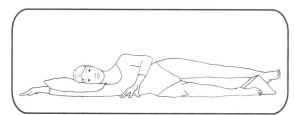

Figure 4.42A   Upper leg lifts – body position.

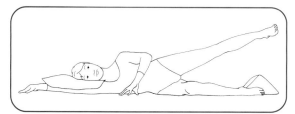

Figure 4.42B   Upper leg lifts – action.

Action

Breathing in – to prepare (Figs 4.42C&D).

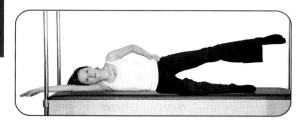

Figure 4.42C   Abductor strengthening.

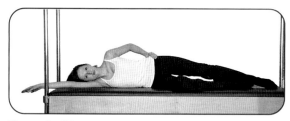

Figure 4.42D   Abductor stretching.

Breathing out – stabilize the pectoral girdle, activate the pelvic floor and lower abdominal muscles. Reach the left leg out of its hip joint and abduct it to approximately hip height. *The hip abducts no more than 45 degrees.*

Breathing in – maintain good abdominal control over the lumbar spine and lower the leg to its starting position.

Breathing out – to begin the next repetition.
Repeat 10 times.
Repeat on the other side.

Modification

Perform with the hip and knee slightly flexed.

Progression

Abductor strengthening/abductor stretching.

Body position

Side lying position (lying on right side). The left foot rests on the floor with the leg aligned with the body.

Action

Breathing in – to prepare.

Breathing out – stabilize the pectoral girdle, activate the pelvic floor and lower abdominal muscles, reach the left leg out of its hip joint and abduct it to approximately hip height.

Breathing in – maintain good abdominal control over the lumbar spine, laterally rotate and extend the left hip a little, moving the leg slightly behind the hip.

Breathing out – maintain lumbar spine stability and lower the left leg to the floor, stretching the upper outer hip structures.

Breathing in – maintaining good abdominal control over the lumbar spine, lift and medially rotate the leg (until the knee faces directly forwards) and realign it with the body at approximately hip height, before lowering it to the floor.

Breathing out – to begin the next repetition.
Repeat three to five times.
Repeat on the other side.

Common problems

- Extension of the cervical, thoracic or lumbar spine and subsequent loss of the correct relationship between the ribs and the pelvis: Place the student against a wall or other back support.
- Twisting from the waist and rotating the pelvis forwards or backwards: Place the student against a wall or other back support.
- Flexing the spine laterally such that the waist drops to the floor: Instruct the student to place a hand on the upper hip together with contracting the lower abdominal muscles more strongly.
- Placing the upper leg in a position of hip extension: Instruct the student to be aware that the upper foot should be lying within their range of peripheral vision when looking straight ahead.

See Table 4.17 for Teaching points.

Specific problems

- Lifting the leg too high (this will involve lateral flexion of the spine; when the hip joint is neither extended nor flexed, the normal range of hip abduction is approximately 45 degrees): Cue for lumbar spine stabilization together with emphasis placed on lengthening rather than lifting the leg.

Table 4.17   Teaching points – Upper leg lifts

Focus on	Examples of visual/verbal cues
Correct side lying alignment with the spinal curves intact	Reach the crown of the head and the sitting bones in opposite directions and allow the breastbone to soften on breathing out
The pelvis and trunk remaining perpendicular to the supporting surface so that the upper hip is aligned directly above to the lower hip	Hollow the lower abdominals towards the spin Stack the upper hip directly above the lower hip and maintain a small space under the waist
Stabilization of the pectoral girdle and the correct relationship between the upper torso and the pelvis	Slide the shoulder blades down the back and funnel the ribs down towards the pelvis
The kneecap of the working leg faces forwards throughout	Imagine a light on the kneecap shining onto a wall in front of you
Lengthening the working leg out of the hip	Reach the heel away from the body to lift the leg
Stabilizing the torso more before lifting the working leg	On breathing out imagine putting on a corset and creating a wasp waist

! Precautions

- Neck and shoulder pathology – modify rest position with appropriate supports.
- Knee pathology – monitor for pain-free activity seek medical advice if unsure.
- Hip pathology and/or surgery – monitor for pain-free activity, seek medical advice if unsure.
- Lower back problems – ensure adequate abdominal muscle control over lumbar spine stability.
- Rheumatoid arthritis – monitor carefully for pain-free activity; ensure adequate abdominal muscle control over lumbar spine stability; consider shortening the lever length of the active leg and a reduced range of adduction motion.

+ Contraindications

- Knee pain during exercise – tight hip abductors together with weak hip adductors and/or tight hamstrings will alter patella tracking and knee mechanics; for onward referral.
- Adolescent knee pain – for onward referral.
- Acute spine, lower back, hip and knee pathology.

Tactile cue suggestions

1. To improve pectoral girdle alignment – use the hands to stroke lightly across the collarbones and direct the scapulae down and across the back.
2. To self-monitor spine alignment and stability and prevent pelvic rotation – instruct the student to place a hand on the upper hip and to perform the exercise lying with their back against a wall.

4

Exercise BCS11 – Lower leg lifts (hip adductor strengthening/hip abductor stretching)

Aim
To collectively activate and equally strengthen the hip adductor muscles.
To stretch the hip abductor muscles.

Equipment
Mat or firm flat bed, pillow or neck support, a small rolled towel for underneath the waist, a triangle or yoga blocks to support the resting leg.

Target muscles

For lumbar spine stability and core control – the pelvic floor and transversus abdominis act together with erector spinae and the oblique abdominals.

For hip adduction – pectineus and adductors brevis, longus and magnus contract concentrically and then eccentrically as the leg returns to the floor.

For pectoral girdle stabilization – gentle activation of latissimus dorsi, teres major and middle and lower fibres of trapezius.

Body position

Side lying position (right side) for exercising the lower left leg (Figs 4.43A&B).

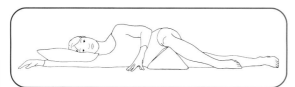

Figure 4.43A   Lower leg lifts – body position.

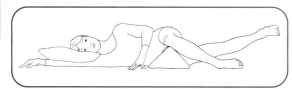

Figure 4.43B   Lower leg lifts – action.

Action

Breathing in – to prepare.

Breathing out – activate the pelvic floor, lower abdominal and pectoral girdle stabilizing muscles. Reach the left leg out of the hip joint and adduct it as far as possible without compromising spine stability.

Breathing in – maintaining abdominal muscle control, pause at the end of the motion to reach the leg out of the hip even more before gently lowering the leg to the floor.

Breathing out – to begin the next repetition.

Repeat 5–10 times.

Repeat on the other side.

Note: Initially aim to raise the leg to approximately the midline of the body. As strength is gained and core stability improves, raise the leg higher.

Modification

Flex the knee of the active leg. Limit the range of adduction.

Progression 1

Maintain medial rotation of the active leg.

Progression 2

Adduction in lateral rotation. Prepare as above, laterally rotate the active leg and perform the sequence with the hip in lateral rotation. Rotate the hip to face the knee forwards before lowering the leg to the floor.

Progression 3

Leg circles. Prepare as in Progression 1.

Action

Breathing in – begin circling the active leg anticlockwise.

Breathing out – complete the circle.

Continue with this breathing pattern to repeat 5–10 times.

Repeat 5–10 times circling the leg in a clockwise direction.

Note: Rotate the hip to face the knee forwards, reach the leg even more out of the hip before lowering the leg to the floor.

Common problems

■ Poor starting alignment: Place student against a wall or other back support.

■ Neck/shoulder tension: Prepare by emphasizing pectoral girdle stabilization together with stronger lower abdominal muscle activation.

■ Poor dynamic leg alignment: Instruct the student to be are aware that the lower foot should be lying within their range of peripheral vision when looking straight ahead.

■ Insufficient core strength: Modify the sequence by flexing the knee of the active leg.

■ Extension of the cervical, thoracic or lumbar spine and subsequent loss of the correct relationship between the ribs and the pelvis: Cue for 'softening the breastbone' and for stronger lower abdominal muscle activation on breathing out; check resting body and leg alignment.

■ Twisting from the waist and rotating the pelvis forwards or backwards: Place student against a wall or other back support.

■ Flexing the spine laterally such that the waist drops to the floor: Instruct the student to place a hand on the upper hip and cue for stronger lower abdominal muscle engagement.

See Table 4.18 for Teaching points.

Table 4.18 Teaching points – Lower leg lifts

Focus on	Examples of visual/verbal cues
Correct side lying alignment with the spinal curves intact	Reach the crown of the head and the sitting bones in opposite directions Stack the upper hip directly above the lower hip and maintain a small space under the waist
Establishing efficient abdominal muscle control before the leg action	Draw up the pelvic floor muscles and hollow the abdominals towards the spine
The pelvis and trunk remaining perpendicular to the supporting surface	Imagine the torso is stretched between two panes of glass Imagine you are lying with your back against a wall
Stabilization of the pectoral girdle throughout	Slide the shoulder blades down and across the back
Directing the kneecap of the active leg to face forwards throughout (basic sequence)	Imagine a light on the kneecap shining onto a wall in front of you
Directing the kneecap of the active leg to face towards the floor (progression in lateral rotation)	Imagine a light on the kneecap shining towards the floor
Lengthening the active leg out of the hip	Reach the heel away from the body

! Precautions
- Neck and shoulder pathology – modify rest position with appropriate supports.
- Knee pathology – for example, Osgood–Schlatter's disease (rest is advised during early stages of management); seek medical advice if unsure.
- Hip pathology and/or surgery – seek medical advice if unsure.
- Lower back problems – ensure adequate abdominal muscle control over lumbar spine stability.
- Rheumatoid arthritis – monitor carefully for pain-free activity; ensure adequate abdominal muscle control over lumbar spine stability; consider shortening the lever length of the active leg and a reduced range of adduction motion.

+ Contraindications
- Knee pain during exercise – tight hip abductors together with weak hip adductors and/or tight hamstrings will alter patella tracking and knee mechanics; for onward referral.
- Adolescent knee pain – for onward referral.
- Hip replacement – seek medical advice.
- Acute spine, lower back, hip and knee pathology.

Tactile cue suggestions

1. To correct pectoral girdle alignment and stability – place the hands firmly over the scapulae to direct them down and across the back.
2. To self-monitor spine alignment and stability and prevent pelvic rotation – instruct the student to place a hand on the upper hip and to perform the exercise lying with their back against a wall.
3. To encourage adductor muscle activity – lightly tap the inside thigh muscles.
4. To promote lengthening the leg out of its hip joint – lightly touch the heel of the active leg.

Exercise BCS12 – Body lengthening (torso stabilization for independent lower limb movement)

Aim
To challenge and improve core stability and control.
To improve the performance of the posterior hip and adductor muscles.
To improve pectoral girdle stability.

Equipment
Mat or firm flat bed, pillow or neck support, a small rolled towel for underneath the waist.

Target muscles
For lumbar spine stability and core control – the pelvic floor, transversus abdominis, oblique abdominals

4

and quadratus lumborum acting together with erector spinae and the lower fibres of gluteus maximus.

For pectoral girdle stabilization – activation of latissimus dorsi, teres major and the middle and lower fibres of trapezius.

For hip stabilization – the posterior hip muscles acting together.

For hip adduction (lower leg) – pectineus and adductors brevis, longus and magnus acting together.

For hip abduction (upper leg) – tensor fasciae latae acting together with gluteus medius and minimus.

Body position

Side lying position, both legs extended. The head rests on a pillow or the extended lower arm. The upper arm is bent so that the hand can be placed on the floor to help stabilize the position (Fig. 4.44A).

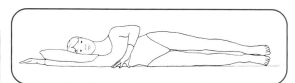

Figure 4.44A   Body lengthening body position.

Action

Breathing in – to prepare.

Breathing out – simultaneously broaden across the front of the chest, stabilize the pectoral girdle and activate the pelvic floor and lower abdominal muscles. (Allow the passive flexion of the spine to release the sternum down and funnel the ribs towards the pelvis to establish a strong connection between the upper torso and the pelvis.)

Lengthen the spine from the crown of the head to the coccyx and lightly activate the lower fibres of the gluteus maximus to stabilize the lumbar spine. Keeping the hips neutral in rotation plantar flex the feet to reach the legs reach away from the body, drawing them together as they lift to align with the body as in standing (Fig. 4.44B).

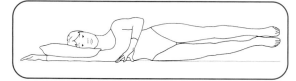

Figure 4.44B   Body lengthening breathing out.

Breathing in – whilst maintaining an elongated stable spine through efficient core control.

Breathing out – increase pectoral girdle stabilization and abdominal muscle control; lengthen more

through the legs, extending them even further away from the body to lower them gradually to the floor (Fig. 4.44C).

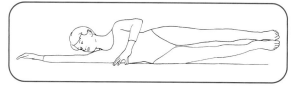

Figure 4.44C   Body lengthening turns the head to the floor.

Return to a stable, correctly aligned side lying position and allow the feet to relax.

Repeat 5–10 times.

Note: As the legs are raised, the head moves to align correctly with the cervical spine (neutral position) before turning slightly towards the floor. The gaze moves with the head so that the eyes continue to look directly forward. The spine curves remain intact and the pelvis is in a neutral position and perpendicular to the floor throughout.

Modification

Perform the sequence with the head resting on a pillow and reduce the range of hip motion.

Progression 1

Breathing in – to prepare.

Breathing out – plantarflex the feet to reach the legs away from the body and draw them together as they lift to align with the body as in standing.

Breathing in – dorsiflex the feet.

Breathing out – plantarflex the feet.

Breathing in – draw the legs more strongly together, reaching them further away from the body.

Breathing out – lower the legs gradually to the floor, returning the body to a stable, correctly aligned side lying position and allow the feet to relax.

Progression 2

Body position

Side lying on the right side. Both knees face directly forwards.

Action

Breathing in – to prepare.

Breathing out – plantarflex the feet to reach the legs away from the body before lifting them to align with the body as in standing.

Breathing in – dorsiflex the feet.

Breathing out – abduct the left leg as far as possible without disturbing pelvic or lumbar spine alignment. During abduction reach through both heels and activate the posterior hip muscles to counteract the abduction motion (this creates resistance as if the leg is moving through water).

Breathing in – simultaneously adduct the left leg and the right leg to bring the legs together (once again creating resistance as if the legs are moving through water).

Repeat the abduction and adduction sequences up to three times before lowering the legs to the floor.

Progression 3

Body position

Side-lying body lengthening with knee flexion.

Action

Breathing in – to prepare.

Breathing out – plantarflex the feet to reach the legs away from the body, drawing them together as they lift to align with the body as in standing.

Breathing in – maintaining a stable pelvis with the lumbar spine in neutral, flex the knees 90 degrees, pointing the toes directly backwards.

Note: To prevent lumbar spine extension during knee flexion, lengthen through the groins, activate the lower gluteal muscles and imagine a hand on the sacrum pushing it forwards.

Breathing out – extend the knees, drawing the legs more strongly together as they reach away from and align with the body.

Breathing in – lower the legs gradually to the floor, returning the body to a stable, correctly aligned side lying position and allow the feet to relax.

Breathing out – to begin the next repetition.

Repeat three to five times.

Common problems

- Twisting from the waist and rotating the pelvis forwards or backwards: Cue for increased spine elongation, stronger abdominal muscle control and for the hips and knees to face directly forwards; place the student against a wall or other back support.
- Flexing the spine laterally such that the waist drops to the floor: Emphasize lengthening the legs away from the body together with stronger abdominal muscle control; cue to align one ASIS directly above the other ASIS to maintain a small space under the waist.
- Pelvic instability as a result of the legs lifting too high: Instruct the student to monitor the leg motion and adjust it according to their ability to stabilize the lumbar spine.
- Neck strain: Use a head support; emphasize pectoral girdle stabilization.
- Lumbar spine extension as the legs lift: Instruct the student to keep the feet within peripheral vision throughout.

- Thoracic spine extension as the legs lift: Emphasize the funnelling of the ribs down towards the pelvis during the preparatory breathing; cue for stronger abdominal muscle control throughout.

See Table 4.19 for Teaching points.

Precautions

- **Neck and shoulder pathology – modify rest position with appropriate supports.**
- **Knee pathology – monitor for pain-free activity, seek medical advice if unsure.**
- **Hip pathology and/or surgery – monitor for pain-free activity, seek medical advice if unsure.**
- **Lower back pathology – ensure adequate abdominal muscle control over lumbar spine stability; seek medical advice if unsure.**
- **Rheumatoid arthritis – monitor carefully for pain-free activity; ensure adequate abdominal muscle control over lumbar spine stability.**

Contraindications

- Knee pain during exercise – tight hip abductors together with weak hip adductors and/or tight hamstrings will alter patella tracking and knee mechanics; for onward referral.
- Adolescent knee pain – for onward referral.
- Acute shoulder, spine, lower back, hip and knee pathology.

Tactile cue suggestions

1. To promote spine elongation – lightly place one hand on the lower back and run the other hand up the spine to rest on the crown of the head.
2. To correct pectoral girdle alignment and stability – place the hands firmly over the scapulae to direct them down and across the back.
3. To monitor spine alignment and stability and prevent pelvic rotation – instruct the student to place a hand on the upper hip (the teacher may slip one hand under the waist to feel the waist curve lifting naturally away from the floor).
4. To self-monitor spine alignment and stability – instruct the student to perform the exercise lying with their back against a wall.
5. To promote lengthening the legs out of the hip joints – lightly touch the heels.

4

Table 4.19 Teaching points – Body lengthening

Focus on	Examples of verbal/visual cues
Correct side lying alignment	Ensure that the front and the back of the body are equally lengthened as you align yourself with the edge of the mat Stack the upper hip bone directly above the lower hip bone Maintain a space under the waist as the legs lift
Stabilization of the pectoral girdle and maintenance of the correct relationship between the upper torso and the pelvis	Broaden across the collarbones, slide the shoulder blades down the back and funnel the ribs down towards the pelvis
Correct dynamic lower limb alignment	Imagine lights on both kneecaps shining forwards
Length through the front of the hips	Imagine your feet are going to touch the wall they are pointing towards
Stabilizing the torso before the lower limbs move	Hollow the abdominals, soften the breastbone and funnel the ribs down towards the pelvis Visualize the muscular connection attaching the ribcage to the pelvis Imagine tightening the strings of a corset and creating a wasp waist
Independent activation of the lower fibres of gluteus maximus	Lightly squeeze the sitting bones together Imagine a drawstring pulling the sitting bones together as the legs open and close
Effective abdominal muscle control	Imagine a seatbelt around the pelvis drawing the abdominal wall to the spine
Appropriate adductor muscle activation	Draw the inner thighs together and reach the legs away as they lower to the floor

4

SPINE, HIP AND SHOULDER STABILIZATION AND MOBILIZATION – QUADRIPED SERIES (EXERCISES BCS13–19)

Exercise BCS13 – Head nodding (craniovertebral joint mobilization)

Aim
To encourage craniovertebral flexion/extension and rotation and improve cervical spine stability.
To improve the performance of the deep cervical spine stabilizing muscles.
To improve pectoral girdle orientation and stability during weight bearing with the upper extremities.
To improve abdominal muscle control over lumbar spine stability during independent cervical spine movement.

Equipment
Mat or firm bed, foam roller.

Target muscles
For lumbar spine stability – erector spinae, the pelvic floor and transversus abdominis.
For pectoral girdle stability – gentle activation of the middle and lower fibres of trapezius, latissimus dorsi and teres major.
For atlanto-occipital flexion – the short muscles between the atlas and occiput, together with the right and left anterior neck muscles (sternomastoid and longus capitis).
For atlanto-occipital extension – the postvertebral muscles.
For atlantoaxial rotation – the suboccipital muscles together with sternomastoid and trapezius.

Body position
Four-point kneeling with the hips flexed 90 degrees, the knees no more than hip distance apart and the feet facing away from the body. The hands are placed approximately in line with or just in front of

the glenohumeral joints (if the arms are comparatively long) and the arms are slightly rotated laterally. The little fingers press lightly into the floor to assist engagement of the pectoral girdle stabilizing muscles. The back of the neck is lengthened with the cervical curve intact and the superficial neck muscles comparatively relaxed. The gaze is between the thumbs (Figs 4.45A&B).

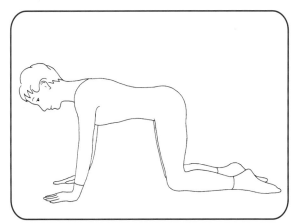

Figure 4.45A Head nodding – body position.

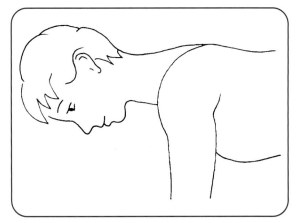

Figure 4.45B Head nodding – cervical spine alignment.

Action
Breathing in – to prepare.
Breathing out – press the little fingers into the floor to increase scapulae stability as the pelvic floor and lower abdominal muscles engage to stabilize the lumbar spine. Maintain the pelvis in neutral, the thoracic and cervical curves intact and lengthen the spine from the crown of the head to the coccyx.
Breathing in – lengthen the back of the neck to flex it, drawing the chin towards the base of the neck (this is very subtle movement, with approximately 10

degrees of flexion). Cue to imagine the chin drawing a line on the floor. The neck should not change its orientation to the floor and gaze moves with the head (Fig. 4.45C).

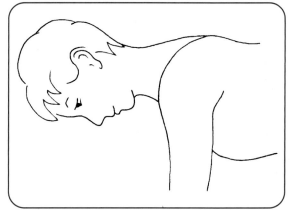

Figure 4.45C Head nodding – flexion.

Breathing out – extend the neck, moving the head through a neutral position to lift the head slightly (this is very subtle movement, with approximately 10 degrees of extension). Cue to imagine the chin first drawing a line on the along the floor before tilting slightly upwards (Fig. 4.45D).

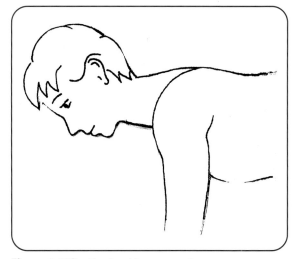

Figure 4.45D Head nodding – extension.

Note: Atlanto-occipital flexion/extension is also likely to involve the few degrees of flexion/extension possible at the atlantoaxial joint, and this increases the observable range of motion during flexion/extension. The superficial neck muscles should appear comparatively relaxed throughout and the gaze moves with the head.
Repeat 5–10 times.

Exercise BCS14 – Head turning (atlantoaxial joint mobilization)

Aim
To encourage atlanto-axial rotation and improve cervical spine mobility.

To improve the performance of the deep cervical spine stabilizing muscles.

To improve pectoral girdle orientation and stability during weight bearing with the upper extremities.

To improve abdominal muscle control over lumbar spine stability during independent cervical spine movement.

Equipment
Mat or firm bed, foam roller.

Target muscles
For lumbar spine stability – erector spinae, the pelvic floor and transversus abdominis.

For pectoral girdle stability – gentle activation of the middle and lower fibres of trapezius, latissimus dorsi and teres major.

For atlantoaxial rotation – the short muscles between the atlas and occiput (suboccipital muscles), together with the right and left sternomastoid and trapezius muscles.

Body position
Four-point kneeling with the hips flexed 90 degrees, the knees no more than hip distance apart and the feet facing away from the body. The hands are placed approximately in line with or just in front of the glenohumeral joints (if the arms are comparatively long) and the arms are slightly rotated laterally. The little fingers press lightly into the floor to assist engagement of the pectoral girdle stabilizing muscles. The back of the neck is lengthened with the cervical curve intact and the superficial neck muscles comparatively relaxed. The gaze is between the thumbs (Fig. 4.46A).

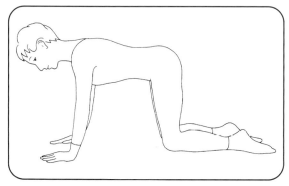

Figure 4.46A

Action
Breathing in – to prepare.

Breathing out – press the little fingers into the floor to increase scapulae stability as the pelvic floor and lower abdominal muscles engage to stabilize the lumbar spine. Maintain the pelvis in neutral, the thoracic and cervical curves intact and lengthen the spine from the crown of the head to the coccyx.

Breathing in – lengthen the back of the neck and rotate the head to the right (this is a very subtle movement with approximately 15 degrees of motion between the first and second cervical vertebrae). Cue to imagine the head and first cervical vertebra moving as a single unit. The neck should not change its orientation to the floor and the gaze moves with the head (Fig. 4.46B).

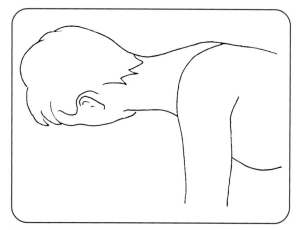

Figure 4.46B Head turning to right.

Breathing out – return the head to neutral.
Repeat on the left side (Fig. 4.46C).

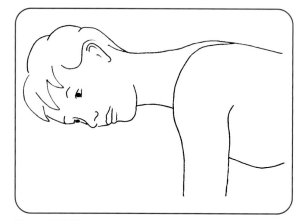

Figure 4.46C Head turning.

Repeat 5–10 times.

Common problems

- Exaggerated cervical spine flexion/extension: Instruct the student to imagine the head/neck as that of a wooden puppet and the head nods and turns on top of an immobile neck.
- Restricted mobility: Ensure correct upper body/pectoral girdle position and stability; cue to release tension in the superficial neck muscles; use the gaze to assist mobility; work within comfortable ranges of motion; practise static exercises for strengthening cervical erector spinae – for example, in the supine position trying to lift the head against the resistance of a hand placed on the forehead or turning the head against the resistance of a hand placed on the side of the face, or pulling the head directly backwards against the resistance of the floor or a wall.

See Table 4.20 for Teaching points.

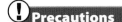

Precautions
- Shoulder pathology – monitor the pectoral girdle position and ensure good stabilization.
- Chronic neck pathology – monitor for pain-free activity seek medical advice if unsure.

Contraindications
- Painful neck pathology – for onward referral.
- Shoulder or knee pathology causing pain on kneeling.

Tactile cue suggestions

1. To promote spine elongation – lightly place one hand on the lower back and run the other hand up the spine to rest on the crown of the head.
2. To correct pectoral girdle alignment and stability – use the hand to direct the shoulder blades down and across the back.
3. To correct the relationship between the upper and lower torso – use the hands to funnel the ribs down towards the pelvis during spine extension.
4. To maintain the superficial neck muscles comparatively relaxed – gently place the thumb and third finger of the left hand just below the occipital tuberosities to direct the head forwards and correct cervical spine alignment. The right hand can assist in supporting and directing the forehead as required (Fig. 4.47).

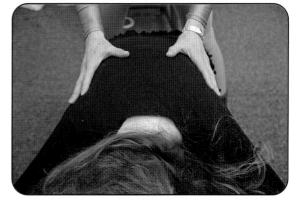

Figure 4.47

Table 4.20 Teaching points – Head nodding and head turning

Focus on	Examples of verbal/visual cues
Efficient abdominal control and core stability throughout	Draw the pelvic floor muscles upwards and the navel back towards the spine
Shoulder alignment and girdle stability	Imagine the shoulder blades sliding down across the back Press the little fingers into the floor
Focus on maintaining the superficial neck muscles comparatively relaxed	Think of floating the head and dropping the chin
Achieving spine elongation and stability	Imagine space between the vertebrae as the tailbone and head move in opposite directions Reach the sitting bones away
Upper cervical spine mobilization	Imagine you are a wooden dog puppet nodding and turning your head on top of the neck

Exercise BCS15 – Rocking (lumbar spine stabilization/hip and glenohumeral joint mobilization)

Aim

To improve pectoral girdle orientation and stability during weight bearing with the upper extremities.

To improve posterior hip muscle flexibility and increase hip range of motion in flexion.

To improve abdominal muscle control over lumbar spine stability during independent hip joint movement.

To improve spine mobility in flexion and extension.

Equipment

Mat or firm bed, foam roller.

Target muscles

For lumbar spine stability – erector spinae, the pelvic floor and transversus abdominis.

For pectoral girdle stability – gentle activation of the middle and lower fibres of trapezius, latissimus dorsi and teres major.

For hip mobilization – pectoral girdle activity moves the torso forwards and backwards in the transverse plane and this has a secondary mobilizing effect on the hip joints. The hip muscles remain comparatively relaxed.

For spine flexion – the oblique abdominals and rectus abdominis.

For spine extension – erector spinae.

Body position

Four-point kneeling (Fig. 4.48A).

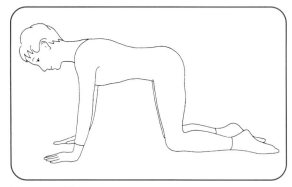

Figure 4.48A   Rocking – body position.

Action

Breathing in – to prepare.

Breathing out – press the little fingers into the floor to increase scapulae stability as the pelvic floor and lower abdominal muscles engage to stabilize the lumbar spine. Maintain the pelvis in neutral, the

thoracic and cervical curves intact and lengthen through the spine from the crown of the head to the sitting bones. Slide the shoulder blades down the back and, keeping the hands still, pull the arms towards the body and draw the body forwards (Fig. 4.48B).

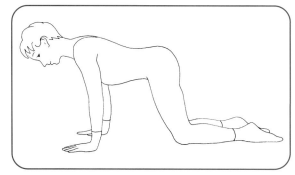

Figure 4.48B   Rocking – hip extension.

Breathing in – maintaining spine stability, slide the shoulder blades further down the back and use pressure through the heels of the hands to rock the body backwards, flexing the hip and glenohumeral joints. Stop at the end of independent hip joint movement (before lumbar spine flexion occurs) (Fig. 4.48C).

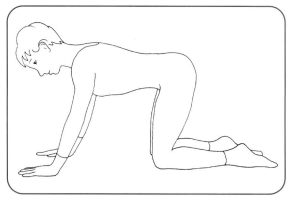

Figure 4.48C   Rocking – hip flexion.

Breathing out – press through the little fingers to assist scapular stability, then use the arms to draw the body forwards, extending the hip and glenohumeral joints.

Repeat the rocking motion 5–10 times.

Progression

Perform with the hands supported on a foam roller.

Table 4.21 Teaching points – Rocking

Focus on	Examples of verbal/visual cues
Efficient abdominal control and core stability throughout	Think of balancing a bowl of water on the back of the pelvis
Shoulder alignment and girdle stability	Imagine the shoulder blades sliding down across the back
Achieving spine elongation throughout	Direct the crown of the head and the sitting bones in opposite directions
Achieving independent hip joint movement	Think of hinging at the hips Imagine a rod between the hips forming an axis as the motion occurs

Common problems

- Incorrect preparatory body position:
  - upper body: instruct the student to press the hands (little fingers) into the floor, draw the front ribs up towards the back ribs and slide the shoulder blades down the back to stabilize the pectoral girdle
  - lower body: instruct the student to visualize the natural spinal curves, engage the pelvic floor and lower abdominal muscles to support the lumbar curve and reach the sitting bones directly backwards.
- Poor proprioception of spine position: Ensure good abdominal muscle control throughout; assist awareness through the use of props such as a stick held to make light contact along the back or by using a mirror; cue to direct the crown of the head forwards and the sitting bones backwards whilst allowing the hips to release.

See Table 4.21 for Teaching points.

Tactile cue suggestions

1. To promote spine elongation – lightly place one hand on the lower back and run the other hand up the spine to rest on the crown of the head.
2. To correct pectoral girdle alignment and stability – use the hand to direct the shoulder blades down and across the back.
3. To assist independent hip joint movement – place the left hand lightly over the sacrum and the right hand in the crease of the groin to indicate where flexion motion occurs.
4. To maintain the superficial neck muscles comparatively relaxed – gently place the thumb and third finger of the left hand just below the occipital tuberosities to direct the head forwards and correct cervical spine alignment. The right hand can assist in supporting and directing the forehead as required.

Precautions

- Wrist and shoulder pathology – monitor the position and use props to reduce the degree of wrist extension as required; ensure correct pectoral girdle alignment and stability.

Contraindications

- Painful neck, wrist, shoulder, back, hip or knee pathology – for onward referral.

Exercise BCS16 – Floating arm and leg series: Arm lifts (lumbar spine stabilization and glenohumeral joint mobilization)

Aim

To improve pectoral girdle orientation and stability during weight bearing with the upper extremities.
To improve abdominal muscle control over lumbar spine stability during independent shoulder flexion.
To improve proprioception of and control over correct spine alignment.

Equipment

Mat or firm bed, foam roller.

Target muscles

For lumbar spine stability – erector spinae, the pelvic floor and transversus abdominis.

For pectoral girdle stability – serratus anterior, the middle and lower fibres of trapezius, latissimus dorsi and teres major.

For shoulder flexion – anterior fibres of deltoid, clavicular head of pectoralis major, coracobrachialis and biceps.

Body position

Four-point kneeling with the hips flexed 90 degrees, the knees no more than hip distance apart and the feet facing away from the body. The hands are placed approximately in line with or just in front of the glenohumeral joints (if the arms are comparatively long) and the arms are slightly rotated laterally. The little fingers press lightly into the floor to assist engagement of the pectoral girdle stabilizing muscles. The back of the neck is lengthened with the cervical curve intact and the superficial neck muscles comparatively relaxed. The gaze is between the thumbs (Fig. 4.49A).

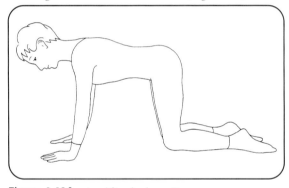

Figure 4.49A Arm lifts – body position.

Action

Breathing in – to prepare.

Breathing out – press the little fingers into the floor to increase scapulae stability as the pelvic floor and lower abdominal muscles engage to stabilize the lumbar spine. Maintain the pelvis in neutral, the thoracic and cervical curves intact and lengthen through the spine from the crown of the head to the coccyx.

Breathing in.

Breathing out – further stabilize the pectoral girdle and flex the left shoulder, reaching the fingers forwards until the left arm aligns with the left ear (Fig. 4.49B).

Breathing in – increase abdominal muscle activation to control spine stability as the hand returns to the floor.

Breathing out – perform on the right side.

Repeat 5–10 times on each side.

Modification 1

Lift the right hand just off the floor. Repeat with the left.

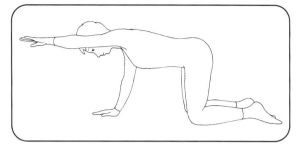

Figure 4.49B Arm lifts – action.

Modification 2

Reduce the range of glenohumeral joint flexion and gradually increase it as spine stability improves.

Progression

Perform with the hands supported on a foam roller or similar unstable support.

Exercise BCS17 – Floating arm and leg series: Leg lifts (lumbar spine stabilization and hip joint mobilization)

Aim

To improve pectoral girdle orientation and stability during weight bearing with the upper extremities.

To improve abdominal muscle control over lumbar spine stability during independent hip extension.

To improve proprioception of and control over correct spine alignment.

Equipment

Mat or firm bed, foam roller.

Target muscles

For lumbar spine stability – erector spinae, the pelvic floor and transversus abdominis.

For pectoral girdle stability – serratus anterior, the middle and lower fibres of trapezius, latissimus dorsi and teres major.

For hip extension – gluteus maximus and hamstrings.

Body position

Four-point kneeling with the hips flexed 90 degrees, the knees no more than hip distance apart and the feet facing away from the body. The hands are placed approximately in line with or just in front of the glenohumeral joints (if the arms are comparatively long) and the arms are slightly rotated laterally. The little fingers press lightly into the floor to assist engagement of the pectoral girdle stabilizing muscles. The back of the neck is lengthened with the cervical curve intact and the superficial neck muscles comparatively relaxed. The gaze is between the thumbs (Fig. 4.50A).

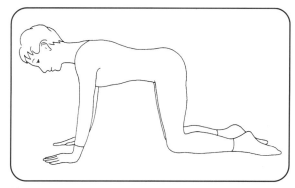

Figure 4.50A Leg lifts – body position.

Action

Breathing in – to prepare.

Breathing out – press the little fingers into the floor to increase scapulae stability as the pelvic floor and lower abdominal muscles engage to stabilize the lumbar spine. Maintain the pelvis in neutral, the thoracic and cervical curves intact and lengthen through the spine from the crown of the head to the coccyx.

Breathing in.

Breathing out – further stabilize the pectoral girdle and increase abdominal muscle activation. Slide the left foot along the floor, extending the left knee and hip to float the left leg up so that the heel aligns with the left ischial tuberosity. The hip remains neutral in rotation (Fig. 4.50B).

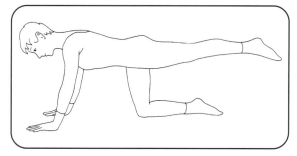

Figure 4.50B Leg lifts – action.

Breathing in – increase abdominal muscle activation to control spine stability as the hip flexes to return the knee to the floor.

Breathing out – perform on the right side.

Repeat 5–10 times on each side.

Modification 1

Lift the right knee just off the floor. Repeat with the left.

Modification 2

Reduce the range of hip joint flexion and gradually increase it as spine stability improves.

Progression

Perform with the hands and knees supported on a foam roller or similar unstable support.

Exercise BCS18 – Floating arm and leg series: Arm and leg lifts (lumbar spine stabilization, shoulder and hip joint mobilization)

Aim

To improve pectoral girdle orientation and stability during weight bearing with the upper extremities.

To improve abdominal muscle control over lumbar spine stability during independent shoulder and hip joint mobilization.

To improve proprioception of and control over correct spine alignment.

Equipment

Mat or firm bed, foam roller.

Target muscles

For lumbar spine stability – erector spinae, the pelvic floor and transversus abdominis.

For pectoral girdle stability – serratus anterior, the middle and lower fibres of trapezius, latissimus dorsi and teres major.

For shoulder flexion – anterior fibres of deltoid, clavicular head of pectoralis major, coracobrachialis and biceps.

For hip extension – gluteus maximus and hamstrings.

Body position

Four-point kneeling with the hips flexed 90 degrees, the knees no more than hip distance apart and the feet facing away from the body. The hands are placed approximately in line with or just in front of the glenohumeral joints (if the arms are comparatively long) and the arms are slightly rotated laterally. The little fingers press lightly into the floor to assist engagement of the pectoral girdle stabilizing muscles. The back of the neck is lengthened with the cervical curve intact and the superficial neck muscles comparatively relaxed. The gaze is between the thumbs (Fig. 4.51A).

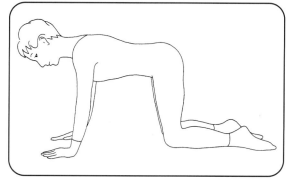

Figure 4.51A Arm and leg lifts – body position.

Action

Breathing in – to prepare.

Breathing out – press the little fingers into the floor to increase scapulae stability as the pelvic floor and lower abdominal muscles engage to stabilize the lumbar spine. Maintain the pelvis in neutral, the thoracic and cervical curves intact and lengthen through the spine from the crown of the head to the coccyx.

Breathing in.

Breathing out – further stabilize the pectoral girdle and flex the left shoulder, reaching the fingers forwards until the left arm aligns with the left ear and simultaneously slide the right foot along the floor, extending the right knee and hip to float the right leg up so that the heel aligns with the right ischial tuberosity. The hips remain neutral in rotation (Fig. 4.51B).

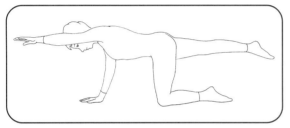

Figure 4.51B   Arm and leg lifts – action.

Breathing in – maintaining spine and pelvic stability, return the limbs to the starting position.

Breathing out – repeat the exercise, flexing the right shoulder joint and the left hip joint.

Repeat five times to each side.

Progression 1

Perform the basic exercise, raising the right arm and right leg simultaneously.

Progression 2

Perform with the hands and knees supported on a foam roller or similar unstable support.

Progression 3

Body position

Perform Progression 1 with torso rotation.

Action

Breathing in – to prepare.

Breathing out – balancing the body weight over the left knee and left hand, rotate the torso to the right, simultaneously reaching the right arm towards the ceiling (directly above the glenohumeral joint) and adducting the right hip. The leg is straight with the hip neutral in rotation so that the knee faces directly forwards.

Breathing in – return to the starting position.

Breathing out – repeat on the other side.

Repeat up to three times each side.

Repeat the sequence 5–10 times.

Common problems

- Incorrect preparatory body position:
  - upper body: instruct the student to press the hands (little fingers) into the floor, draw the front ribs up towards the back ribs and slide the shoulder blades down the back to stabilize the pectoral girdle
  - lower body: instruct the student to visualize the natural spinal curves, engage the pelvic floor and lower abdominal muscles to support the lumbar curve and reach the sitting bones directly backwards.
- Insufficient core control: Cue for stronger pelvic floor and lower abdominal muscle engagement; assist awareness through the use of props such as a stick held to make light contact along the back; cue to reach the crown of the head and the sitting bones in opposite directions.
- Scapular instability during independent shoulder mobilization: Cue to broaden across the collarbones and press the little fingers into the floor to engage the pectoral girdle muscles.
- Spine and/or pectoral girdle instability during independent hip mobilization: Cue for stronger abdominal muscle control together with spine elongation; cue to reach the crown of the head and the sitting bones in opposite directions as the hip releases to initiate hip extension; cue to imagine a bowl of water balancing on the pelvis throughout the motion.

See Table 4.22 for Teaching points.

> **⊘ Precautions**
> - Wrist and shoulder pathology – monitor the position and use props to reduce the degree of wrist extension as required; ensure correct pectoral girdle alignment and stability.
> - Hip pathology – ensure sufficient abdominal muscle control over lumbar spine stability and monitor hip range of motion and leg alignment.

> **✚ Contraindications**
> - Painful neck, wrist, shoulder, back, hip or knee pathology – for onward referral.

Table 4.22 Teaching points – Floating arm and leg series

Focus on	Examples of verbal/visual cues
Efficient abdominal control and core stability throughout	Draw the pelvic floor muscles upwards and the navel back towards the spine
Shoulder alignment and girdle stability	Imagine the shoulder blades sliding down across the back
Achieving independent glenohumeral joint movement	Lengthen the spine as the hand floats away from the floor Imagine the little finger slowly moving through water as the hand floats upwards
Achieving spine elongation throughout	Visualize light or space between the vertebrae
Achieving independent hip joint movement	Release and lengthen through the front of the hip to reach the leg away Imagine the leg floating up as if being lifted by a hot air balloon

Tactile cue suggestions

1. To promote spine elongation – lightly place one hand on the lower back and run the other hand up the spine to rest on the crown of the head.
2. To promote spine/pelvic stabilization – rest a stick along the spine throughout the motion.
3. To correct pectoral girdle alignment and stability – use the hands to direct the shoulder blades down and across the back.
4. To correct the relationship between the upper and lower torso – use the hands to funnel the ribs down towards the pelvis during spine extension.
5. To correct dynamic alignment – lightly touch the back of the hand or the heel.
6. To promote lengthening the leg out of the hip joint – lightly touch the heel of the active leg.
7. To maintain the superficial neck muscles comparatively relaxed – gently place the thumb and third finger of the left hand just below the occipital tuberosities to direct the head forwards and correct cervical spine alignment. The right hand can assist in supporting and directing the forehead as required.

Exercise BCS19 – Cat (spine mobilization)

Aim
To promote spine elongation and segmental mobilization.
To improve vertebral column mobility in flexion/extension.
To improve abdominal muscle control over spine mobilization.
To improve pectoral girdle orientation and stability during weight bearing with the upper extremities.

Equipment
Mat or firm bed, foam roller.

Target muscles
For lumbar spine stability – the pelvic floor and transversus abdominis.
For pectoral girdle stability – gentle activation of the middle and lower fibres of trapezius, latissimus dorsi and teres major.
For spine mobilization in flexion – rectus abdominis and the oblique abdominals.
For spine mobilization in extension – erector spinae.

Body position
Four-point kneeling (Fig. 4.52A).

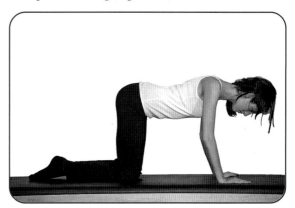

Figure 4.52A

Action
Breathing in – to prepare.
Breathing out – press the little fingers into the floor to increase scapulae stability as the pelvic floor and lower abdominal muscles engage.
Breathing in – maintain abdominal muscle activation and begin by flexing the lumbar spine, directing the ischial tuberosities towards the backs of the knees (Fig. 4.52B).

4

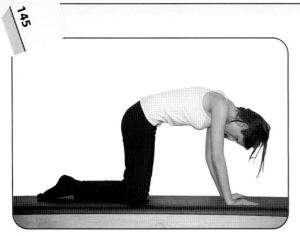

Figure 4.52B

Continue spine mobilization, allowing the thoracic
spine to move into flexion to create an elongated
bow shape from the crown of the head to the
coccyx. Allow the neck to hang from the shoulders
and the head to hang from the neck. The gaze
moves with the head (Fig. 4.52C).

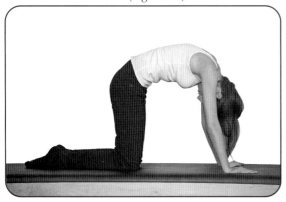

Figure 4.52C

Breathing out – deepen abdominal muscle engagement
to begin spine extension, first reaching the ischial
tuberosities towards the heels before directing them
backwards and up (Fig. 4.52D).

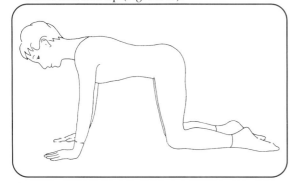

Figure 4.52D Cat – moving into extension.

Simultaneously reach the crown of the head forwards
as the sternum moves forwards and upwards as if

to shine a light on a wall in front of the body. As
the spine extends, maintain the cervical curve intact
and move the gaze with the head whilst
lengthening the spine from the crown of the head
to the sitting bones to create an elongated curve
(Fig. 4.52E).

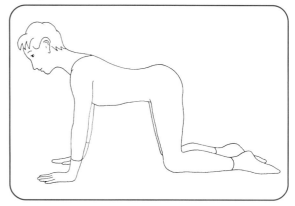

Figure 4.52E Cat – spine extension.

Breathing in – to continue the motion with spine
flexion and progress as before.

Repeat the sequence 5–10 times.

Common problems

- Exaggerated thoracic spine flexion: Instruct the
  student to initiate the motion by directing the
  sitting bones towards the heels and then to drop
  them towards the backs of the knees as spine
  flexion progresses; emphasize spine elongation;
  use tactile cues to mobilize restricted areas.
- Exaggerated lumbar spine extension: Emphasize
  stronger pelvic floor and abdominal muscle
  activation together with spine elongation.
- Poor spine articulation: Begin with small ranges of
  motion and ensure good abdominal muscle control
  throughout; use tactile cues to mobilize restricted
  areas.

See Table 4.23 for Teaching points.

Precautions

- Wrist and shoulder pathology – monitor the
  position and use props to reduce the degree of
  wrist extension as required; ensure correct
  pectoral girdle alignment and stability.
- Chronic neck pathology – work within
  comfortable ranges of motion; practise static
  exercises for strengthening cervical erector
  spinae together with craniovertebral
  atlantoaxial mobilization exercises; seek
  medical advice if unsure.
- Chronic spine or lower back pathology – for
  example, arthritis, spinal stenosis, facet joint or

⊘ Precautions—cont'd

sacroiliac problems that may have symptoms brought on by spine extension; seek medical advice if unsure.
- Osteoporosis – flexion is contraindicated and spine elongation must be promoted during spine extension; seek medical advice if unsure.

✚ Contraindications

- Painful neck, wrist, shoulder, knee, lower back or spine pathology – for onward referral.

Tactile cue suggestions

1. To promote spine elongation – lightly place one hand on the lower back and run the other hand up the spine to rest on the crown of the head.
2. To correct pectoral girdle alignment and stability – use the hand to direct the shoulder blades down and across the back.
3. To correct the relationship between the upper and lower torso, particularly during spine extension – use the hands to funnel the ribs down towards the pelvis.
4. To promote spine articulation – lightly move the fingers along the spine anticipating joint mobilization.
5. To assist spine extension – place the left hand on the sternum, gently directing it forwards and upwards, and the right hand on the back opposite the left hand, directing the spine to lengthen and move inward.

Tactile cue suggestions—cont'd

6. To maintain the superficial neck muscles comparatively relaxed – gently place the thumb and third finger of the left hand just below the occipital tuberosities to direct the head forwards and correct cervical spine alignment. The right hand can assist in supporting and directing the forehead as required.

SUPINE SPINE MOBILIZATION (EXERCISES SSM20–22)

Exercise SSM20 – Pelvic tilt (lumbar spine mobilization)

Aim
To facilitate controlled segmental lumbar spine mobilization in flexion and extension.
To improve the performance of the abdominal muscles.

Equipment
Exercise mat, box, bolster for between thighs, gym ball; head supports to correct head/neck alignment and prevent neck tension.

Target muscles
For pelvic tilt control – levator ani, coccygeus, transversus abdominis.
For trunk flexion – iliopsoas flexes the hip joint and assists pelvic tilt. Rectus abdominis and the oblique abdominal muscles act together to draw the pelvis towards the thoracic cage.

Body position
Supine with 90 degrees of hip and knee flexion and the lumbar spine in neutral (Fig. 4.53A).

Table 4.23 Teaching points – Cat

Focus on	Examples of verbal/visual cues
Efficient abdominal control and core stability throughout	Draw the pelvic floor muscles upwards and hollow the abdominals towards the spine
Shoulder alignment and girdle stability	Imagine the shoulder blades sliding down across the back.
Achieving spine elongation and even vertebral column mobilization during spine flexion	Imagine space between the vertebrae as the tailbone and head move in opposite directions Maintain length in the lower back and reach the sitting bones away as they begin moving down towards the backs of the knees
Achieving spine elongation and even vertebral column mobilization during spine extension	Lengthen and curl the upper spine from just under the bra strap Move the spine between the shoulder blades towards the breastbone as the spine lengthens

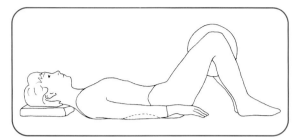

Figure 4.53A   Pelvic tilt – body position.

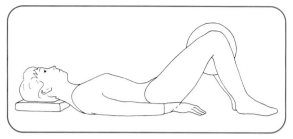

Figure 4.53B   Pelvic tilt – action.

Action

Breathing in – to prepare.

Breathing out – tighten the pelvic floor and transversus abdominis muscles to tilt the pelvis, directing the sacrum forwards and up, lengthening and flattening the lumbar vertebral curve. This is a very small movement and the posterior-superior iliac spine (PSIS) should not lift away from the floor (Fig. 4.53B).

Breathing in – maintain the abdominal muscle contraction.

Breathing out – Pull the abdominal muscles more deeply back towards the spine as it lengthens and rolls back to the neutral position.

Repeat up to 10 times.

Progression 1

Enlarge the range of motion by following the posterior pelvic tilt with an anterior tilt.

Progression 2

The breathing cycles can be reversed to encourage spinal elongation and stability.

Common problems

■ Breathing and abdominal work not coordinated: Allow the student to find their own breathing rhythm.

■ Movement restricted by lumbar spine or sacroiliac pathology, or by tight glutei and other lower back structures: Consider elevating the feet with a half barrel or small box.

See Table 4.24 for Teaching points.

> **Precautions**
> ■ Discomfort or pain in the hips, back or pelvic area; facet joint strain; sacroiliac strain; spinal stenosis; lumbar disc prolapse; osteopaenia.

Table 4.24   Teaching points – Pelvic tilt

Focus on	Examples of verbal/visual cues
Correct head and neck alignment without neck tension	Relax the tongue in the throat and imagine the muscles of the face melting away
Correct pectoral girdle alignment and stability	Feel the collarbones spreading apart so that the shoulder blades can slide diagonally down towards the centre of the back
Using pelvic floor and abdominal muscle activation to initiate the posterior pelvic tilt	Tighten the pelvic floor and lower abdominal muscles Imagine the pelvis as bowl of water and then tilt to spill just one drop towards the navel
Using pelvic floor and abdominal muscle activation to initiate the anterior pelvic tilt	Imagine the pelvis as bowl of water and then tilt to spill just one drop towards the heels
Relaxing and lengthening the whole back as the lumbar spine flattens and the tail bone curls upwards	Allow the back muscles to release Imagine the tail bone is painting a vertical line towards the ceiling
Lengthening and articulating the vertebral column as the pelvis returns to a neutral position	Think of unrolling a carpet Imagine space between each vertebra as the spine unfolds

➕ **Contraindications**

- Back, pelvis or hip pain; facet joint strain; acute lumbar disc prolapse; osteoporosis – for onward referral.
- Pelvic tilts can be appropriate at various stages of the rehabilitation process – for safe practice always seek medical advice.

Tactile cue suggestions

1. To increase breadth across the front of the chest – use the hands to stroke the collarbones from the sternum to their lateral aspects.
2. To correct pectoral girdle alignment and stability – use the hands to guide the shoulder blades down the back.
3. To activate the transversus abdominis – before exercising, instruct the student to place two fingers of each hand on the top of the hip and trace a line towards the centre of body until the fingers are still approximately 10 cm apart. Then instruct to press slightly inwards and upwards, and encourage the student to draw the abdominal wall away from the fingers.

Exercise SSM21 – Pelvic curls (lumbar and thoracic spine mobilization)

Aim
To facilitate controlled, segmental mobilization of the lumbar and thoracic spine in flexion and extension.

Equipment
Exercise mat, box, roller, bolster for between thighs, gym ball; head supports to correct head/neck alignment and prevent neck tension.

Target muscles
For lumbar spine stability – levator ani, coccygeus, transversus abdominis acting together.

For trunk flexion – rectus abdominis and the oblique abdominal muscles act concentrically to draw the pelvis towards the ribcage.

For pectoral girdle stability – the middle and lower fibres of trapezius, latissimus dorsi and teres major muscles are engaged.

For hip stability and controlled hip extension – the posterior muscles of the hip and the adductors work together.

Body position
Supine with 90 degrees of hip and knee flexion with the lumbar spine in neutral (Fig. 4.54A).

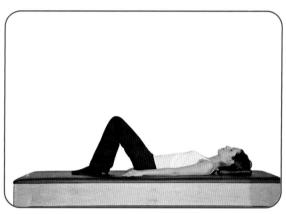

Figure 4.54A

Action
Breathing in – to prepare.

Breathing out – simultaneously engage the pelvic floor and transversus abdominis muscles to initiate a posterior tilt of the pelvis (Fig. 4.54B).

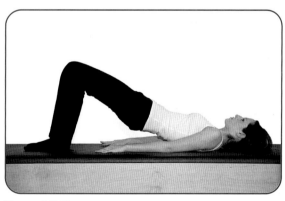

Figure 4.54B

Direct the ischial tuberosities towards the backs of the knees, lengthening and flattening the lumbar vertebral column. Continue to lengthen the spine, sequentially peeling the vertebrae from the floor to establish the shoulder bridge position. This is approximately at mid scapulae level.

4

Breathing in – maintain abdominal control whilst in the elevated position. Broaden across the collar bones and slide the shoulder blades down the back, reaching the fingers towards the heels.

Note: The whole body is lengthened, the thoracic curve of the spine remains intact and the pelvis is in a slight posterior tilt. This facilitates the correct relationship and a strong muscular connection between the upper torso and pelvis.

Breathing out – relax the upper back and allow passive flexion of the thoracic spine to release the sternum downwards. Lengthen the C-shape of the spine by directing the sitting bones towards the backs of the knees, deepening the abdominal muscle contraction and allowing the vertebrae to return sequentially to the floor. The pelvis then levels to re-establish the neutral position.

Repeat up to 10 times.

Modification

Pelvic lift. For students recovering from spine pathology, substitute a pelvic lift until the student has been pain free for at least 3 weeks.

Body position

Feet on the gym ball, legs extended and pressed together (Fig. 4.54C).

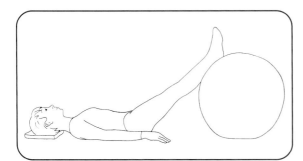

Figure 4.54C   Pelvic lift – body position.

Action

Breathing in – to prepare.

Breathing out – engage the abdominal muscles, flatten the lumbar spine, reach the legs away, squeeze the gluteals to float the pelvis away from the floor (at the end of the movement there should be a strong muscular connection between the lower ribs and the pelvis).

Breathing in.

Breathing out – engage the abdominal muscles more deeply and hinge at the hips to lower the whole body back to the floor, through the flattened lumbar spine position, ending in neutral.

Progression 1

Reverse the breathing.

Progression 2

Perform the basic exercise lying along a roller with the feet elevated on a small box. The roller helps to fire the pelvic floor and lower abdominal muscles.

Progression 3

Perform the basic exercise with the heels resting on a gym ball, legs extended in parallel and inner thighs squeezed together.

Progression 4

Perform the basic exercise with the feet resting on a gym ball, with approximately 90 degrees of hip/knee flexion.

Progression 5

Spine mobilization – hip drops.

Body position

Shoulder bridge position.

Action

Allow the right hip to drop slightly whilst keeping the left hip still.

Note: This is a small movement with minimal rotation of the pelvis. Imagine that both hips are suspended by strings from the ceiling – one string releases a little to drop one hip, then tightens to draw it back up.

Use the abdominal muscles to control the pelvis as the right hip lifts back to its starting position.

Repeat the hip drop and lift commencing with the left hip.

Roll the spine down one vertebra and repeat the sequence.

Continue repetitions at each vertebral joint as the spine mobilizes back to the floor. Work towards achieving a minimum of 10 repetitions.

Progression 6

Lateral spine mobilization – pelvic shifts.

Body position

Shoulder bridge position.

Action

Shift the pelvis towards the right then towards the left at each vertebral level. Roll the spine down one vertebra and repeat the sequence.

Note: This exercise achieves lateral mobilization and can selectively target restricted areas. The movements are small and confined to the spine. Stabilize the pectoral girdle and use the abdominal muscles to control the relationship between the upper torso and the pelvis. Think of reaching the knees over the toes, keeping them as still as possible.

Progression 7

Pelvic circles.

Body position

Shoulder bridge position.

Action

Allow the right hip to drop slightly whilst keeping the left hip still (this is a small movement with minimal rotation of the pelvis: imagine that both hips are suspended by strings from the ceiling – one string releases a little to drop one hip).

Allow the left hip to drop to align horizontally with the right hip.

Return the right hip to its starting position.

Return the left hip to its starting position.

Lower the spine one vertebra and repeat the sequence.

Repeat at each level of the spine as it rolls down to the floor.

Note: This exercise mobilizes the spine in different planes. Be sure to stabilize the pectoral girdle and use the abdominal muscles to control the relationship between the upper torso and the pelvis.

Common problems

- Breathing and abdominal work not coordinated: Allow the student to find their own breathing rhythm.
- Overextending the spine when in the shoulder bridge position: The sternum should be dropped to allow the ribs to funnel down towards the pelvis with the pelvis in a slight posterior tilt so that the groins and lumbar spine are lengthened.
- Overactivity of the hamstrings and gluteal muscles that results in pushing the pelvis away from the floor (dominant or tight hamstrings may result in cramping): Cue to initiate the tilt through pelvic floor and deep abdominal action whilst maintaining the gluteal muscles comparatively relaxed; consider raising the feet on a small box to slightly increase hip flexion and lengthen the hamstring and lower gluteal muscles (this tends to prevent their dominance as the action begins).
- If the feet arc too far away from the pelvis when resting (the knees flexed more than 90 degrees), the hamstrings may be dominant and cramp

during the hip extension motion: Ensure that the feet are correctly positioned approximately in line with the hip joints and the knees are flexed no less than 90 degrees.
- Trying too hard: Cue to encourage a slower, more relaxed approach.
- Immobility at particular vertebral joints: Refer to Progressions 5–7.
- Loss of lower limb alignment: Use a bolster between the knees.
- Students with a pronounced thoracic kyphosis: Use appropriate head and neck support. Monitor the head and upper spine position for comfort.

See Table 4.25 for Teaching points.

Precautions

- Discomfort or non-specific pain in the knees, hips, back or pelvic area; facet joint strain; sacroiliac strain; spinal stenosis; cervical and lumbar spine pathology.
- Hypertension.
- Pelvic tilts can be appropriate at various stages of the rehabilitation process – for safe practice always seek professional medical advice.

Contraindications

- Pain in the back, pelvis, hips or knees; facet joint strain; acute sacroiliac strain or spine pathology; osteoporosis.

Exercise SSM22 – Pelvic curls with arm lifts (spine mobilization with shoulder flexion)

Aim

To improve controlled segmental mobilization of the spine.

Equipment

Exercise mat, roller, box, gym ball, bolster for between the knees to assist leg alignment.

Target muscles

For vertical arm extension – concentric contraction of latissimus dorsi, teres major and posterior deltoid.

For pectoral girdle stability – the pectoral girdle muscles act together to maintain the scapulae in a relatively stable position: trapezius, levator scapulae, rhomboids, serratus anterior, pectoralis minor and subclavius.

Body position

Supine with 90 degrees of hip and knee flexion with the lumbar spine in neutral.

Table 4.25   Teaching points – Pelvic curls

Focus on	Examples of verbal/visual cues
Correct head and neck alignment without neck tension	Relax the tongue in the throat and imagine the muscles of the face melting away
Vertebral column length	Reach the crown of the head and the sitting bones in opposite directions
Correct pectoral girdle alignment and stability	Feel the collarbones spreading apart and visualize the shoulder blades sliding diagonally down across the back
Correct lower limb/feet placement	Align the knees with the second and third toes Spread the toes and imagine the feet imprinting in warm sand
Coordinating the breath and the movement	Allow the out breath to enhance the initial abdominal muscle work Allow the in breath to lengthen the spine
Correct initial direction for the movement	Curl the tailbone between the legs
Facilitating spinal elongation and smooth controlled mobilization of the vertebral column as the spine flexes and extends	Reach the sitting bones to the back of the knees as the spine peels from the floor Imagine the spine as a string of pearls dropping one by one as the back unfolds to the floor

4

Tactile cue suggestions

1. To increase breadth across the front of the chest – use the hands to stroke the collar bones from the sternum to their lateral aspects.
2. To correct pectoral girdle alignment and stability – use the hands to guide the shoulder blades down the back.
3. To activate the lower abdominal muscles – before exercising, instruct the student to place two fingers of each hand on the top of the hips and to trace a line towards the centre of body until the fingers are still approximately 10 cm apart. Then instruct to press slightly inwards and upwards and encourage the student to draw the abdominal wall away from the fingers.
4. To promote spine elongation during lumbar flexion – use the hands to direct the pelvis up and away towards the knees (thumbs are placed approximately at the level of the anterior-superior iliac spine (ASIS), fingers around and towards the back of the pelvis).
5. To promote spine articulation during spine extension – walk the fingers down the spine, anticipating joint mobilization.

Action
Breathing in – to prepare (Fig. 4.55A).

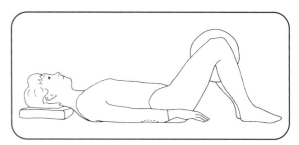

Figure 4.55A   Pelvic curls – breathing in.

Breathing out – articulate the spine up into the shoulder bridge position (Figs 4.55B–D).

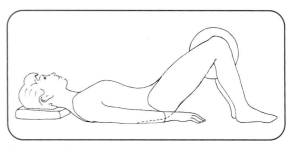

Figure 4.55B   Pelvic curls – breathing out.

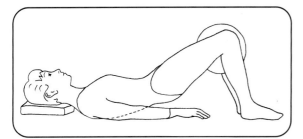

Figure 4.55C   Pelvic curls with arm lifts – mid curl.

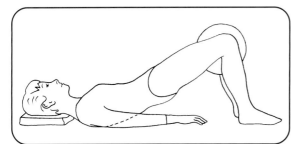

Figure 4.55D   Pelvic curls with arm lifts – shoulder bridge position.

Breathing in – maintain the shoulder bridge position. Gently draw the shoulder blades down and across the back. Flex the glenohumeral joints, lifting the arms to a vertical position above the shoulders, reaching the fingers for the ceiling (Fig. 4.55E).

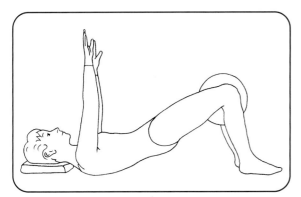

Figure 4.55E   Pelvic curls with arm lifts – stretching the upper back.

Still reaching the fingertips to the ceiling, allow the shoulder blades to rotate forwards around the ribcage to stretch the upper back.

Breathing out – broaden across the collarbones and allow the passive flexion of the thoracic spine to release the sternum down, enhancing the stretch across the upper back. Still reaching the fingers to the ceiling, allow the shoulders blades to rotate

back around the ribcage as the shoulder blades glide down and across the back to re-establish pectoral girdle neutrality and stability (Fig. 4.55F).

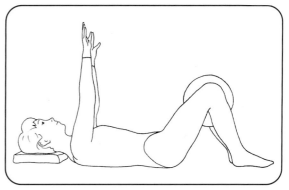

Figure 4.55F   Pelvic curls with arm lifts – re-establishing the body position.

Breathing in – still reaching the fingers to the ceiling.

Breathing out – relax the upper back and allow passive flexion of the thoracic spine to release the sternum downwards. Lengthen the C-shape of the spine by directing the sitting bones towards the heels, deepening the abdominal muscle contraction and allowing the vertebrae to return sequentially to the floor.

Breathing in – the pelvis levels to re-establish the neutral position.

Breathing out – relax the back and take the arms over the head to rest on the floor (Fig. 4.55G).

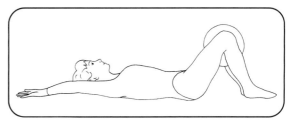

Figure 4.55G   Pelvic curls with arm lifts – breathing out.

Breathing in – bring the arms back down to the sides of the body to prepare for the next repetition.

Common problems
- Overactivity of the upper trapezius during glenohumeral joint flexion: Cue for breadth across the front of the chest, relaxation of the throat and neck muscles and space between the ears and the upper arms.

- Loss of lower limb alignment: Use a bolster between the knees.
- For students with a pronounced thoracic kyphosis: Use appropriate head and neck support; monitor the head and upper spine position carefully.

See Table 4.26 for Teaching points.

Precautions
- Discomfort or non-specific pain in the neck, shoulders, knees, hips, back or pelvic area; facet joint strain; sacroiliac strain; spinal stenosis; cervical and lumbar spine pathology.
- Hypertension.

Contraindications
- Pain in the shoulder, back, pelvis, hips or knees; facet joint strain; acute sacroiliac strain or spine pathology; osteoporosis.
- Pelvic tilts can be appropriate at various stages of the rehabilitation process – for safe practice always seek professional medical advice.

Table 4.26 Teaching points – Pelvic curls with arm lifts

Focus on	Examples of verbal/ visual cues
Breadth across the collarbones and correct pectoral girdle stabilization as the shoulders flex	Broaden across the collarbones Imagine the shoulder blades are sliding down and across the back into pockets on the opposite back hip
Allowing the breastbone to drop towards the spine as spine extension is initiated	Soften the breastbone
Good scapula mobilization	Imagine holding a stick and first reaching it towards the ceiling then drawing it back towards the body

Tactile cue suggestions

1. To increase breadth across the front of the chest – use the hands to stroke the collarbones from the sternum to their lateral aspects.
2. To correct pectoral girdle alignment and stability – use the hands to guide the shoulder blades down the back.
3. To activate the lower abdominal muscles – before exercising, instruct the student to place two fingers of each hand on the top of the hip and to trace a line towards the centre of the body until the fingers are still approximately 10 cm apart. Then instruct to press slightly inwards and upwards and encourage the student to draw the abdominal wall away from the fingers.
4. To promote spine elongation during lumbar flexion – use the hands to direct the pelvis up and away towards the knees (thumbs are placed at approximately the level of the ASIS, fingers around and towards the back of the pelvis).
5. To promote spine articulation during spine extension – walk the fingers down the spine anticipating joint mobilization.
6. To correct dynamic arm alignment – guide the fingers through the motion.

SUPINE UPPER ABDOMINAL MUSCLE STRENGTHENING (EXERCISES SAS23–24)

Exercise SAS23 – Sit ups (anterior abdominal wall muscles strengthening)

Aim
To increase lower abdominal muscle control over the lumbar spine during upper torso flexion.
To improve rectus abdominis and oblique abdominal muscle strength and performance.

Equipment
Mat, firm bed, half barrel, box, gym ball.

Target muscles
For lumbar spine stability – the pelvic floor and transversus abdominis.
For pectoral girdle stability – the isometric activity of latissimus dorsi and teres major, together with the middle and lower fibres of the trapezius muscle acting isometrically.
For trunk flexion – rectus abdominis and the internal oblique abdominal muscles work concentrically to

draw the ribcage towards the pelvis. They act eccentrically during the return from flexion.

Body position

Supine position with 90 degrees of hip and knee flexion. The arms are bent with the hands behind the head, the fingers interlocked so that the hands can cradle the head. The elbows are slightly forward and just within peripheral vision. The upper trapezius muscles are comparatively relaxed (Fig. 4.56A).

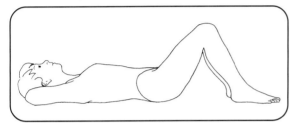

Figure 4.56A Sit ups – body position.

Preparatory action

Tighten the pelvic floor and lower abdominal muscles, hollowing them towards the spine. Simultaneously broaden across the collarbones, stabilize the scapulae to support the head in the hands and lift it just off the floor.

Note: The chin is dropped slightly so that the back of the neck is lengthened and the superficial neck muscles remain comparatively relaxed.

Action

Breathing in.

Breathing out – Further stabilize the scapulae and allow the passive flexion of the thoracic spine to drop the breastbone down and inwards, bringing the ribs nearer to the pelvis. Increase lower abdominal muscle activation and begin to peel the upper body away from the floor (Fig. 4.56B).

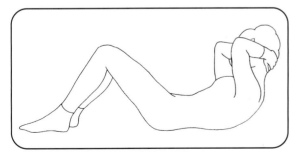

Figure 4.56B Sit ups – spine flexion.

Note: Maintain the same head/cervical spine alignment, moving the head with the upper body and the gaze with the head

Continue spine flexion, allowing the lower back muscles to relax as the lumbar spine flattens.

Note: Maintain the pelvis neutral and stable and stop the motion before tension occurs in the groins.

Breathing in – maintaining good lower abdominal muscle control over the lumbar spine, lengthen and roll the thoracic spine vertebra by vertebra back towards the floor to the starting position.

Breathing out – repeat spine flexion.

Repeat 5–10 times.

Modification 1

Perform beginning with the lumbar spine flattened, and the pelvis in a slight posterior tilt and with the feet raised on a small box or half barrel.

Modification 2

Reduce the range of spine flexion by preparing for the exercise with the upper body curled slightly forwards, supported from behind with a pillow or triangle, and stopping the spine flexion motion earlier.

Progression 1

Perform with the feet resting on a gym ball with the knees and hips flexed approximately 70 degrees.

Progression 2

Perform the basic exercise without returning the upper thoracic spine to the floor between repetitions. Maintain correct cervical alignment throughout.

Progression 3

Assisted Roll-Down.

Body position

Sitting with the back in neutral, the pectoral girdle correctly aligned and the front of the chest open. The knees are hip distance apart and flexed approximately 90 degrees. The hands are placed lightly on the backs of the thighs.

Action

Breathing in – keeping the gaze directly ahead, stabilize the pectoral girdle and simultaneously activate the pelvic floor and lower abdominal muscles. Hollow the abdominals to initiate lumbar spine flexion (Figs 4.57A–C).

Breathing out – nod the head forwards (craniovertebral flexion), taking the gaze down as spine flexion progresses. Continue the motion, reaching the ischial tuberosities towards the heels, progressing spine flexion and lifting the feet from the floor, taking the legs to act as a counterbalance with the body as it moves to balance between a central point

4

4

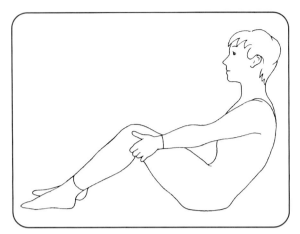

Figure 4.57A

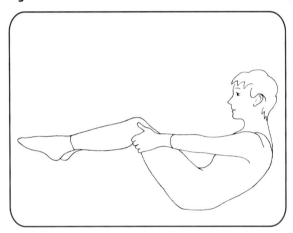

Figure 4.57B

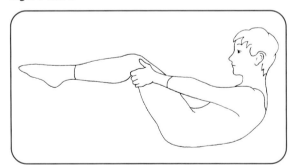

Figure 4.57C

over the base of the sacrum. Stabilize the hips and deepen the abdominal contraction to control sequential spine mobilization. Roll the body to the floor and rest in a supine position with approximately 90 degrees of hip/knee flexion (Fig. 4.57D).

Relax. Roll over to the side and sit up to repeat again. Repeat 5–10 times.

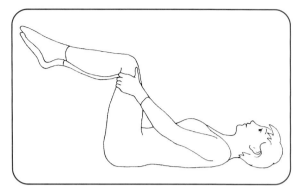

Figure 4.57D

Progression 4

Assisted Roll-Up.

Body position

Supine with the knees and hips flexed approximately 90 degrees. The feet are softly plantarflexed and the hands are on the backs of the thighs.

Action

Breathing in – strongly stabilize the pectoral girdle, activate the pelvic floor and hollow the lower abdominal muscles back to the spine. Maintaining an elongated spine, allow the head to nod, with the gaze moving towards the pubic bone, and initiate spine flexion.

Breathing out – further slide the shoulder blades down the back and broaden across the front of the chest. Increase spine flexion, moving the torso forwards as the backs of the thighs push lightly into the hands. Using the legs as a counterweight, peel the spine vertebra by vertebra away from the floor, moving through a central point over the base of the sacrum between which the upper body and legs balance. The motion continues until the legs and torso have achieved a sitting position with the feet on the floor.

Reach through the crown of the head to lengthen the spine and complete the motion. The gaze has moved with the head during the motion and is now directly forward.

Note: To achieve continuous, smooth motion, beginners may need to extend and flex the knees a little once or twice to increase momentum.

Roll onto the side and return to the semi-supine position to repeat.

Repeat 5–10 times.

Progression 5

Perform Progressions 2 and 3 consecutively.

Progression 6

Roll-Down.

Body position

Sitting upright with the spine in neutral and the front of the chest open and broad. The legs are extended in front of the body, drawn together with the knees facing the ceiling. The shoulders are flexed with the arms reaching forwards and the palms of the hands facing each other (Fig. 4.58A).

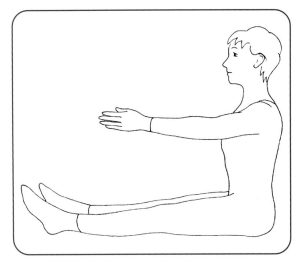

Figure 4.58A   Roll-Down – body position.

Action

Breathing in – with the gaze directly ahead, maintain breadth across the collarbones, stabilize the pectoral girdle, activate the pelvic floor muscles and hollow the abdominals back to the spine, elongating and flexing the spine.

Breathing out – drop the chin, flexing the head on top of the spine, and allow the gaze to move with the head. Allow the sternum to drop down and inwards as spine flexion progresses, sending the ischial tuberosities towards the heels and rolling the spine vertebra by vertebra to the floor. As the body rolls down the arms remain parallel with the floor until scapular contact is made. At this point allow the arms to float up to the ceiling and then over behind the head as the head descends to the floor (Figs 4.58B&C).

Breathing in and out – release the upper back into the floor, allowing the sternum to drop down and inwards as the cervical spine re-establishes its neutral position. The chin is slightly dropped and the superficial neck muscles should appear relaxed. The gaze is directly ahead.

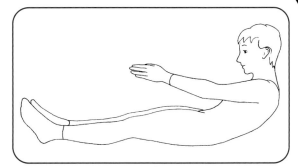

Figure 4.58B   Roll-Down – mid action.

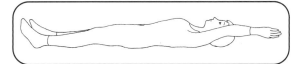

Figure 4.58C   Roll-Down – end of action.

Reverse shoulder flexion, moving the arms back through an arc to rest beside the hips. Relax. To repeat, roll over to one side and sit up. Repeat 5–10 times.

Progression 7

Roll-Up.

Body position

Supine. The legs are extended in front of the body, drawn together with the knees facing the ceiling. The shoulders are flexed with the arms extended over the head to rest on the floor. The elbows are soft, the palms face each other and the arms frame the face (Fig. 4.59A).

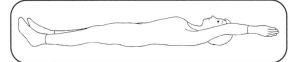

Figure 4.59A   Roll-up – body position.

Action

Breathing normally – stabilize the scapulae and bring the arms back to 90 degrees of shoulder flexion to reach the fingers for the ceiling. Further stabilize the pectoral girdle, activate the pelvic floor and hollow the lower abdominal muscles back to the spine.

Breathing in – flex the neck, nodding the head on top of the spine and moving the gaze with the head. Begin peeling the shoulders and upper torso away from the floor, maintaining 90 degrees of shoulder flexion and keeping the gaze ahead between the arms (Fig. 4.59B).

4

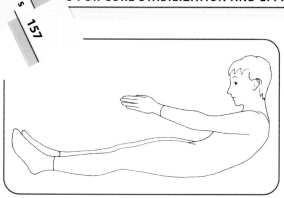

Figure 4.59B   Roll-Up – peeling the shoulders and upper torso away.

Improve pectoral girdle stability, then progress spine flexion to the sitting position by peeling the vertebra one by one away from the floor (Fig. 4.59C).

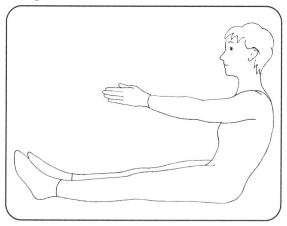

Figure 4.59C   Roll-Up – moving into upright position.

Breathing out – continue spine flexion to achieve an extended C-curve with the arms parallel with the floor and framing the face as the crown of the head reaches forward over the legs. The gaze has moved with the head and is now towards the legs.

Breathing in and breathing out – allow the arms to rest beside the legs. Breathe into the back, stretching the back muscles.

Breathing in – stabilize the scapulae to reach the arms forwards over the legs. Engage the pelvic floor and abdominal muscles and begin stacking the vertebrae one on top of the other above the sacrum.

Breathing out – continue spine extension, elongating the spine from above the sacrum to the base of the skull until the upright sitting position is achieved. Bring the arms forwards to reach in front of the body in preparation for the Roll-Down (Fig. 4.59D).

Common problems

■ Neck/shoulder tension: Cue for stronger pectoral girdle stabilization for the hands to support the

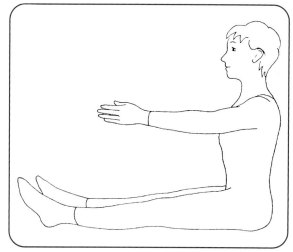

Figure 4.59D   Roll-Up – preparing for the next Roll-Down.

weight of the head. Consider moving the elbows slightly further forward.

■ Insufficient abdominal muscle control over lumbar spine stability: Cue for stronger lower abdominal muscle engagement and consider performing the exercise with the lumbar spine flattened, or with the legs further apart or further from the body.

■ Incorrect head/thoracic spine alignment: Cue to maintain length at the back of the neck and for the gaze to follow the movement of the head.

■ Unstable lower limb alignment: Place supports between the thighs and/or use visual imagery to encourage better leg alignment.

■ Tension in the groins, legs and feet: Consider performing the exercise with the lumbar spine flattened throughout and cue to release body tension.

See Table 4.27 for Teaching points.

> **Precautions**
> ■ **Chronic neck pathology** – cue for stronger pectoral girdle stabilization for the hands to give greater support to the weight of the head; consider moving the elbows slightly further forward.
> ■ **Back pathology** – ensure efficient abdominal muscle control over lumbar spine stability (see Modifications); seek medical advice if unsure.
> ■ **Pregnancy** – this may be an appropriate exercise for fit students in early pregnancy but always ensure good lower abdominal muscle control over lumbar spine stability.

Table 4.27   Teaching points – Sit ups

Focus on	Examples of verbal/visual cues
Correct pectoral girdle alignment and stabilization	Imagine the shoulder blades as snowboards sliding diagonally down towards the centre of the back Broaden across the collarbones
Achieving correct head and neck alignment without neck tension	Imagine you a holding a soft peach under the chin Cradle the head in the hands and feel how heavy it is
Relaxation of the face, throat and muscles of the back	Imagine you are going to drool
Lower limb/feet placement	Imagine strings from the ceiling suspending the knees in an upright position
Correct lower abdominal muscle activation	Hollow the abdominals towards the spine
Lumbar spine flattening during thoracic spine flexion	Allow the lower back to relax as the upper body curls
Achieving segmental vertebral column mobilization in spine flexion and extension	Imagine the spine peeling from the floor bone by bone as the upper body curls forwards Imagine the spine unravelling like a carpet roll as it returns to the floor

4

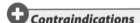

Contraindications

- Poor lower abdominal muscle strength.
- Advanced stages of pregnancy.
- Recent abdominal surgery.
- Abdominal, pelvic or back pain.
- Neck or shoulder pain.
- Osteoporosis.

Tactile cue suggestions

1. To cue and assist thoracic spine flexion – use one hand to gently but firmly press the base of the breastbone downwards and back towards the spine and the other to encourage thoracic spine flexion.
2. To assist spine mobilization during spine flexion/extension – anticipate vertebral mobilization with the fingers, walking them lightly along the spine.
3. To correct pectoral girdle alignment and stability – place the hands firmly over the scapulae to direct them down and across the back.

Exercise SAS24 – Sit ups with twist (oblique abdominal muscle strengthening)

Aim
To increase abdominal muscle control over the lumbar spine during upper torso flexion and rotation.
To improve rectus abdominis and oblique abdominal muscle strength and performance.

Equipment
Mat, firm bed, half barrel, box, gym ball.

Target muscles
For lumbar spine stability – the pelvic floor and transversus abdominis acting together isometrically.
For trunk flexion – rectus abdominis and the internal oblique abdominal muscles work concentrically to draw the ribcage towards the pelvis. They act eccentrically during the return from flexion.
For spine rotation to the left – the left internal obliques, the right external obliques, right multifidus and right rotator acting concentrically.
Note: Multifidus can produce rotation, lateral flexion and extension at all levels of the vertebral column whereas the rotatores can produce rotation in the thoracic spine only. As well as producing movement, both multifidus and the rotatores assist vertebral column stability during spine

mobilization where they act as extensible ligaments, adjusting their length to stabilize adjacent vertebrae irrespective of the position of the vertebral column.

For spine rotation to the right – the right internal obliques, left external obliques, left multifidus and left rotator acting concentrically.

For pectoral girdle stability – the isometric activity of latissimus dorsi and teres major, together with the middle and lower fibres of trapezius.

Body position

Supine with 90 degrees of hip and knee flexion and the spine in neutral. The arms are bent with the hands behind the head, the fingers interlocked so that the hands can cradle the head. The elbows are slightly forward and just within peripheral vision. The upper trapezius muscles are comparatively relaxed. This position is maintained throughout.

Preparatory action

Broaden across the collarbones and stabilize the scapulae. Activate the pelvic floor and hollow the lower abdominal muscles towards the spine.

Action

Breathing in.

Breathing out – further stabilize the scapulae and allow the passive flexion of the thoracic spine to drop the breastbone down and inwards, bringing the ribs nearer to the pelvis. Increase lower abdominal muscle activation and peel the upper body away from the floor (Fig. 4.60A).

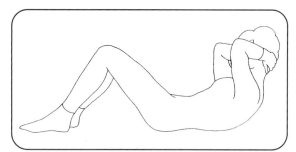

Figure 4.60A Sit ups with twist – spine flexion.

Note: Maintain the same head/cervical spine alignment, moving the head with the upper body and the gaze with the head.

Progress flexion and, as the lumbar spine flattens, rotate the upper torso to the left, facing the ribs towards the left hip.

Continue spine flexion/rotation, directing the right shoulder first towards the left knee then towards

the left hip as the lower ribs draw nearer to the hips. Stop when the end of range of independent thoracic spine flexion/rotation is reached.

Note: This can be monitored by recognizing tension beginning to occur in the groins, lower limbs or feet or by the body weight distribution changing under the back of the hips.

Breathing in – maintain good lower abdominal muscle control over the lumbar spine and reverse the motion, lengthening the spine as it rotates and the vertebrae roll one by one to the floor.

Breathing out – repeat to the right side.

Repeat 5–10 times to each side.

Modification

Perform beginning with the lumbar spine imprinted and the pelvis in a slight posterior tilt.

Progression 1

Perform with arm variation 1 – the right arm behind the head and the left arm reaching to the left as the body rotates to the left (Fig. 4.60B).

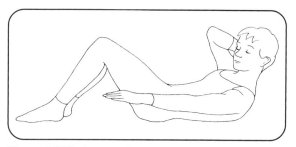

Figure 4.60B Sit ups with twist – progression 1.

Perform with arm variation 2 – the left arm behind the head and the right arm reaching across the body as the body rotates to the right (Fig. 4.60C).

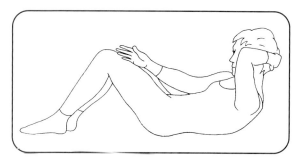

Figure 4.60C Sit ups with twist – progression 2.

Perform with arm variation 3 – the shoulders flexed forwards, the arms softly extended with the hands clasped together and palms facing the chest. As the body rotates to the left the hands reach to the left, then the right arm rotates medially as the left arm rotates laterally, further activating the pectoral girdle stabilizers. Repeat to alternate sides.

Progression 2

Perform with the feet resting on a gym ball with the knees and hips flexed approximately 70 degrees.

Progression 3
Body position

Perform with the right foot resting on a gym ball, the knee and hip flexed approximately 70 degrees and the left leg extended on the floor in line with the left hip.

Action

As the torso flexes and rotates to the right, increase hip flexion; as the torso moves out of flexion and rotation, reduce hip flexion. The left arm is behind the head with the right arm reaching to the right side or both hands remain behind the head.

Repeat several times to the right without allowing the upper back to return to the floor and increase hip and knee flexion/extension with each repetition. Repeat to the left side.

Common problems

- Neck/shoulder tension: Cue for stronger pectoral girdle stabilization for the hands to support the weight of the head; consider moving the elbows slightly further forward.
- Insufficient abdominal muscle control over lumbar spine stability: Cue for stronger lower abdominal muscle engagement and consider performing the exercise with the lumbar spine flattened, or with the legs further apart or further from the body.
- Incorrect head/thoracic spine alignment: Cue to maintain length at the back of the neck and for the gaze to follow the movement of the head.
- Compromised spine mobility: Practise exercises to increase ranges of motion in side flexion and rotation.
- Unstable lower limb alignment: Place supports between the thighs and/or use visual imagery to encourage better leg alignment.
- Tension in the groins, legs and feet: Consider performing the exercise with the lumbar spine flattened throughout and cue to release body tension.

See Table 4.28 for Teaching points.

⚠ Precautions

- Chronic neck pathology – cue for stronger pectoral girdle stabilization for the hands to give greater support to the weight of the head; consider moving the elbows slightly further forward.
- Back pathology – ensure efficient abdominal muscle control over lumbar spine stability (see Modifications); Seek medical advice if unsure.
- Pregnancy – this may be an appropriate exercise for fit students in early pregnancy but always ensure good lower abdominal muscle control over lumbar spine stability.

➕ Contraindications

- Poor lower abdominal muscle strength.
- Advanced stages of pregnancy.
- Recent abdominal surgery.
- Abdominal, pelvic or back pain.
- Neck or shoulder pain.
- Osteoporosis.

4

Tactile cue suggestions

1. To cue and assist thoracic spine flexion – use one hand to gently but firmly press the base of the breastbone downwards and back towards the spine and the other to encourage thoracic spine flexion.
2. To assist spine mobilization during spine flexion/extension – anticipate vertebral mobilization with the fingers, walking them lightly along the spine.
3. To correct pectoral girdle alignment and stability – place the hands firmly over the scapulae to direct them down and across the back.
4. To assist spine rotation – direct the shoulder towards the opposite knee.

PRONE SPINE MOBILIZATION (EXERCISES PSM25–26)

Exercise PSM25 – Cobra (spine mobilization in extension)

Aim

To correct head and cervical spine alignment.
To improve thoracic spine mobility in extension.

Table 4.28 Teaching points – Sit ups with twist

Focus on	Examples of verbal/visual cues
Correct pectoral girdle alignment and stabilization	Imagine the shoulder blades as snowboards sliding diagonally down towards the centre of the back Broaden across the collarbones
Achieving correct head and neck alignment without neck tension	Imagine you a holding a soft peach under the chin Cradle the head in the hands and feel how heavy it is
Relaxation of the face, throat and muscles of the back	Imagine you are going to drool
Lower limb/feet placement	Imagine strings from the ceiling suspending the knees in an upright position
Correct lower abdominal muscle activation	Visualize the pelvic floor muscles as an elevator moving to the top floor of a skyscraper
Lumbar spine flattening during thoracic spine flexion	Allow the lower back to relax as the upper body curls
Achieving segmental vertebral column mobilization in spine flexion and extension	Imagine the spine peeling from the floor bone by bone as the upper body curls forwards Imagine the spine unravelling like a carpet roll as it returns to the floor
Achieving thoracic spine rotation and flexion	Think of rotating from above the waist to twist the upper body As you twist the upper body, funnel the ribs down towards the pelvis As you twist and curl the upper body to the right, whisper with your left shoulder to your right hip

To improve abdominal muscle control over lumbar spine stability during thoracic spine extension.

To improve the flexibility of the rectus abdominis and oblique abdominal muscles.

Equipment

Mat or firm bed, foam roller.

Target muscles

For lumbar spine stability – the pelvic floor and transversus abdominis.

For pectoral girdle stability – gentle activation of the middle and lower fibres of trapezius, latissimus dorsi and teres major.

Body position

Prone with the arms beside the body, the hands placed approximately in line with the glenohumeral joints, the elbows reaching towards the heels. The back of the neck is lengthened with the chin slightly dropped towards the sternum so that the cervical curve is reduced and the neck muscles appear relaxed. The gaze is between the thumbs (Fig. 4.61A).

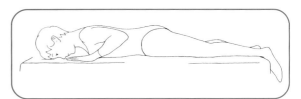

Figure 4.61A Cobra – body position.

Action

Breathing in – to prepare.

Breathing out – stabilize the scapulae and activate the pelvic floor and lower abdominal muscles to reach the elbows further towards the heels. Extend the neck, moving the head into correct head/thoracic spine alignment with the normal cervical curve intact (Fig. 4.61B).

Breathing in – maintaining abdominal muscle activation, slide the shoulder blades further down the back, moving the elbows towards the floor as if placing them in back pockets (Fig. 4.61C).

Breathing out – gently elongate and extend the thoracic spine simultaneously with elbow extension until

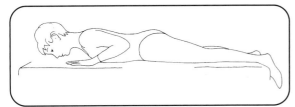

Figure 4.61B   Cobra – elongating the thoracic spine.

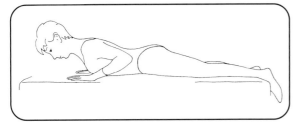

Figure 4.61C   Cobra – moving into spine extension.

the arms are straight and the hips and upper thighs are off the floor. The thoracic spine articulates sequentially as the upper body moves away from the floor to create a bow shape, extending from the crown of the head to the heels (Fig. 4.61D).

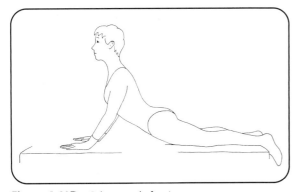

Figure 4.61D   Cobra – end of action.

The head maintains its neutral position throughout, moving only as an extension of the cervical and thoracic spine. The cervical spine curve remains intact and the gaze follows where the head leads.
Note: Initially thoracic back extension range of movement may be limited with the arms not fully extending.
Breathing in – maintaining scapulae stability and abdominal muscle control over the lumbar spine, further lengthen the spine to articulate it back to its starting position. At the end of the motion the cervical spine flexes to relax the neck muscles and drops the chin a little towards the sternum.
Breathing out – to begin the next repetition.
Repeat five to eight times.

Modification
Body position
Prone as in cobra but with the arms slightly abducted and the hands further forward. The palms face the floor and the elbows reach towards the heels. The back of the neck is lengthened with the chin slightly dropped towards the sternum so that the cervical curve is intact. The gaze is between the thumbs.

Action
Breathing in – reach through the crown of the head to lengthen the back of the neck.
Breathing out – keeping the forearms in contact with the floor and the pelvis in neutral, activate the pelvic floor and abdominal muscles and slide the shoulder blades down the back to move the thoracic spine into extension. The cervical curve remains intact and the gaze is to the floor (Fig. 4.62).

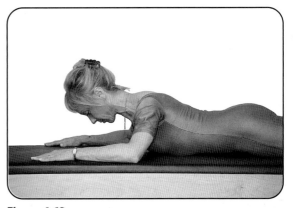

Figure 4.62

Breathing in – maintaining this position and abdominal muscle control, expand the back and sides of the ribcage, increasing spine length and thoracic extension. The chin may drop slightly to further lengthen the back of the neck (atlanto-occipital flexion).
Breathing out – lengthen through the crown of the head to articulate the spine back to its starting position.

Progression
Body position
Prone with the arms reaching over a foam roller (Fig. 4.63).

Action
Breathing in – reach through the crown of the head to lengthen the back of the neck.
Breathing out – keeping the cervical spine curve intact and the gaze to the floor, activate the pelvic floor and lower abdominal muscles to stabilize the

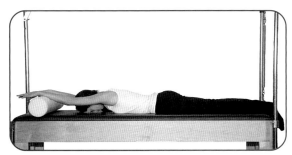

Figure 4.63

lumbar spine. Rotate the arms laterally so that the little finger moves towards the floor and slide the shoulder blades down the back. Feel that the arms are well supported by the roller and move it towards the body, extending the thoracic spine and lifting the upper torso away from the floor. Stop the movement when the end range of independent thoracic spine motion is reached.

Breathing in – maintaining this position and abdominal muscle control, expand the back and sides of the ribcage, increasing spine length and thoracic extension. The chin may drop slightly to further lengthen the back of the neck (atlanto-occipital flexion).

Breathing out – lengthen through the crown of the head and maintain scapular stability to begin medially rotating the arms, moving the roller away and articulating the spine back to its starting position.

Common problems

- Neck tension: Encourage lengthening through the back of the neck and engagement of the scapulae stabilizing muscles.
- Exaggerated lumbar spine extension: Cue for stronger pelvic floor and abdominal muscle activation, correct head/cervical spine alignment and spine elongation to release the lower back muscles; reduce the range of thoracic extension motion by not completing elbow extension.
- Exaggerated cervical spine extension: Instruct for correct use of gaze and cue to maintain space between the ears and tips of the shoulders.
- Poor spine mobility: Emphasize spine elongation and begin with a small range of extension motion; practise alternative exercises to mobilize the spine in side flexion and rotation.
- Insufficient pectoral girdle/upper limb strength to move into full spine extension: Practise alternative exercises for upper limb strength, emphasize pectoral girdle stabilization and reduce the range of spine extension by performing the motion lying over a half barrel or gym ball.

- Painful wrists during body weight bearing: Place the hands on yoga blocks so that the fingers drop forwards over the blocks and the angles of the wrists are reduced.

See Table 4.29 for Teaching points.

ⓘ Precautions
- Discomfort in the back during exercising – ensure alignment is correct with good abdominal muscle control throughout; spine pathology such as arthritis and facet joint problems can be irritated by spine extension; seek medical advice if unsure.
- Osteoporosis – beware loaded lumbar spine extension as this carries the risk of vertebral fracture.
- Prevention of lumbar spine loading – ensure a well-supported and elongated spine throughout; limit the range of thoracic spine extension if required to prevent hyperextension of the lumbar spine; seek medical advice if unsure.
- Lower back/spine pathology or surgery – seek medical advice if unsure.
- Shoulder pathology.

✚ Contraindications
- Painful wrist, shoulder lower back or spine pathology – for onward referral.
- Advanced stages of osteoporosis.
- Advanced stages of pregnancy.

Tactile cue suggestions

1. To increase breadth across the front of the chest – use the hands to stroke the collarbones as the spine moves into extension.
2. To promote spine elongation – lightly place one hand on the lower back and run the other hand up the spine to rest on the crown of the head.
3. To encourage the superficial neck muscles to remain comparatively relaxed – gently place the thumb and third finger of the left hand just below the occipital tuberosities to direct the head forwards and correct cervical spine alignment. The right hand can assist in supporting and directing the forehead as required.

4. To correct pectoral girdle alignment and stability – use the hands to direct the shoulder blades down and across the back.
5. To correct the relationship between the upper and lower torso during spine extension – use the hands to funnel the ribs down towards the pelvis.
6. To promote spine articulation – lightly move the fingers along the spine, anticipating joint mobilization.
7. To assist spine extension – place the left hand on the sternum, gently directing it forwards and upwards and the right hand on the back opposite the left hand directing the spine to lengthen and move inward.

Exercise PSM26 – Arrow (thoracic spine mobilization and strengthening)

Aim
To correct head and cervical spine placement.
To improve thoracic spine mobility in extension.
To improve the resting alignment of the pectoral girdle.
To improve the stability of the pectoral girdle.
To improve abdominal muscle control over spine stability during thoracic spine extension.

To improve the performance of the erector spinae muscles.

Equipment
Mat or firm bed, a small support for the forehead.

Target muscles
For lumbar spine stability – the pelvic floor and transversus abdominis.
For pectoral girdle stability – gentle activation of the middle and lower fibres of trapezius, latissimus dorsi and teres major.
For spine extension and return from spine extension – erector spinae acting concentrically during spine extension and eccentrically on the return from extension.

Body position
Prone with the arms medially rotated resting beside the body. The shoulders are relaxed, the elbows are extended and the palms face the ceiling. The forehead may rest on a small support to correct cervical spine alignment. The chin is slightly dropped towards the sternum so that the back of the neck is lengthened. The crown of the head reaches away from the top of the spine (Fig. 4.64A).

Action
Breathing in – lift the outer tips of shoulders away from the floor and broaden across the front of the

Table 4.29 Teaching points – Cobra

Focus on	Examples of verbal/visual cues
Efficient abdominal control throughout	Tighten the pelvic floor muscles and hollow the lower abdominal area
Length through the front of the hip as the spine extends	Release the front of the hip and reach the legs away
Shoulder alignment and girdle stability	Imagine the shoulder blades sliding down across the back
Extending the neck to move the head into a neutral position (cranio/vertebral flexion)	Imagine rolling a golf ball along the floor with your chin Stop when you feel that the cervical spine is lengthened and that you could hold a soft peach between your chin and collarbones
Correct spine length at the beginning of spine extension	Imagine a light on the breastbone shining first on the floor under you then along the floor to where the floor and wall meet in front of you
Correct dynamic alignment of the head and cervical spine	Move the gaze along the floor in front of the body and then up the wall in front as the spine extends
Correct spine articulation	Imagine light or air between the vertebrae as the spine peels away from the floor bone by bone

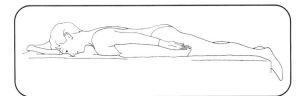

Figure 4.64A Arrow – body position.

chest to correctly align the pectoral girdle. Lift the
arms to align beside the body.

Breathing out – reach the fingers for the heels and
stabilize the scapulae, moving them down the back
as if placing them in back hip pockets.
Simultaneously activate the pelvic floor and lower
abdominal muscles together with gentle lower
gluteus maximus engagement.

Slide the shoulder blades further down the back,
lifting the arms higher and reach through the
crown of the head as the thoracic spine moves into
and completes its full range of extension motion
(Fig. 4.64B).

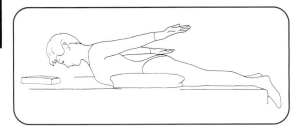

Figure 4.64B Arrow – end of extension action.

Note: The pelvis should remain in neutral with the
lumbar spine lengthened and stable. Where
possible, the thoracic kyphosis is reversed as the
thoracic spine reaches its end range of extension
motion. The chin is still softly dropped towards the
sternum with the gaze to the floor (craniovertebral
flexion), the neck muscles being comparatively
relaxed as the crown of the head reaches forwards
and the arms reach backwards.

Breathing in – lengthen more through the crown of the
head and slide the shoulder blades further down
the back, possibly lifting the arms and sternum a
little higher.

Breathing out – renew abdominal muscle activation as
required for lumbar spine stability to lengthen and
articulate the spine back to its starting position.

Rest, allowing the shoulders to release forwards to the
floor.

Repeat initially up to five times and build towards 10
repetitions.

Modification 1

Prepare by performing the sequence without lifting
the body from the floor.

Modification 2

Perform with a reduced range of extension motion.

Modification 3

Body position

Kneeling with the front torso resting over a gym ball
as in a modified cat position. The hips are flexed
approximately 80–90 degrees.

Note: This position is extremely useful for students
with tight hip flexors and/or poor thoracic spine
mobility. The ball facilitates independent thoracic
spine movement and prevents lumbar spine and
hip extension.

Action

Perform as in the basic exercise and monitor the range
of thoracic extension motion.

Modification 4

Perform with a small (tennis ball sized), reasonably
firm but compliant ball placed under the chest at
the level of the body of the sternum. Roll the ball
forwards as the spine moves into extension.

Progression 1

Perform as in the basic exercise and, as spine
extension completes, take the extended arms to
reach overhead with the palms of the hands facing
the floor. Hold for one or two breathing cycles
before returning to the starting position.

Progression 2

Preparation for swimming: Perform Progression 1 and,
whilst maintaining spine extension with the arms
reaching overhead and keeping the hips neutral in
rotation, lengthen the legs out of the hip joints and
float the legs away from the floor. Hold for one or
two breathing cycles before returning to the starting
position.

Common problems

- Neck tension: Instruct the student to keep the gaze
to the floor.
- Exaggerated lumbar spine extension: Encourage
stronger pelvic floor and abdominal muscle
activation, together with lengthening through the
crown of the head.
- Lumbar spine instability: Instruct the student to
activate the lower fibres of gluteus maximus as
required; reduce the range of thoracic extension
motion.
- Poor spine articulation: Begin with a small range of
extension motion and ensure that good pectoral

girdle alignment and stabilization are achieved throughout.

■ Poor erector spinae performance: Practise modifications and the quadriped exercise series.

See Table 4.30 for Teaching points.

Tactile cue suggestions

1. To increase breadth across the front of the chest – use the hands to stroke across the collarbones as the spine moves into extension.
2. To encourage the superficial neck muscles to remain comparatively relaxed – gently place the thumb and third finger of the left hand just below the occipital tuberosities to direct the head forwards and correct cervical spine alignment. The right hand can assist in supporting and directing the forehead as required.
3. To promote spine elongation – lightly place one hand on the lower back and run the other hand up the spine to rest on the crown of the head.
4. To correct pectoral girdle alignment and stability – use the hands to direct the shoulder blades down and across the back.
5. To correct the relationship between the upper and lower torso during spine extension – use the hands to direct the ribs down towards the pelvis.
6. To promote spine articulation – lightly move the fingers along the spine, anticipating joint mobilization.
7. To assist spine extension – place the left hand on the sternum, gently directing it forwards and upwards and the right hand on the back opposite the left hand directing the spine to lengthen and move inward.
8. To assist lumbar spine stability – encourage lower gluteal muscle activation by gently tapping with the fingers or by directing the gluteal creases to move towards each other.

SIDE LYING SPINE MOBILIZATION (EXERCISE SLM27)

Exercise SLM27 – Chest opener with spine twist (shoulder and thoracic spine mobilization)

Aim

To promote spine elongation.

To improve abdominal muscle control over lumbar spine stability during thoracic spine mobilization.

To increase thoracic spine mobility in rotation.

To improve pectoral girdle alignment and stability.

To stretch the anterior chest muscles.

Equipment

Mat or raised bed, head support as required for correct alignment and comfort, pillow or other support for behind the upper back or under the arm to monitor spine rotation.

Target muscles

For shoulder flexion – pectoralis major, coracobrachialis and the anterior fibres of the deltoid.

For shoulder abduction – the deltoid and supraspinatus assisted by infraspinatus and the long head of biceps.

For shoulder adduction – pectoralis major, latissimus dorsi and teres major assisted by teres minor, short head of biceps and coracobrachialis.

Table 4.30 Teaching points – Arrow

Focus on	Examples of verbal/visual cues
Efficient abdominal control and core stability throughout	Tighten the pelvic floor and hollow the abdominal muscles Draw the sitting bones together
Length through the front of the hip as the spine extends	Release the front of the hip and reach the legs away
Limiting neck tension	Keep the gaze towards the floor Imagine a delicate object being held between the chin and the collarbones
Strong engagement of the pectoral girdle stabilizing muscles	Face the palms of the hands towards the ceiling and imagine placing them in someone's hands as they lift Lengthen through the crown of the head and reach through the little fingers to slide the shoulder blades down across the back
Lengthening the thoracic spine as spine extension begins and progresses	Imagine a light on the breastbone first shining along the floor and then a little way up a wall in front of you as the chest lifts away from the floor
Thoracic spine mobilization	Curl the spine in from just under the bra strap (women only) Move the spine between the shoulder blades towards the breastbone

4

For scapular stability – all three parts of trapezius act together to pull the scapula towards the midline. It is assisted by the rhomboids, latissimus dorsi and teres major.

For maintaining lumbar spine stability – the combined action of the pelvic floor and transverse and oblique abdominals.

For thoracic spine rotation to the right – the right internal obliques, left external oblique abdominals and left erector spinae act together concentrically to initiate rotation then eccentrically to counteract the effects of gravity as the upper torso turns towards the ceiling.

For return to side lying from rotation to the right – the left external oblique abdominals and left erector spinae, together with the right internal oblique abdominals, act concentrically to counteract the effects of gravity.

Body position

Side lying on the right side, with the arms flexed and resting on the floor in front of the body slightly below shoulder height. The glenohumeral joints are neutral in rotation and adducted so that the left palm faces and rests on the right (Fig. 4.65A).

Action

Breathing in – to prepare.

Breathing out – activate the pelvic floor and lower abdominal muscles and elongate the spine,

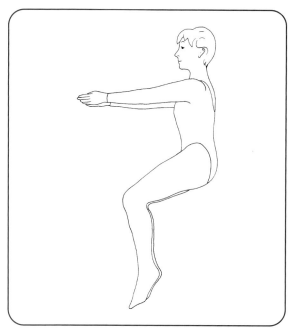

Figure 4.65A Side lying spine mobilization – body position.

reaching from the crown of the head through to the ischial tuberosities whilst maintaining the normal spinal curves.

Breathing in – broaden across the front of the chest, stabilize the left scapula, moving it down the back as if placing it in the right back hip pocket, maintain abdominal muscle control and rotate the upper torso to the left. Move the left arm as a unit with the body until it reaches to the ceiling directly above the left glenohumeral joint (Fig. 4.65B).

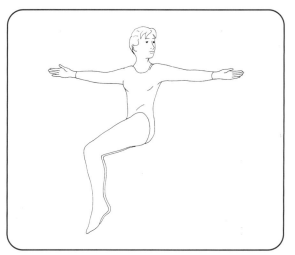

Figure 4.65C   Side lying spine mobilization – end range of action.

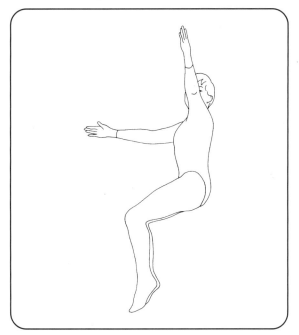

Figure 4.65B   Side lying spine mobilization – mid action.

Note: The head moves with the spine and the eyes move with the head, then the gaze follows the line of the arm to its fingers as they reach for the ceiling.

Breathing out – maintaining abdominal muscle control, continue rotating the torso and arm as a unit until the arm rests on the floor or, if spine rotation is limited, on a suitable support (Fig. 4.65C).

Note: The eyes continue to gaze at the fingers as the arm moves towards the floor.

Breathing in – maintaining abdominal muscle control, reverse the motion, keeping the upper torso and left arm as a unit until the left arm once again reaches for the ceiling.

Note: The eyes continue to gaze at the fingers.

Breathing out – further engage the abdominal muscles and continue rotating the torso and arm as a unit back to the starting position.

Repeat three to five times on each side.

Common problems

■ For spine alignment and stability problems: Focus on correct starting alignment with the normal spinal curves intact; cue to engage the abdominal muscles before the action begins and to rotate the

upper torso from above the waist; cue to move the arm and upper torso as one unit; monitor the range of thoracic spine rotation by placing supports for the upper back or arm to rest on.

■ Poor thoracic spine mobility in rotation: Use visual imagery cues to initiate spine rotation from the thoracic vertebrae; practise in conjunction with spine mobilizing exercises in lateral flexion – for example, sitting side bending and mermaid.

■ Inability to sequence the breathing with the motion: Cue for a relaxed breathing cycle and focus on abdominal muscle control throughout.

See Table 4.31 for Teaching points.

! Precautions

■ Discomfort in the lower back during exercising – ensure sufficient abdominal control to prevent lumbar spine extension.

■ Shoulder pathology – monitor the pectoral girdle position and consider performing with the elbow flexed and the hand on the shoulder; use supports behind the upper back for the arm to rest on as the chest turns to the ceiling.

■ Osteoporosis – monitor carefully and ensure rotation motion occurs in the thoracic and not the lower lumbar spine.

■ Pregnancy – always know the stage of pregnancy and ensure position and motion are comfortable and without side effects.

■ Lower back/spine pathology/surgery – ensure the motion is pain free; know where movement does not occur as in cases of spinal fusion or rod insertion; seek medical advice if unsure.

Table 4.31 Teaching points – Side lying spine mobilization

Focus on	Examples of verbal/visual cues
Maintaining a well-aligned spine and the correct relationship between the upper and lower torso as the spine rotates	Reach the crown of the head and the sitting bones in opposite directions Maintain spine length as the chest turns to the ceiling
Good abdominal muscle control over the lumbar spine	Before moving, draw up the pelvic floor muscles and tighten the lower abdominal muscles
Moving the arm and upper body as one unit	Think of moving the upper body and arm in one piece
Rotation in the thoracic spine only stretching the anterior chest muscles	Turn the ribcage from above the waist
Coordinated head and arm motions	As the arm moves towards the floor, feel a stretch from the collarbone to the little finger Follow the fingers with the eyes

4

✚ *Contraindications*

- Painful shoulder, upper limb, lower back or spine pathology – for onward referral.
- Advanced stages of pregnancy.

Tactile cue suggestions

1. To encourage spine elongation – place one hand lightly on the top of the head to direct it up and away from the spine.
2. Before the ribcage turns – walk the fingers up the spine and rest them approximately where spine rotation is to occur.
3. To correct the relationship between the upper torso and the pelvis – use the hands to direct the ribs to funnel down towards the pelvis.
4. To assist pectoral girdle stability – use the hand to direct the shoulder blades to slide down and across the back.
5. To correct the arms – dynamic alignment guides each one through its motion.

KNEE STRENGTHENING (EXERCISE KS28)

Exercise KS28 – Quadriceps strengthening

Aim

To address imbalances within the quadriceps group of muscles and improve their overall performance.
To specifically improve the performance of vastus medialis.

Equipment

Mat or firm flat bed, pillows or a triangle to support the head and curl the upper back, a small rolled towel or triangle to support the back of the knee.

Target muscles

For core control – the pelvic floor and transversus abdominis.
For knee extension – the quadriceps.
For the final 10–20 degrees of knee extension – vastus medialis.

Body position

Lying on the back with the upper body flexed so that the back and head lie supported on a triangle or pillows. The inactive leg is extended and the active leg is flexed by placing a small towel or triangle at the back of the knee. The hip is neutral in rotation with the knee facing the ceiling and the feet are relaxed (Fig. 4.66A).

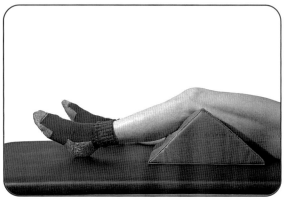

Figure 4.66A

Action

Breathing in – to prepare.

Breathing out – activate the pelvic floor and lower abdominal muscles just sufficiently to stabilize the lumbar spine and trunk. Gently dorsiflex the foot of the active leg and begin to extend the knee. Reach the toes for the ceiling and extend the leg without pushing the knee backwards into its support (Fig. 4.66B).

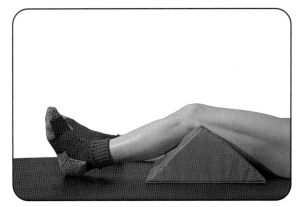

Figure 4.66B

Breathing in – maintaining abdominal control, plantarflex the foot.

Breathing out – increasing abdominal action, dorsiflex the foot.

Breathing in – maintaining abdominal control, plantarflex the foot.

Breathing out – increasing abdominal action, dorsiflex the foot and gently control knee flexion to allow the heel to return.

Variation

Perform with the active leg in lateral rotation and focus on vastus medialis action during the final 10–20 degrees of extension (Figs 4.66C&D).

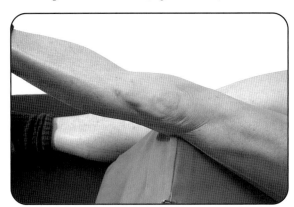

Figure 4.66C

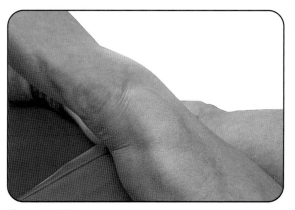

Figure 4.66D

Progression 1

Body position

Perform with the active leg in lateral rotation.

Action

Breathing in – to prepare.

Breathing out – activate the pelvic floor and lower abdominal muscles just sufficiently to stabilize the lumbar spine and trunk. Gently dorsiflex the foot of the active leg and begin to extend the knee. Reach the toes for the ceiling and extend the leg without pushing the knee backwards into its support. Reach the heel away and focus on vastus medialis action during the final 10–20 degrees of extension.

Breathing in.

Breathing out – increase pelvic floor and lower abdominal muscle activation to further stabilize the trunk, then lift the extended leg slightly off its supporting surface.

Breathing in – maintaining abdominal muscle control, gently return the leg to its starting position.

Progression 2

Perform Progression 1 until the leg is fully extended, then abduct the leg as it lifts away from its supporting surface.

Progression 3

Perform Progressions 1 and 2 using light leg weights.

Common problems

- Loss of trunk stability: Use sufficient back supports to adequately flexed the trunk for efficient abdominal muscle control; where required, cue for stronger abdominal muscle control.
- Inability to fully extend the knee: Cue to reach through the back of the knee and for the heel to

4

Table 4.32 Teaching points – Quadriceps strengthener

Focus on	Examples of verbal/visual cues
Correct starting position	Ensure that and head, back and leg are sufficiently supported for comfort
Stabilizing the torso before the lower limb moves	Lightly activate the pelvic floor and gently hollow the lower abdominals
Maintaining torso stability throughout	Maintain abdominal muscle control and allow the sitting bones to drop onto the floor as the knee extends
Correct dynamic lower limb alignment	Imagine the kneecap as a light shining on the ceiling Align the second and third toes with the centre of the knee Observe the big toe reaching for the ceiling as the knee extends
Vastus medialis action as the knee moves towards full extension	Observe the upper inner knee area and draw the muscles upwards as the leg extends
Length through the back of the leg	Imagine your heel is going to touch the wall as it reaches away

reach away as the knee extends; consider hamstring and calf muscle flexibility as well as tight structures at the back of the knee.

■ Inability to fully engage vastus medialis: Cue to pull the inner knee muscles up as the leg moves towards full extension.

■ Loss of foot alignment during plantarflexion and extension: Cue to align the second and third toes with the centre of the knee joint and the axis of the hip joint.

See Table 4.32 for Teaching points.

Precautions

■ Ongoing knee pathology – monitor for pain-free activity seek medical advice if unsure.
■ The use of leg weights – monitor for pain-free activity seek medical advice if unsure.

Contraindications

■ Knee pain during exercise – tight hip abductors together with weak hip adductors and/or tight hamstrings will alter patella tracking and knee mechanics; for onward referral.
■ Adolescent knee pain – for onward referral.

Tactile cue suggestions

1. To assess vastus medialis activation – instruct the student to place a hand on the upper inner knee to locate vastus medialis as the knee moves towards extension.
2. Length through the back of the knee – the teacher or student may lightly stroke the back of the knee as it extends.
3. To promote lengthening the leg out of the hip joint – lightly touch the heel as the leg reaches away.

References

Oliver J 1999 Back in line. Butterworth-Heinemann, Oxford
Sahrmann SA 2002 Diagnosis and treatment of movement impairment syndromes. Mosby, St Louis

Chapter 5

Anatomy review – the upper limb

PECTORAL GIRDLE

BONES AND JOINTS

The pectoral girdle on each side comprises three bones – the scapula, clavicle and coracoid – together with the three sternoclavicular, acromioclavicular and glenohumeral joints:

- The clavicle links the scapula to the sternum by means of the acromio- and sternoclavicular joints, respectively. The scapula is also slung by several powerful muscles from the skull, vertebral column and thoracic cage – the so-called scapulothoracic articulation.
- The coracoid, poorly developed in humans, exists only as a small process joined to the scapula close to its glenoid rim.
- The humerus articulates with the glenoid fossa of the scapula at the glenohumeral joint.

It is this arrangement – involving the three joints, together with the attachments of the whole girdle to the skull, vertebral column and thoracic cage – that gives the upper limb such an extensive range and freedom of movement. However, such mobility can only come at the expense of stability when the upper limb is used for weight bearing and other such physical activities.

The powerful muscles attaching the pectoral girdle to the upper body achieve shoulder stability. In addition, this musculature acts as a shock absorber when weight bearing with the upper limbs, whilst the clavicle can act as a strut to steady and brace the pectoral girdle, especially during abduction of the upper limb.

Scapula

Normal alignment

The scapula lies against the posterior thoracic cage overlying the second to the seventh ribs inclusive, its medial border parallel to, and about three fingers breadth from, the middle of the back. It lies flat against the thorax, rotated 30 degrees anterior to the frontal plane, in contact with the curvature of the ribcage.

The scapulothoracic articulation

The scapula moves by gliding over the underlying ribs and muscles of the posterolateral surface of the thoracic cage. The specific movements involved are elevation, depression, medial and lateral rotation. Scapular elevation and depression have an approximate linear range of 10–12 cm and these movements are usually accompanied by some degree of rotation. With scapular elevation the glenoid fossa tends to face more upwards and, with depression, downwards.

The scapula rotates around an axis located just below the medial end of its spine over a range of about 60 degrees. This involves a lateral displacement of its inferior angle of 10–12 cm, and a medial displacement of the superolateral angle of 5–6 cm.

Humerus

The humerus is the proximal long bone of the upper limb, connecting the pectoral girdle with the forearm.

Normal alignment

When viewed from the side, less than one-third of the humeral head should normally protrude in front of the acromion process. The antecubital crease at the elbow joint faces anteriorly during neutral rotation whilst the olecranon process faces posteriorly and the palm of the hand faces the side of the body. The proximal and distal ends of the humerus should be in the same vertical plane when viewed from the side, the front or the back (Sahrmann 2002, p. 198).

Glenoid fossa and glenohumeral joint

Normal alignment

The shoulders should be positioned slightly below the horizontal axis through T1 in the front and back view. In the side view, the plumb line should bisect the acromion (Sahrmann 2002, p. 194).

The glenoid fossa is a shallow, saucer-shaped articular depression at the lateral border of the scapula, deepened only slightly by a fibrous rim. The ball and socket arrangement of the glenohumeral joint allows movement to occur around innumerable axes intersecting at the head of the humerus. This makes it the most mobile joint in the body and its movements are described as flexion, extension, abduction, adduction, and medial and lateral rotation, but, like the whole pectoral girdle, this inherently unstable arrangement requires the support of powerful musculature.

Scapulohumeral rhythm

When upper limb movement also begins to involve scapular rotation, the glenoid fossa travels in an arc of which the clavicle forms the radius and the relative positions of clavicle and scapula change at both the acromio- and sternoclavicular joints.

During the first 60 degrees of shoulder flexion and 30 degrees of shoulder abduction the movement of the scapula is highly variable. Inman et al (1994) termed this

the *setting phase*. After the *setting phase* the humerus and scapula move in a constant ratio. A ratio of 2 degrees of glenohumeral motion for 1 degree of scapulothoracic motion results in 120 degrees of glenohumeral joint motion and 60 degrees of scapula motion at the completion of shoulder flexion. More recent studies have reported variability in the exact timing of that motion (Sahrmann 2002, p. 202).

MUSCLES THAT STABILIZE AND MOVE THE SCAPULA AND PECTORAL GIRDLE AS A WHOLE

Scapula stabilization

This is achieved through the combined action of trapezius, the rhomboids, levator scapulae, serratus anterior and pectoralis minor.

The *trapezius* has an important function in stabilizing the scapula as a base for upper limb movements. Its middle horizontal fibres pull the scapula towards the midline and its upper and lower fibres can produce a resolved force towards the midline by contracting together.

The upper fibres of trapezius elevate the pectoral girdle and maintain the level of the shoulders against the effects of gravity or when a weight is being carried in the hand.

When both left and right muscles contract together they can produce neck extension and when acting alone the upper fibres produce lateral neck flexion. The lower fibres pull down the medial part of the scapula and lower the shoulder, especially against resistance – for example when getting out of a chair. The upper and lower fibres acting together produce lateral rotation of the scapula.

The *rhomboids* are important stabilizers for the scapula when other muscles are active. They also retract the scapula and are active in medial rotation of the pectoral girdle.

Levator scapulae act together with trapezius to produce elevation and retraction of the pectoral girdle or to counteract its downward movement as when carrying a weight in the hand. They also help to stabilize the scapula and are active in resisting its medial rotation.

Serratus anterior is a major protractor of the pectoral girdle and is involved in all thrusting, pushing and punching movements where the scapula is driven forwards, carrying with it the upper limb. During upper limb flexion, or when a weight is carried in front of the body, serratus anterior acts to maintain the contact between the medial border of the scapula and the chest wall.

Pectoralis minor acts anteriorly whilst the rhomboids and levator scapulae act posteriorly to stabilize the scapula during upper limb extension. When leaning on the hands it helps to transfer the weight of the trunk to the upper limb. In addition, its insertion into the coracoid process allows it to pull the scapula forwards and downwards during punching and pushing movements and to help produce medial rotation against resistance (Palastanga et al 2002, p. 62, 65–66).

Pectoral girdle stabilization

This is achieved through the actions of latissimus dorsi, teres major and pectoralis major, together with the muscles involved in scapular stabilization.

Latissimus dorsi is a strong extensor of the flexed arm and a strong adductor and medial rotator of the humerus at the shoulder joint. If the humerus is fixed relative to the scapula it protracts the pectoral girdle. Latissimus dorsi is also attached to the inferior angle of the scapula and this allows it to assist scapular stability during upper limb movements.

Teres major acts with latissimus dorsi to adduct and medially rotate the humerus at the shoulder joint and also helps to extend the flexed arm. It also assists shoulder joint stability together with latissimus dorsi and pectoralis major.

Pectoralis major is a powerful adductor and medial rotator of the humerus at the shoulder joint. In addition, its clavicular head can flex the humerus approximately 60 degrees whilst its sternocostal head can then extend the flexed humerus. As one of the main muscles for climbing, it pulls the trunk upwards when the arms are fixed above the head. It also acts during pushing, punching and throwing to move the humerus powerfully forwards as the pectoralis minor and serratus anterior protract the pectoral girdle.

Muscles such as subscapularis counterbalance pectoralis major to align and stabilize the humerus in the glenoid fossa.

Summary of muscles that stabilize the scapula and the pectoral girdle

- Protraction – serratus anterior and pectoralis minor.
- Retraction – rhomboid minor, rhomboid major and trapezius and, if the humerus is fixed relative to the scapula, latissimus dorsi.
- Elevation – trapezius (upper fibres) and levator scapulae.
- Depression – trapezius (lower fibres) and serratus anterior (lower fibres).

- Lateral rotation – trapezius and serratus anterior.
- Medial rotation – rhomboids major and minor, pectoralis minor and levator scapulae.

MUSCLES THAT STABILIZE AND MOVE THE HUMERUS IN THE GLENOID FOSSA

The glenohumeral joint is stabilized by the tone and proximity to the joint of the rotator cuff muscles and by the muscles that pass between the pectoral girdle and the humerus, such as the long heads of biceps and triceps.

Rotator cuff muscles

Supraspinatus initiates humeral abduction up to approximately 20 degrees, placing the humerus into a position that allows the deltoid to continue with the motion. During this action it braces the humeral head firmly against the glenoid fossa, thus preventing an upwards dislocation of the humeral head. This stabilizing action continues as abduction progresses.

Infraspinatus laterally rotates the humerus in the glenoid fossa and, together with the other rotator cuff muscle tendon units, assists glenohumeral joint stability by its close proximity to the joint. Their combined actions also firmly brace the humeral head against the glenoid fossa during upper limb weight bearing.

Teres minor is a lateral rotator of the humerus; when the arm is in an abducted position it acts to both laterally rotate and adduct the arm. Together with the other rotator cuff muscles it also produces glenohumeral joint stability.

Subscapularis is a strong medial rotator of the humerus and it may be active during upper limb adduction. During upper limb movement it also helps to maintain the humeral head within the glenoid fossa and during deltoid and biceps activity it helps to prevent an upward displacement of the humeral head.

Coracobrachialis is a weak glenohumeral joint flexor and is active during resisted upper limb adduction.

The *deltoid* is the main glenohumeral joint abductor after the supraspinatus has initiated the motion by approximately 20 degrees. The anterior fibres of deltoid flex and medially rotate the humerus; the posterior fibres extend and laterally rotate the humerus. During resisted upper limb adduction the posterior fibres counteract the medial rotation produced by pectoralis major and latissimus dorsi.

Biceps brachii is a powerful elbow joint flexor and supinator of the forearm. It also flexes and helps to stabilize the arm at the glenohumeral joint.

The *triceps* extends the elbow joint and its long head can adduct the arm and extend it from a flexed position.

5

Summary of muscles involved in specific movements of the glenohumeral joint

- Flexion – anterior fibres of deltoid, clavicular head of pectoralis major, coracobrachialis and biceps.
- Extension – posterior fibres of deltoid, teres major and latissimus dorsi. When active extension is performed from a flexed position this also involves the long head of triceps and the sternal fibres of pectoralis major. Passive extension from flexion is essentially due to the eccentric action of the shoulder flexors.
- Abduction – supraspinatus initiates abduction and the deltoid continues the motion.
- Adduction – under the influence of gravity this is produced by the eccentric contraction of serratus anterior, trapezius, deltoid and supraspinatus. During resisted adduction pectoralis minor, teres major, latissimus dorsi and coracobrachialis are active.
- Medial rotation – subscapularis, pectoralis major, latissimus dorsi, teres major and the anterior fibres of the deltoid.
- Lateral rotation – infraspinatus, teres minor and the posterior fibres of the deltoid.

ELBOW JOINT

5

BONES, MOVEMENTS AND THE MUSCLES INVOLVED

The elbow joint lying between the arm and the forearm comprises the articulating surfaces of the distal humeral trochlea and the trochlear notch of the proximal end of the ulna. It is a hinge joint that allows movement for flexing and extending the forearm.

Elbow movements and the main muscles involved

The elbow joint is a simple hinge joint and its movements are flexion and extension – increasing the angle at the elbow to move the forearm towards, and decreasing the angle to move the forearm away from the shoulder, respectively.

The radioulnar joint is a separate unit that, by allowing the radial head to rotate within the radial notch of the ulna, allows pronation and supination of the forearm. When the elbow is flexed during pronation, the palm of the hand moves from facing upwards to facing downwards, and during supination the palm of the hand moves from facing downwards to facing upwards.

Elbow flexion

- Biceps brachii
- Brachialis
- Brachioradialis.

Biceps brachii has two heads, the long head originating from above the superior lip of the glenoid fossa and the short head from the coracoid process of the scapula and the upper lip of the glenoid fossa. The two heads become two fleshy muscle bellies that merge into one muscle just below the middle of the arm. Its insertion is into the posterior part of the radial tuberosity and the bicipital aponeurosis, a strong membranous band that attaches to the deep fascia on the ulnar side of the forearm.

Biceps brachii is a powerful elbow joint flexor and forearm supinator, its actions being enhanced when flexing the elbow with the forearm supinated and when supinating the forearm with the elbow flexed.

Brachialis originates from the lower half of the anterior aspect of the arm and attaches to the coronoid process and tuberosity of the ulna. Its single attachment to the non-rotating ulna makes it the main elbow joint flexor as it produces pure flexion irrespective of forearm pronation or supination.

Brachioradialis is a superficial muscle that extends from its origin from the distal two-thirds of the humerus to its insertion into the distal lateral aspect of the radius. It is an important elbow stabilizer and acts to bring about elbow flexion when the forearm is midway between pronation and supination. It also assists forearm pronation to supination as far as the neutral position.

Elbow extension

- Triceps brachii
- Anconeus.

Triceps brachii has three heads, the long head arising from below the inferior lip of the glenoid fossa of the scapula, the lateral head from the upper, posterior aspect of the humerus and the medial head from the lower posterior aspect of the humerus. The three muscles form the palpable bulk at the back of the arm and their attachments merge to form one tendon that inserts into the olecranon process of the ulna. Triceps brachii is the main extensor of the elbow and its long head also adducts and extends the arm at the glenohumeral joint.

Anconeus is a small triangular muscle lying just behind the elbow joint. It originates from the posterior surface of the lateral humeral condyle and is inserted into the posterior surface of the ulnar olecranon process. Anconeus contracts together with triceps brachii to produce elbow extension, and is also thought to abduct and extend the ulna so as to assist rotation of the radius around the distal end of the ulna during pronation.

Forearm pronation

- Pronator teres
- Pronator quadratus
- Brachioradialis.

Pronator teres has two heads originating from the distal, medial aspect of the humerus and the proximal, medial aspect of the ulna, and their muscles fibres pass downwards and laterally to finally merge as a flattened tendon that is inserted into the middle third of the lateral surface of the radius. The muscle is comparatively easy to palpate and can be felt running along the medial border of the antecubital fossa at the elbow, particularly during resisted pronation. To produce pronation it pulls the radius forwards and medially to swing it over the ulna. Pronator teres also plays a minor role during elbow flexion.

Pronator quadratus lies in the distal quarter of the forearm, deep within the flexor compartment. It originates from the anterior aspect of the ulna and the fibres pass transversely to insert into the anterior aspect of the radius. The transverse fibres help to stabilize and maintain the relationship between the radius and ulna, and protect the distal radioulnar joint during weight bearing with the hand. Pronator quadratus initiates forearm pronation and, when acting with the triceps as it extends the elbow, it will produce forearm pronation.

Brachioradialis assists forearm pronation to supination as far as the neutral position.

Forearm supination

- Supinator
- Biceps brachii
- Brachioradialis.

The *supinator* muscle surrounds the upper head of the radius, deep within the muscular structures of the proximal forearm. It arises by a humeral head attached to the lateral, distal aspect of the humerus and an ulnar head attached to the neighbouring posterior part of the ulna. The fibres pass downwards and laterally and are inserted into the proximal, lateral surface of the radius just below the radial head. Actions that comprise supination with the elbow extended such as turning a screwdriver require supinator activity.

Biceps brachii is a powerful supinator of the forearm, its actions being enhanced when flexing the elbow with the forearm supinated and when supinating the forearm with the elbow flexed.

Brachioradialis supinates the forearm from the pronated position to neutral.

WRIST JOINT

BONES, MOVEMENTS AND THE MUSCLES INVOLVED

The wrist and hand together contain 29 bones including the distal radius and ulna. There are numerous joints, muscles, ligaments and nerves that allow the fine, controlled hand movements required for many everyday activities. Wrist joint movement mainly occurs at the radiocarpal joint, formed between the articular surfaces of the distal end of the radius and the scaphoid, lunate and triquetrum bones of the proximal carpal row. It is a condyloid joint and allows up to 90 degrees of flexion, 85 degrees of extension, 40 degrees of adduction and 25 degrees of abduction.

The numerous bones of the hand include the remaining carpal and metacarpal bones and the phalanges. The joints include the intercarpal joints between the individual carpal bones and the midcarpal joint between the proximal and distal rows of carpal bones. The intercarpal joints provide only small motions that accompany and enhance radiocarpal and midcarpal joint action. The midcarpal joint acts as a single unit that, like the wrist joint, allows flexion, extension, abduction and adduction around axes passing through the head of the capitate bone, but to a much lesser degree.

The complicated arrangement of more than 30 muscles that move the wrist and hand comprises those that move the wrist but not the fingers, those that primarily move the fingers but also assist wrist function, and the small intrinsic muscles within the hand that move the fingers and thumb independently. In this text the main flexors and extensors of the wrist itself have been selected for discussion as they are brought into play during all activities that involve wrist mobilization and stabilization for upper limb weight bearing. Wrist movements range from the fine, controlled motions for handwriting and keyboard work to the large, powerful actions needed when playing tennis or golf. Joint stabilization is important during wrist mobilization and essential for efficient weight bearing with the upper limbs.

Muscles that flex, extend, adduct and abduct the wrist joint

Flexion, abduction, adduction

- Flexor carpi ulnaris
- Flexor carpi radialis
- Palmaris longus.

Flexor carpi ulnaris lies along the medial border of the forearm. It is a superficial muscle that can be identified and palpated in the upper medial forearm during wrist

5

flexion against resistance. It originates from the radius and ulna and attaches via tendons into the palmar surfaces of the pisiform, hamate and fifth metatarsal bones. It acts with flexor carpi radialis and palmaris longus to flex the wrist and, together with extensor carpi ulnaris, produces wrist adduction.

Flexor carpi radialis lies along the lateral aspect of the forearm. It is also a superficial muscle that can be identified as the most lateral of the tendons on the anterior aspect of the wrist during wrist flexion with abduction. It originates from the medial epicondyle of the humerus and is inserted into the bases of the second and third metacarpal bones. It acts powerfully with flexor carpi ulnaris and palmaris longus to flex the wrist and produces abduction together with extensor carpi radialis longus and extensor carpi radialis brevis.

Palmaris longus, not always present, is a small superficial muscle running down the middle of the forearm. It originates from the medial epicondyle of the humerus and is attached to the palmar superficial flexor retinaculum and the aponeuroses of the second, third, fourth and fifth metacarpals. It assists flexor carpi ulnaris and flexor carpi radialis during wrist flexion.

Extension, abduction, adduction

- Extensor carpi radialis longus
- Extensor carpi radialis brevis
- Extensor carpi ulnaris.

Extensor carpi radialis longus lies in the posterior compartment of the lateral forearm. It originates from the lateral supracondylar ridge and lateral epicondyle of the humerus and is inserted into the posterior surface of the base of the second metacarpal. It acts with extensor carpi radialis brevis and extensor carpi ulnaris to produce wrist extension, and they all act together with flexor carpi radialis to produce wrist abduction.

Extensor carpi radialis brevis lies in the posterior compartment of the forearm, near to and possibly fused with extensor radialis longus. It originates from the lateral epicondyle of the humerus and is inserted into the posterior surface of the base of the third metacarpal bone. It acts with extensor carpi radialis longus and extensor carpi ulnaris to produce wrist extension, and they all act together with flexor carpi radialis to produce wrist abduction.

Extensor carpi ulnaris originates from the lateral epicondyle of the humerus and inserts into the medial side

of the base of the fifth metacarpal. It acts with extensor carpi radialis longus and extensor carpi radialis brevis to produce wrist extension and it acts with flexor carpi ulnaris to produce wrist adduction.

Muscles that primarily move the fingers but also assist with wrist function

- *Flexor digitorum superficialis* flexes the fingers at the metacarpophalangeal and proximal interphalangeal joints; it assists wrist flexion.
- *Flexor digitorum profundus* flexes the fingers at the metacarpophalangeal, proximal and distal interphalangeal joints; it assists wrist flexion.
- *Flexor pollicis longus* of the thumb flexes the carpometacarpal, metacarpophalangeal and interphalangeal joints; it assists wrist flexion.
- *Extensor digitorum* extends the fingers at the metacarpophalangeal joints and assists interphalangeal joint extension; it assists wrist extension.
- *Extensor digiti minimi* extends the little finger at the metacarpophalangeal joint; it assists wrist extension.
- *Extensor indicis* extends the index finger at the metacarpophalangeal joint enabling it to be used independently; it assists wrist extension.
- *Extensor pollicis longus* extends all the joints of the thumb; it assists wrist extension and abduction.
- *Extensor pollicis brevis* extends the thumb at the metacarpophalangeal joints; it possibly assists wrist extension and abduction against resistance.
- *Abductor pollicis longus* abducts the thumb at the carpometacarpal joint; it possibly assists wrist abduction.

There are many other small muscles that enable the complex mechanisms required for various intricate hand movements but as this text is mainly concerned with correct exercise techniques for addressing postural faults these muscles are not considered individually here.

References

Inman VT, Saunders JB, Abbott LC 1994 Observations of the function of the shoulder joint. J Bone Joint Surg Am 32:1–30
Palastanga N, Field D, Soames R 2002 Anatomy and human movement, 4th edn. Butterworth-Heinemann, Oxford
Sahrmann SA 2002 Diagnosis and treatment of movement impairment syndromes. Mosby, St Louis

5

Chapter 6

Upper body, stretching and overall joint mobilization exercises

The pectoral girdle is the most mobile set of articulating surfaces in the body allowing, with respect to the trunk, approximately 180 degrees of shoulder flexion, abduction and rotation, and 90 degrees of shoulder extension. However, this mobility is to some degree at the expense of shoulder stability, which is nevertheless essential for providing a firm base for upper limb movement and weight bearing.

Shoulder stability is facilitated by correct pectoral girdle alignment and the following exercises aim to improve alignment as well as overall function. This is to help prevent shoulder injuries during everyday activities and provide a sound foundation for the Pilates and comparable exercise systems. The series begins with basic scapular movements and then progresses to cover more complex sequences, but the order of these may be rearranged as required.

As discussed in Chapter 1, poor pectoral girdle alignment and its consequences are both associated with postural faults, and they must always be considered together when dealing with defective pectoral girdle function.

EXERCISE LIST

BASIC UPPER BODY EXERCISES

Supine pectoral girdle mobilization (Exercises UBE1–5)

UBE1	Shoulders forwards and back
UBE2	Shoulder shrugs
UBE3	Bilateral arm arcs
UBE4	Chest opener
UBE5	Arm arcs with arms in opposition, arm arcs with half circles, arm circles

Sitting pectoral girdle mobilization (Exercises UBE6–7)

UBE6	Shrugs
UBE7	Chest opener

Sitting spine and pectoral girdle mobilization (Exercises UBE8–10)

UBE8	Spine twist
UBE9	Side bending
UBE10	Spine curls

Prone pectoral girdle mobilization and stabilization (Exercises UBE11–12)

UBE11   Batman
UBE12   Sphinx

*Side lying pectoral girdle stabilization and
strengthening (Exercise UBE13)*
UBE13   Side lifts

STRETCHING, JOINT MOBILIZATION AND EXERCISES TO IMPROVE FOOT ALIGNMENT, MOBILITY AND STRENGTH

*Improving foot alignment, mobility and strength
(Exercises FM1–3)*
FM1   Exercising the forefoot
FM2   Ankle mobilization
FM3   Exercising the lower limb and foot

*Stretching the posterior hip and lower limb
(Exercises ST1–18)*
ST1   Calf muscle stretch
ST2   Hamstring muscle stretch
ST3   Tensor fasciae latae stretch
ST4   Gluteal and hamstring stretch
ST5   Iliopsoas stretch
ST6   Quadriceps stretch
ST7   Adductor stretch
ST8   Supine back stretch
ST9   Spine stretch
ST10   Neck stretch
ST11   Neck, shoulder and upper back
         stretch
ST12   Sitting back stretch
ST13   Prone back stretch
ST14   Standing back stretch
ST15   Spine roll down and up
ST16   Spine curl
ST17   Hip rolls with stretch
ST18   Front of chest stretch

BASIC UPPER BODY EXERCISES

SUPINE PECTORAL GIRDLE MOBILIZATION (EXERCISES UBE1–5)

Exercise UBE1 – Shoulders forwards and back (scapular protraction and retraction)

Aim
To protract and retract the scapulae.
To improve the resting alignment of the scapulae.
To increase scapular and shoulder joint mobility.
To enhance scapular stability.
To improve abdominal muscle control over lumbar
    spine stability during independent upper limb
    movement.

Equipment
Mat or firm flat bed, pillow or neck support, a small
    rolled towel or chi ball for between the knees.

Target muscles
For shoulder flexion – pectoralis major (up to 60 degrees
    then the deltoid takes over), coracobrachialis and
    the anterior fibres of the deltoid.
For scapular protraction (abduction) – serratus anterior
    acting to draw the scapula forwards and
    downwards over the underlying ribcage; pectoralis
    minor helps to produce medial rotation of the
    scapula against resistance, thereby drawing its
    upper lateral border downwards onto the ribcage.
For scapular retraction (adduction) – the middle fibres of
    trapezius acting to draw the medial border of the
    scapula towards the spine, the rhomboids acting to
    draw the scapulae towards each other.
For scapular stability – all three parts of trapezius acting
    together to pull each scapula towards the midline,
    assisted by the rhomboids, latissimus dorsi and
    teres major.
For maintaining lumbar spine stability – the combined
    action of the pelvic floor and transversus
    abdominis.

Body position
Supine, the legs hip distance apart with approximately
    90 degrees of hip/knee flexion. The shoulders are
    flexed approximately 90 degrees with the fingers
    reaching for the ceiling and the palms of the hands
    facing each other. The scapulae are drawn gently
    downwards over the lower ribs and the anterior
    chest muscles are released, allowing the shoulders
    to drop back to the floor (Fig. 6.1).

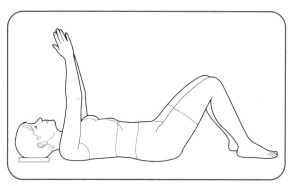

Figure 6.1   Body position – shoulders forwards and back.

Action
Breathing in – to prepare.
Breathing out – gently activate the pelvic floor and
    lower abdominal muscles to stabilize the lumbar
    spine.

Breathing in – maintaining breadth across the front of the chest, protract the pectoral girdle, allowing the scapulae to abduct and glide forwards around the ribcage.

Breathing out – adduct the scapulae and glide them back to their starting position, allowing the shoulders to release back to the floor.

Breathing in – to begin the next repetition.

Repeat 5–10 times.

Note: The fingers reach softly for the ceiling and the lumbar spine/pelvis remain neutral and stable throughout.

Common problems

■ Upper body/neck tension: Ensure sufficient head and neck support for correct alignment and comfort. On the exhalation, cue for the neck muscles to release, the thoracic cage to relax and monitor abdominal muscle control over lumbar spine stability.

■ Insufficient abdominal muscle control over lumbar spine stability: Consider performing the exercise with an imprinted lumbar spine and raising the feet; cue for improved pelvic floor and lower abdominal muscle action.

■ Poor lower limb alignment: Place a chi ball or other soft support between the knees.

Note: if there is impaired scapular alignment and mobility associated with postural faults (e.g. exaggerated thoracic kyphosis), consider:

■ improving thoracic spine mobility, particularly in extension

■ manually assisting scapular depression during shoulder flexion

■ increasing flexibility in levator scapulae, upper trapezius and the pectoral muscles

■ improving the performance of the lower and middle fibres of trapezius, the rhomboids and latissimus dorsi.

See Table 6.1 for Teaching points.

Precautions
■ Neck and shoulder pathology – provide sufficient support for comfort; monitor to ensure that the range of movement is appropriate and pain free; seek medical/ physiotherapy advice if unsure.
■ Back or spine pathology – consider performing the exercise with an imprinted lumbar spine and/or raising the feet and cue for improved pelvic floor and lower abdominal muscle activation; perform in an upright position.

Contraindications
■ Painful neck or shoulder pathology – for onward referral.

Tactile cue suggestions

1. To cue transversus abdominis muscle activation – before exercising, instruct the student to place the fingers on the lower portion of the anterior abdominal wall just above the pubic bone, to feel the area tightening as the pelvic floor and lower abdominal muscles contract. Then instruct the student to place the hands around the waist to feel that the oblique abdominal muscles remain comparatively relaxed as the lower abdominal muscles are activated.

2. To correct the relationship between the upper and lower torso – before exercising, instruct the student to place the thumbs over the lowest floating ribs and the little fingers over the anterior superior iliac spine (ASIS) to feel the space between these two landmarks. Explain that this space should be maintained as the pectoral girdle muscles are activated and the upper limbs move. The teacher may use their hands to direct the ribs in and down towards the pelvis.

3. To improve scapular mobility and dynamic alignment – the teacher's hands may be used to guide each scapula through abduction, adduction and return to starting position.

Exercise UBE2 – Shoulder shrugs (scapular elevation and depression)

Aim
To elevate and depress the scapulae.
To improve the resting alignment of the scapulae.
To increase scapulae and shoulder joint mobility.
To enhance scapula stability.
To improve abdominal muscle control over lumbar spine stability during independent upper limb movement.

Equipment
Mat or firm flat bed, pillow or neck support, a small rolled towel or bolster for between the knees.

Target muscles
For scapular elevation – upper fibres of trapezius, the rhomboids and levator scapulae.

6

Table 6.1 Teaching points – Shoulders forwards and back

Focus on	Examples of verbal/visual cues
Relaxation of the neck and upper body	Imagine you are going to drool Imagine the body imprinting itself in warm sand
Vertebral column length	Reach the crown of the head and the sitting bones away from each other
Correct resting scapular alignment	Release the front of the shoulders and allow the shoulder blades to sink back to the floor Imagine the shoulder blades imprinting their images into the floor
Length through the arms as they reach for the ceiling	Imagine the arms begin where the breastbone and collarbones join Imagine a ball of energy circling between the ears and the shoulders as the fingers reach for the ceiling
Maintaining a stable lumbar spine	Imagine the pelvic floor as a magic carpet lifting gently Imagine the pelvis as a bowl of water and the surface of the water is absolutely level and still
Scapular mobility during protraction	Imagine the shoulder blades gliding forwards around the ribcage
Scapular mobility during retraction	Imagine the shoulder blades gliding around and hugging the ribcage as they move back and down to rest on the floor
Lower limb stability	Imagine the knees are suspended from the ceiling by strings

For scapular depression – lower fibres of trapezius acting to pull the medial border of the scapula downwards; the lower fibres of serratus anterior acting to draw the lower, lateral border of the scapula downwards and forwards; pectoralis minor acting to pull the upper part of the scapula downwards onto the ribcage.

For scapular stability – all three parts of trapezius acting together to pull each scapula towards the midline, assisted by the rhomboids, latissimus dorsi and teres major.

For maintaining lumbar spine stability – the combined action of the pelvic floor and transversus abdominis.

Body position

Supine, the legs hip distance apart with approximately 90 degrees of hip/knee flexion. The arms rest beside the body with the palms facing the floor. The scapulae are drawn gently downwards over the lower ribs and the anterior chest muscles are released, allowing the shoulders to drop back to the floor (Fig. 6.2A).

Action

Breathing in – to prepare.

Breathing out – gently activate the pelvic floor and lower abdominal muscles to stabilize the lumbar spine.

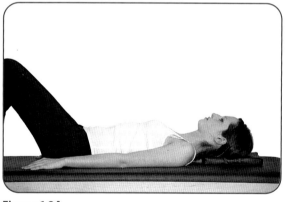

Figure 6.2A

Breathing in – maintaining the anterior chest muscle release so that the backs of the shoulders still make contact with the floor, raise the shoulders towards the ears (Fig. 6.2B).

Breathing out – release the shoulders and allow the scapulae to glide down the back to the starting position (Fig. 6.2C).

Breathing in – maintaining the anterior chest muscle release, lightly press the little fingers into the floor and depress the shoulders. Reach the hands for the heels and allow the scapulae to slide over the floor as they draw down towards the centre of the back.

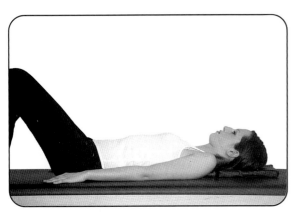

Figure 6.2B

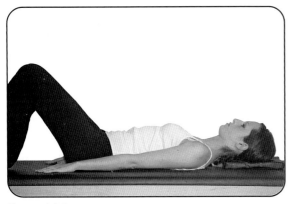

Figure 6.2C

Breathing out – release shoulder depression and
allow the scapulae to glide back to their starting
position.
Repeat 5–10 times.

Common problems

■ Upper body/neck tension: Provide sufficient
head/neck support for correct alignment and
comfort. On the exhalation, cue for the neck
muscles to release, the thoracic cage to relax
and monitor abdominal muscle control over the
lumbar spine stability.
■ Insufficient abdominal muscle control over lumbar
spine stability: Consider performing the exercise
with an imprinted lumbar spine and raising the
feet and cue for improved pelvic floor and lower
abdominal muscle activation.
■ Poor lower limb alignment: Place a chi ball or other
soft support between the knees.

See Table 6.2 for Teaching points.

(!) Precautions

■ Neck and shoulder pathology – provide
sufficient support for comfort; monitor
to ensure that the range of movement is
appropriate and pain free; seek medical/
physiotherapy advice if unsure.
■ Back or spine pathology – consider performing
the exercise with an imprinted lumbar spine
and/or raising the feet and cue for improved
pelvic floor and lower abdominal muscle
activation.

(+) Contraindications

■ Painful neck or shoulder pathology – for
onward referral.

Tactile cue suggestions

1. To cue transversus abdominis muscle
activation – before exercising, instruct the
student to place the fingers on the lower
part of the anterior abdominal wall just above
the pubic bone to feel the area tightening as
the pelvic floor and lower abdominal muscles
contract. Then instruct the student to place
the hands around the waist to feel that the
oblique abdominal muscles remain
comparatively relaxed as the lower
abdominal muscles are activated.
2. To correct the relationship between the upper
and lower torso – before exercising, instruct
the student to place the thumbs over the
lowest floating ribs and the little fingers over
the ASIS to feel the space between these two
landmarks. Explain that this space should be
maintained as the pectoral girdle muscles are
activated and the upper limbs move. The
teacher may use the hands to direct the ribs in
and down towards the pelvis.
3. To improve scapular mobility and dynamic
alignment – the teacher's hands may be
used to guide the scapulae through elevation,
depression and return to starting position.

Exercise UBE3 – Bilateral arm arcs (shoulder joint flexion)

Aim

To improve trapezius and deltoid muscle performance.
To increase scapular and shoulder joint mobility.

6

Table 6.2   Teaching points – Scapula elevation and depression

Focus on	Examples of verbal/visual cues
Relaxation of the neck and upper body	Imagine you are going to drool Imagine the body imprinting itself in warm sand
Breadth across the front of the torso	Broaden across the collarbones and allow the shoulders to drop back to the floor. Maintain this contact throughout
Spine elongation	Lengthen from the crown of the head through to the sitting bones
Length through the arms with the shoulders dropping back towards the floor	Imagine the arms begin where the breastbone and collarbones join before reaching the fingers for the toes
Maintaining a stable lumbar spine	Hollow the lower abdominal area Imagine the pelvis as a bowl of water and the surface of the water is absolutely level and still
Scapular mobility during elevation	Imagine the outer tips of the shoulders touching the posterior portion of the ear lobes
Scapular mobility during depression	Imagine the shoulder blades as skis gliding down and across the back to the opposite sides
Lower limb stability	Imagine the knees are suspended from the ceiling by strings

To enhance scapular stability during upper limb movement.

To improve abdominal muscle control over lumbar spine stability during independent upper limb movement.

Equipment

Mat or firm flat bed, pillow or neck support, a small rolled towel or bolster for between the knees; a beach ball, small gym ball or magic circle to hold in the hands.

Target muscles

For shoulder lateral rotation – infraspinatus, teres minor and the posterior fibres of the deltoid.

For shoulder flexion – pectoralis major (up to 60 degrees then the deltoid takes over), coracobrachialis and the anterior fibres of the deltoid.

For scapular stability – all three parts of trapezius acting together to pull each scapula towards the midline, assisted by the rhomboids, latissimus dorsi and teres major.

For maintaining lumbar spine stability – the pelvic floor and transversus abdominis acting together.

Body position

Supine, the legs hip distance apart with approximately 90 degrees of hip/knee flexion. The glenohumeral joints are medially rotated and flexed approximately 90 degrees. The elbows are slightly flexed and the hands are approximately

shoulder width apart holding a small gym ball or magic circle above the sternum. The anterior chest muscles are released, allowing the shoulders and upper back to release back to the floor. The scapulae are drawn gently down across the back (Fig. 6.3A).

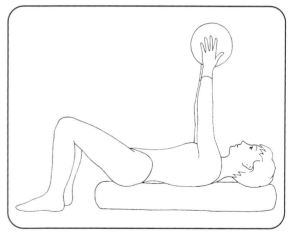

Figure 6.3A   Bilateral arm arcs – body position using a bolster.

Action

Breathing in – to prepare.

Breathing out – gently activate the pelvic floor and lower abdominal muscles and allow the sternum to drop downwards with the passive spinal flexion that occurs during exhalation. Maintaining the upper back in contact with the floor, increase shoulder flexion to carry the hands over the head to the end range of independent shoulder joint flexion (Fig. 6.3B).

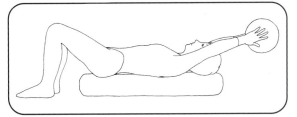

Figure 6.3B Arm arcs – end range of shoulder flexion.

Breathing in – rest for a moment.
Breathing out – improve abdominal muscle engagement and begin gently extending the elbows, allowing the scapulae to abduct.
Breathing in – rest for a moment to stretch the scapular adductors.
Breathing out – reverse the motion, allowing the scapulae and arms to return to the starting position.
Repeat three to five times and build to 10 repetitions, aiming to increase the range of scapula motion with each repetition.

Progression 1

Perform standing approximately one foot length away from a wall with the knees slightly flexed and the spine in neutral supported by the wall.

Progression 2

Perform Progression 1, emphasizing depression of the scapulae during shoulder flexion.

Common problems
- Limited range of independent shoulder joint movement (observed by the occurrence of lumbar spine extension during shoulder joint flexion): Reduce the range of flexion by blocking the overhead motion of the arm with a stack of yoga blocks, a triangle or pillow placed near the head; cue to maintain the relationship between the lower ribs and the pelvis and for stronger pelvic floor and lower abdominal engagement.
- Upper body/neck tension: Provide sufficient head and neck support for correct alignment and comfort. On the exhalation, cue for the throat to soften, the thoracic cage to relax and monitor abdominal muscle control over lumbar spine stability.
- Insufficient abdominal muscle control over lumbar spine stability: Consider raising the feet, performing

the exercise with a flattened lumbar spine throughout and cue for improved lower pelvic floor and lower abdominal muscle activation.
- Poor lower limb alignment: Place a chi ball or other soft support between the knees.

See Table 6.3 for Teaching points.

 Precautions
- Neck and shoulder pathology – provide sufficient support for comfort; monitor to ensure that the range of movement is appropriate and pain free; seek medical/physiotherapy advice if unsure.
- Back or spine pathology – consider performing the exercise with an imprinted lumbar spine and raising the feet, and cue for improved pelvic floor and lower abdominal muscle activation; alternatively, perform sitting with the back supported against a wall or foam roller.

✚ Contraindications
- Painful neck or shoulder pathology – for onward referral.

Tactile cue suggestions

1. To cue transversus abdominis muscle activation – before exercising, instruct the student to place the fingers on the lower part of the anterior abdominal wall just above the pubic bone to feel the area tightening as the pelvic floor and lower abdominal muscles contract. Then instruct the student to place the hands around the waist to feel that the oblique abdominal muscles remain comparatively relaxed as the lower abdominal muscles are activated.
2. To correct the relationship between the upper and lower torso – before exercising, instruct the student to place the thumbs over the lowest floating ribs and the little fingers over the ASIS to feel the space between these two landmarks. Explain that this space should be maintained as the pectoral girdle muscles are activated and the upper limbs move. Use the hands to direct the lower ribs in and down towards the pelvis.
3. To improve scapular stability – before exercising, instruct the student to flex the right

6

shoulder approximately 90 degrees so that the right arm is raised, with the elbow softly bent. The teacher's left hand should be placed over the right scapula to hold and stabilize it (the thumb forward in the armpit and the fingers on the back just below the spine of the scapula). The right hand is placed over the shoulder with the fingers just medial to the acromion process. As the right shoulder increases flexion, the hands are used firmly to assist scapula depression (Fig. 6.3C).

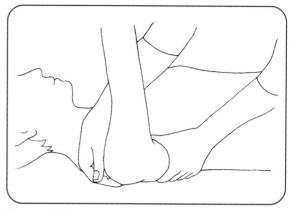

Figure 6.3C Assisting scapula depression.

Exercise UBE4 – Chest opener (shoulder joint flexion, abduction and adduction)

Aim

To improve the performance and flexibility of the pectoral muscles.

To increase shoulder joint mobility.

To enhance scapular stability during upper limb movement.

To improve abdominal muscle control over lumbar spine stability during independent upper limb movement.

Equipment

Mat or firm flat bed, pillow or neck support, a small rolled towel or bolster for between the knees, light hand weights (0.5–1 kg/1.1–2.2 lb).

Table 6.3 Teaching points – Bilateral arm arcs

Focus on	Examples of verbal/visual cues
Relaxation of the neck and upper back	Imagine the body imprinting itself in warm sand
A correctly aligned and lengthened spine	Imagine holding a soft peach between the chin and the sternum Lengthen through the back of the neck Reach the sitting bones towards the heels and the crown of the head away from the shoulders
Maintaining a stable lumbar spine and the correct relationship between the upper torso and the pelvis throughout	Tighten the pelvic floor muscles Imagine the pelvis as a bowl of water and the surface of the water is absolutely level and still On breathing out, imagine the ribs closing together and funnelling down towards the pelvis as the breastbone drops back towards the spine
Breadth across the front and back of the torso	Broaden across the collarbones and the back of the chest
Length through the arms	Imagine the arms begin where the collarbones join the breastbone before reaching the arms away. As the arms lift, allow the arm bones to drop down into the shoulder joints and visualize the shoulder blades gliding down the back
Scapular depression at the end range of flexion	As the arms move to the ear, imagine the shoulder blades sliding down the back
Lower limb stability	Imagine the feet are sinking in warm sand Imagine holding a small, soft beach ball between the knees

Target muscles

For shoulder flexion – pectoralis major, coracobrachialis and the anterior fibres of the deltoid.

For shoulder abduction – the deltoid and supraspinatus, assisted by infraspinatus and the long head of biceps.

For shoulder adduction – pectoralis major, latissimus dorsi and teres major, assisted by teres minor, short head of biceps and coracobrachialis.

For scapular stability – all three parts of trapezius acting together to pull each scapula towards the midline, assisted by the rhomboids, latissimus dorsi and teres major.

For maintaining lumbar spine stability – the combined action of the pelvic floor and transversus abdominis.

Body position

Supine with the legs hip distance apart. The chest is open with breadth across the clavicles, the upper back is relaxed and the scapulae are drawing gently down the back. The glenohumeral joints are flexed to 90 degrees. The elbow joints are slightly flexed so that the arms create a rounded position as if hugging a large ball. The palms of the hands face toward the sternum with the fingers in a neutral position (Figs 6.4A&B).

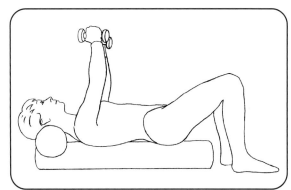

Figure 6.4A

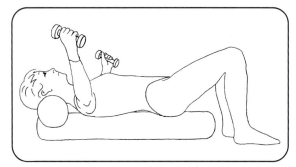

Figure 6.4B

Action

Breathing in – to prepare.

Breathing out – gently activate the pelvic floor and lower abdominal muscles to stabilize the lumbar spine. Maintaining elbow flexion, increase scapular stabilization before abducting the arms fully or until a stretch is felt across the front of the chest.

Breathing in – maintaining breadth across the clavicles and, with the upper back in contact with the floor, return the arms along the same pathway to the starting position.

Breathing out – to begin the next repetition.

Repeat 5–10 times.

Modification 1

Perform with the pelvis in a slight posterior tilt and the lumbar spine imprinted.

Modification 2

Reduce the range of shoulder joint abduction.

Progression 1

Reverse the breathing.

Progression 2

Use hand weights to increase exercise intensity.

Progression 3

Perform lying along a foam roller. Although this progression requires greater mental concentration and core control, the instability of the roller also increases pelvic floor and lower abdominal muscle action.

Common problems

- Upper body/neck tension: Ensure sufficient head and neck support for correct alignment and comfort. On the exhalation, cue for the throat to soften, the thoracic cage to relax and for pectoral girdle stabilization.
- Impaired scapular stability: Consider reducing the range of motion and cue for increased breadth across the front of the chest and for stronger pectoral girdle muscle engagement.
- Poor dynamic alignment: Cue to trace the arms through the same arc in space.
- Insufficient abdominal muscle control over lumbar spine stability: Consider raising the feet, performing the exercise with an imprinted lumbar spine

6

throughout and cue for improved pelvic floor and lower abdominal muscle action.

■ Poor lower limb alignment: Place a chi ball or other soft support between the knees.

See Table 6.4 for Teaching points.

! Precautions

■ **Neck and shoulder pathology – provide sufficient support for comfort; monitor to ensure that the range of movement is appropriate and pain free; seek medical advice if unsure.**

■ **Back or spine pathology – provide sufficient support for comfort; ensure sufficient abdominal muscle control over lumbar spine stability; consider raising the feet or performing with the lumbar spine flattened.**

■ **Recent neck, shoulder or elbow injury – seek medical advice about the stage of recovery and the suitability of specific shoulder girdle exercises.**

✚ Contraindications

■ Painful neck or shoulder pathology – for onward referral.

Tactile cue suggestions

1. To cue transversus abdominis muscle activation – before exercising, instruct the student to place the fingers on the lower part of the anterior abdominal wall just above the pubic bone to feel the area tightening as the pelvic floor and lower abdominal muscles contract. Then instruct the student to place the hands around the waist to feel that the oblique abdominal muscles remain comparatively relaxed as the lower abdominal muscles are activated.

2. To correct the relationship between the upper and lower torso – before exercising, instruct the student to place the thumbs over the lowest floating ribs and the little fingers over the ASIS to feel the space between these two landmarks. Explain that this space should be maintained as the pectoral girdle muscles are activated and the upper limbs move. Use the hands to direct the lower ribs in and down towards the pelvis.

3. To improve scapular mobility and dynamic alignment – the teacher's hands may be used to guide the student's arms through their correct dynamic alignment or to assist scapular motion and stability as required.

Table 6.4   Teaching points – Chest opener

Focus on	Examples of verbal/visual cues
Relaxation of the neck and upper body	Imagine you are going to drool Imagine the body imprinting itself in warm sand
Vertebral column length	Reach the crown of the head and the sitting bones away from each other
Maintaining a stable lumbar spine	Imagine the pelvis as a bowl of water and the surface of the water is absolutely level and still
Breadth across the front and back of the torso	Broaden across the collarbones Visualize the front and back of the chest being equally wide
Length through the arms	Imagine the arms begin where the collarbones join the breastbone as the arms curve as if around a large ball
Scapular stability throughout	Allow the arm bones to drop into the shoulder joints Imagine the shoulder blades skiing down the back and the little fingers drawing through water as the arms open and close
Lower limb stability	Imagine the feet are sinking in warm sand Imagine the knees are suspended from the ceiling by strings

Exercise UBE5 – Arm arcs with arms in opposition, arm arcs with half circles, arm circles (shoulder flexion, abduction, adduction and circumduction)

Aim

To improve the performance and flexibility of the pectoral muscles.

To increase shoulder joint mobility.

To enhance scapulae stability during upper limb movement.

To improve abdominal muscle control over lumbar spine stability during independent upper limb movement.

Equipment

Mat or firm flat bed, pillow or neck support, a small rolled towel or bolster for between the knees.

Target muscles

For shoulder medial rotation/flexion – the anterior fibres of the deltoid.

For shoulder flexion – pectoralis major (up to 60 degrees then the deltoid takes over), coracobrachialis and the anterior fibres of the deltoid.

For shoulder abduction – the deltoid and supraspinatus, assisted by infraspinatus and the long head of biceps.

For shoulder adduction – pectoralis major, latissimus dorsi and teres major, assisted by teres minor, short head of biceps and coracobrachialis.

For scapular stability – all three parts of trapezius acting together to pull each scapula towards the midline, assisted by the rhomboids, latissimus dorsi and teres major.

For maintaining lumbar spine stability – the combined action of the pelvic floor and transversus abdominis.

Body position

Supine with the legs hip distance apart. The chest is open with breadth across the clavicles, the upper back relaxed and the scapulae drawing gently down the back. The arms lie beside the body and are medially rotated so that the palms of the hands face the floor (Fig. 6.5A).

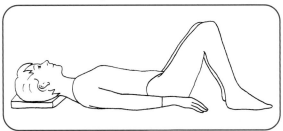

Figure 6.5A   Arm arcs – body position.

Action

Breathing in – to prepare.

Breathing out – gently activate the pelvic floor and lower abdominal muscles and allow the back muscles to release so that the sternum drops down and in towards the spine, stabilize the pectoral girdle and flex both glenohumeral joints to approximately 90 degrees (Fig. 6.5B).

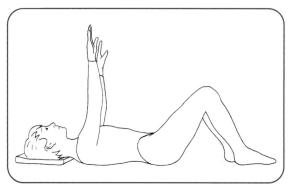

Figure 6.5B   Arm arcs – bilateral shoulder flexion.

Breathing in – maintaining pectoral girdle stability, broaden across the collarbones and reach the little fingers towards the ceiling.

Breathing out – arc the arms in opposite directions until the left arm is aligned beside the left hip and the right arm is aligned with the right ear (approximately 180 degrees of shoulder joint flexion) (Fig. 6.5C).

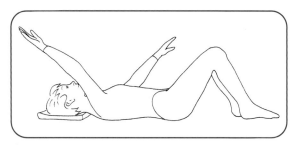

Figure 6.5C   Arm arcs – moving arms in opposite directions.

Breathing in – reverse the motions, returning both arms to 90 degrees of shoulder flexion.

Breathing out – repeat the arm arcing motions in opposite directions, taking the right arm to lie beside the body and the left arm to reach beside the ear (Fig. 6.5D).

Repeat the sequence up to 10 times, aiming to increase the glenohumeral joint range of motion with each repetition.

6

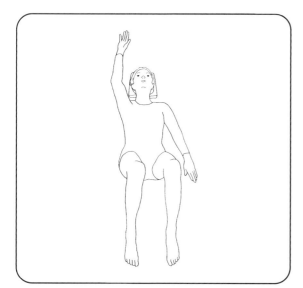

Figure 6.5D   Arm arcs – right arm at end range of shoulder flexion.

Modification 1

Perform with the pelvis in a slight posterior tilt and the lumbar spine imprinted.

Modification 2

Perform with the elbows slightly flexed to shorten the lever length of the arms.

Modification 3

Reduce the range of flexion by blocking the overhead motion of the arm with a stack of yoga blocks, a triangle or pillow placed near the head.

Progression 1

Perform lying along a foam roller. Although this progression requires mental concentration and core control, the instability of the roller increases pelvic floor and lower abdominal muscle action.

Progression 2

Arm circles with shortened levers.

Body position

Supine with the legs hip distance apart. The chest is open with breadth across the clavicles, the upper back relaxed and the scapulae drawing gently down the back. The arms lie beside the body and are medially rotated so that the palms of the hands face the floor. Flex the elbows and place the fingers lightly on the shoulders. Create space in the glenohumeral joints by reaching the elbows away from the body.

Action

Breathing in – to prepare.
Breathing out – gently activate the pelvic floor and lower abdominal muscles, relax the back allowing the sternum to drop back towards the spine, activate the pectoral girdle stabilizing muscles and flex both glenohumeral joints to approximately 90 degrees, pointing the elbows to the ceiling.
Breathing in – reaching the elbows away from the body, further flexing the glenohumeral joints.
Breathing out – maintain lumbar spine stability and move the arms through abduction and adduction, allowing them to rotate naturally to return to a neutral position beside the body.
Breathing in – continuing the motion, flex the glenohumeral joints and move the arms overhead to begin the next repetition.

Progression 3

Perform as for Progression 2 with extended arms.

Progression 4

Arm arcs with half circles.

Body position

Supine with the legs hip distance apart. The chest is open with breadth across the clavicles, the upper back relaxed and the scapulae drawing gently down the back. The arms lie beside the body and are medially rotated so that the palms of the hands face the floor.

Action

Breathing in – to prepare.
Breathing out – gently activate the pelvic floor and lower abdominal muscles, relax the back allowing the sternum to drop back towards the spine, stabilize the pectoral girdle and flex both glenohumeral joints to approximately 90 degrees.
Breathing in – maintaining pectoral girdle stability, broaden across the collarbones and reach the little fingers towards the ceiling.
Breathing out – arc the arms in opposite directions to align the left arm beside the left hip and the right arm with the right ear (Fig. 6.6A).
Breathing in – continue moving the arms in opposite directions, the right arm adducting and the left arm abducting until the arms are reaching away from the body in line with the shoulders (Figs 6.6B&C).
Breathing out – continue moving the arms in opposite directions, allowing them to rotate naturally until the left arm is beside the left ear and the right arm is beside the right hip. The palm of the left hand now faces the ceiling and the palm of the right hand faces the floor (Fig. 6.6D).
Breathing in – repeat the arm arcs.

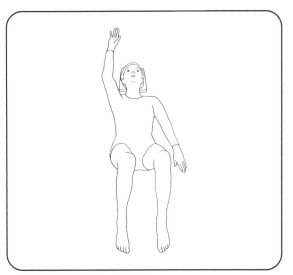

Figure 6.6A The windmill position 1.

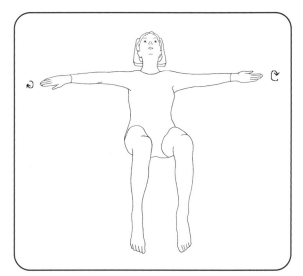

Figure 6.6C The windmill position 3.

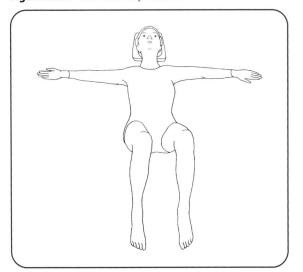

Figure 6.6B The windmill position 2.

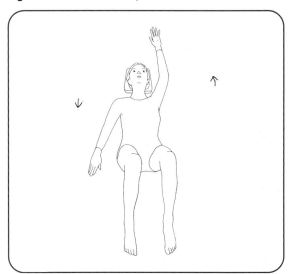

Figure 6.6D The windmill position 4.

6

Breathing out – again move the arms in opposite directions through abduction and adduction.
Repeat the sequence three to five times in each direction.
Note: Incorporate the breathing patterns as required for lumbar spine stability and the correct relationship between the upper and lower torso.

Progression 5

The Windmill. Perform Progression 4 with *two* arm arcs between each half circle.

Common problems

- Upper body/neck tension: Ensure sufficient head and neck support for correct alignment and comfort. On the exhalation, cue for the throat to soften, the thoracic cage to relax and for pectoral girdle stabilization.
- Lumbar spine extension as the arms move overhead (loss of independent shoulder movement): Cue to improve pelvic floor and lower abdominal engagement; consider performing the exercise with an imprinted lumbar spine or with the feet elevated; cue to relax the upper back and maintain the correct relationship between the ribcage and the pelvis.
- Poor dynamic alignment: Cue to trace the arms through imaginary lines in space.
- Poor lower limb alignment: Place a chi ball or other soft support between the knees.

■ Impaired scapular stability: Consider reducing the range of motion and cue for increased breadth across the front of the chest and for stronger pectoral girdle muscle engagement.

See Table 6.5 for Teaching points.

Precautions
- Neck and shoulder pathology – provide sufficient support for comfort; monitor to ensure that the range of movement is appropriate and pain free; seek medical advice if unsure.
- Severely limited shoulder joint range of motion – seek medical advice.
- Back or spine pathology – provide sufficient support for comfort; ensure sufficient abdominal muscle control over lumbar spine stability; consider raising the feet or performing with the lumbar spine flattened.
- Recent neck, shoulder or elbow injury – seek medical advice about the stage of recovery and the suitability of specific exercises.

Contraindications
- Painful neck, arm or shoulder pathology – for onward referral.

Tactile cue suggestions

1. To correct the relationship between the upper and lower torso – before exercising, instruct the student to place the thumbs over the lowest floating ribs and the little fingers over the ASIS to feel the space between these two landmarks. Explain that this space should be maintained as the pectoral girdle muscles are activated and the upper limbs move. Use the hands to direct the ribs in and down towards the pelvis (Fig. 6.6E).

2. To improve scapular stability – before exercising, instruct the student to flex the right shoulder approximately 90 degrees so that the right arm is raised, with the elbow softly bent. The teacher's left hand should be placed over the right scapula to hold and stabilize it (the thumb forward in the armpit and the fingers on the back just below the spine of the scapula). The right hand is placed over the shoulder with the fingers just medial to the acromion process. As the right shoulder increases flexion, the hands are used firmly to assist scapula depression.

3. To improve scapular mobility and dynamic alignment – the teacher's hands may be used to guide the student's arms through their correct dynamic alignment or to assist scapular motion and stability as required.

Table 6.5 Teaching points – Arm arcs

Focus on	Examples of verbal/visual cues
A correctly aligned head/cervical spine	Imagine holding a soft peach between the chin and the sternum
Maintaining a stable lumbar spine	Imagine the pelvis as a bowl of water and the surface of the water is absolutely level and still
Breadth across the front and back of the torso	Broaden across the collarbones and the back of the chest
Length through the arms	Imagine the arms begin where the collarbones join the breastbone as the arms reach away
Scapular stability throughout	As the arms lift, allow the arm bones to drop back into the shoulder joints Imagine the shoulder blades sliding down the back
Scapular depression at the end range of flexion	As the arm moves to the ear, imagine the shoulder blade sinking downwards
Achieving correct dynamic arm alignment	Imagine the hands painting repeated patterns in space
Lower limb stability	Imagine holding a small, soft beach ball between the knees

6

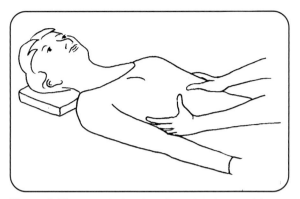

Figure 6.6E   Using the hands to direct the ribs in and down towards the pelvis.

SITTING PECTORAL GIRDLE MOBILIZATION (EXERCISES UBE6–7)

Exercise UBE6 – Shrugs (scapular elevation and depression)

Aim
To enhance postural awareness.
To improve the resting alignment and stability of the scapulae.
To increase scapular mobility.
To increase shoulder joint mobility in extension.
To improve lumbar spine stability during independent upper limb movement.

Equipment
Stool or chair, bolster or chi ball for between the legs, support for feet as required.

Target muscles
For scapular elevation – the upper fibres of trapezius, levator scapulae and the rhomboids.
For scapular return to neutral from elevation – the upper fibres of trapezius, levator scapulae and the rhomboids acting eccentrically.
For scapular depression – the lower fibres of trapezius pull the medial border of the scapula downwards; the lower fibres of serratus anterior draw the lower part of the lateral border of the scapula downwards and forwards; pectoralis minor pulls the upper part of the scapula downwards onto the ribcage.
For adduction, medial rotation and extension – teres major, latissimus dorsi.
For scapular stability – all three parts of trapezius acting together to pull each scapula towards the midline, assisted by the rhomboids, latissimus dorsi and teres major.
For maintaining spine stability – the combined action of the pelvic floor, anterior abdominal wall muscles and erector spinae.

Body position
Sitting erect with the spine elongated, the legs hip distance apart and thighs fully supported on the stool or chair. The feet are on the floor or raised to achieve approximately 90 degrees of hip/knee flexion. The glenohumeral joints are neutral in rotation so that the arms hang from the shoulders to align beside the body with the thumbs facing directly forwards (Fig. 6.7A).

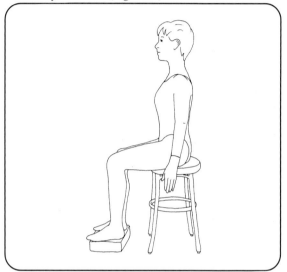

Figure 6.7A   Shrugs – body position.

Action
Breathing in – gently engage the pelvic floor and lower abdominal muscles, broaden across the front of the chest and raise the shoulders towards the ears (Fig. 6.7B).

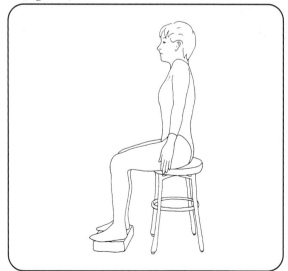

Figure 6.7B   Shrugs – scapula elevation.

6

Breathing out – increase pelvic floor muscle action and further lengthen the spine as the shoulders release. Allow the scapulae to glide down the back to the starting position (Fig. 6.7C).

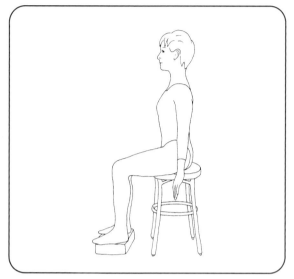

Figure 6.7C   Medial rotation of the glenohumeral joints.

Breathing in – maintaining breadth across the collarbones, medially rotate the arms and depress the scapulae, reaching the fingers to the floor.

Breathing out – continue reaching the fingers towards the floor and extend the glenohumeral joints, stretching the front chest muscles as the arms move behind the body (Fig. 6.7D).

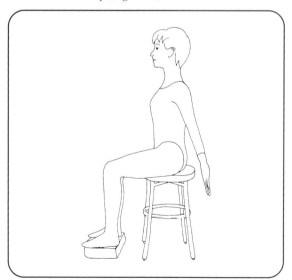

Figure 6.7D   Extension of the glenohumeral joints.

Pause – return the arms to the starting position.
Repeat the sequence 5–10 times.
Note: The lumbar spine/pelvis should remain neutral and stable throughout.

Common problems

- Neck extension as the shoulders elevate: Cue for reaching the crown of the head to the ceiling, lengthen through the back of the neck with the chin softly dropped.
- Lumbar spine extension as the shoulders elevate: Cue for stronger pelvic floor and lower abdominal muscle action and to maintain the connection between the ribcage and the pelvis.
- Spine sag as the shoulders release and depress: Cue for stronger pelvic floor muscle engagement and to reach the crown of the head towards the ceiling.
- Pectoral girdle protraction as the shoulders shrug or release: Cue for breadth across the front of the chest and improved pectoral girdle stability; consider pectoral muscle flexibility.

See Table 6.6 for Teaching points.

Precautions
- **Neck and shoulder pathology – seek medical advice if unsure.**

Contraindications
- Painful neck or shoulder pathology – for onward referral.

Tactile cue suggestions

1. To correct spine alignment and promote spine elongation – lightly run the fingers from above the sacrum up along the spine towards the skull to rest with the thumb and forefinger supporting the base of the skull gently directing the spine upwards. Lightly touch the crown of the head to direct it upwards.
2. To correct the relationship between the upper and lower torso – use the hands to improve spine elongation and alignment. Correct the relationship between the upper torso and the pelvis by directing the lower ribs in and down towards the pelvis.
3. To release unwanted shoulder and neck tension – sweep the hands lightly down the sides of the neck to the tips of the shoulders as if 'dusting' the neck and shoulders.

4. To assist scapular depression and improve scapular stability – place the hands over the shoulders, fingers forwards and thumbs on the spines of the scapulae, then use the fingers to draw the collarbones away from each other as the thumbs depress the scapular spines. Follow this by moving the hands down so that they wrap around the inferior angles of the scapulae and sides of the ribcage, thumbs behind, fingers forwards. Continue to direct the scapulae down and across the back.

Exercise UBE7 – Chest opener (lateral rotation of the glenohumeral joint)

Aim
To enhance postural awareness.
To improve pectoral girdle alignment and stability.
To increase shoulder joint mobility in lateral rotation.
To improve lumbar spine stability during independent upper limb movement.

Equipment
Stool or chair, bolster or chi ball for between the thighs, support for feet as required.

Target muscles
For lateral rotation – infraspinatus, teres minor and the posterior fibres of the deltoid.

For return to neutral – subscapularis, latissimus dorsi, teres major, pectoralis major and the anterior fibres of the deltoid.
For scapular stability – all three parts of trapezius acting together to pull each scapula towards the midline, assisted by the rhomboids, latissimus dorsi and teres major.
For maintaining spine stability – the combined action of the pelvic floor, anterior abdominal wall muscles and erector spinae.

Body position
Sitting erect with the spine elongated, the legs hip distance apart and with the thighs supported on the stool or chair. The feet are on the floor or raised to achieve approximately 90 degrees of hip/knee flexion. The glenohumeral joints are neutral in rotation so that the arms hang from the shoulders to align beside the body with the thumbs facing directly forwards. The elbows are flexed 90 degrees so that the palms of the hands face each other, maintaining the glenohumeral joints neutral in rotation (Fig. 6.8A).

Action
Breathing in – to prepare.
Breathing out – gently activate the pelvic floor and lower abdominal muscles and lengthen the spine from the sacrum through to the crown of the head. Maintaining breadth across the front and back of the chest, stabilize the scapulae and laterally rotate the glenohumeral joints to open the forearms (Fig. 6.8B).

Table 6.6   Teaching points – Shrugs

Focus on	Examples of verbal/visual cues
Correct head/cervical spine placement with the back of the neck lengthened	Imagine wearing long, dangling earrings hanging above the shoulders
Vertebral column length and correct spine alignment	Imagine a string suspending the crown of the head from the ceiling Balance the upper torso over the pelvis and the head on top of the spine
Good scapular mobility as the shoulder are raised	Imagine the outer tips of the shoulders touching the posterior portion of the ear lobes
Correct scapulae alignment as the shoulders depress	As the shoulder blades release, imagine them gliding diagonally downwards towards the spine
Length through the arms as the shoulders extend	Imagine the fingers softly trailing along the floor as the arms reach down and move backwards
Maintaining a stable lumbar spine	As the arms reach back, imagine the lower front ribs and the hip bones are lightly stitched together
Lower limb stability	Imagine the feet are sinking in warm sand Imagine holding a small, soft ball between the knees

6

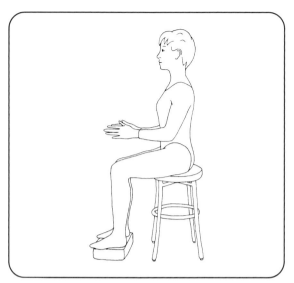

Figure 6.8A   Chest opener – body position.

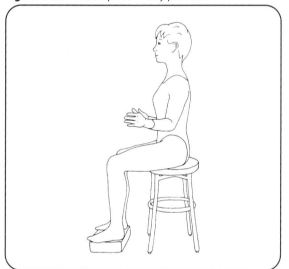

Figure 6.8B   Chest opener – lateral rotation of glenohumeral joints.

Breathing in – return the arms along the same pathway back to the starting position.

Breathing out – begin the next repetition.

Repeat 5–10 times.

Note: The upper limb movement is confined to the glenohumeral joints and the lumbar spine/pelvis remain neutral and stable throughout.

Progression 1

Perform with the palms of the hands facing the floor.

Progression 2

Perform with palms of the hands facing the ceiling and allow the glenohumeral joints to slightly abduct during lateral rotation.

Common problems

- Lumbar spine extension as the shoulder joints mobilize: Cue for stronger pelvic floor and lower abdominal muscle engagement and to maintain the connection between the ribcage and the pelvis.
- Spine sag as the arms return to the starting position: Cue for stronger pelvic floor muscle engagement and further spine elongation.
- Pectoral girdle protraction as the glenohumeral joints mobilize: Cue for breadth across the front of the chest and improved scapular stabilization.

See Table 6.7 for Teaching points.

Precautions
- **Neck and shoulder pathology – monitor for pain-free activity seek medical advice if unsure.**

Contraindications
- Painful neck or shoulder pathology – for onward referral.

Tactile cue suggestions

1. To correct spine alignment and promote spine elongation – lightly run the fingers from above the sacrum up along the spine towards the skull to rest with the thumb and forefinger supporting the base of the skull gently directing the spine upwards. Lightly touch the crown of the head to direct it upwards.
2. To correct the relationship between the upper and lower torso – use the hands to improve spine elongation and alignment. Correct the relationship between the upper torso and the pelvis by directing the lower ribs in and down towards the pelvis.
3. To release unwanted shoulder and neck tension – sweep the hands lightly down the sides of the neck to the tips of the shoulders as if 'dusting' the neck and shoulders.
4. To assist scapular depression and improve scapular stability – place the hands over the shoulders, fingers forwards and thumbs on the spines of the scapulae, then use the fingers to draw the collarbones away from each other as the thumbs depress the scapular spines. Follow this by moving the hands down so that they wrap around the inferior angles of the scapulae and sides of the ribcage, thumbs behind, fingers forwards. Continue to direct the scapulae down and across the back (Fig. 6.8C).

Table 6.7 Teaching points – Chest opener

Focus on	Examples of verbal/visual cues
Correct head/cervical spine placement with the back of the neck lengthened and the superficial neck muscles comparatively relaxed	Imagine wearing long, dangling earrings hanging almost to the shoulders Imagine the shoulders are made of warm butter that is melting and dripping to the floor
Correct spine alignment	Balance the pelvis over the tips of the sitting bones and tighten the pelvic floor muscles Balance the upper torso over the pelvis and the head on top of the spine
Vertebral column length	Imagine a string suspending the crown of the head from the ceiling
Correct upper limb preparatory position	Allow the arms to hang from the shoulders then bend the elbows so that the palms of the hands face each other
Breadth across the front and back of the torso	Think of broadening across the chest as the arms open and return to the staring position
Good scapular stability as the shoulder joint rotates	As the arm rotates, imagine the shoulder blades gliding diagonally downwards towards the spine
The left and right arms moving simultaneously through the same ranges of motion	Imagine the elbows resting and pivoting on poles With the eyes looking straight ahead, allow your peripheral vision to observe the forearms moving together
Lower limb stability	Imagine the feet are sinking in warm sand Imagine holding a small, soft ball between the knees

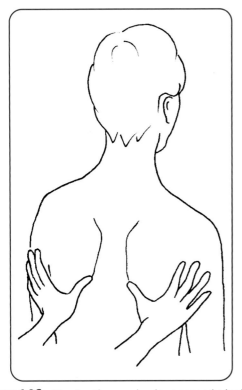

Figure 6.8C   Directing the scapulae down across the back.

SITTING SPINE AND PECTORAL GIRDLE MOBILIZATION (EXERCISES UBE8–10)

Exercise UBE8 – Spine twist (thoracic spine rotation)

Note: Spine twist and side bending should be repeated sequentially to improve mobility in both rotation and lateral flexion.

Aim
To enhance postural awareness.
To promote spine elongation.
To improve lumbar spine stability during thoracic spine mobilization.
To increase thoracic spine mobility in rotation.
To improve pectoral girdle alignment and stability.

Equipment
Stool or chair, back support or wall as required, bolster or chi ball for between the thighs, support for feet as required, small theraball to hold in front of the body as required.

Target muscles
For scapular stability – all three parts of trapezius acting together to pull each scapula towards the midline, assisted by the rhomboids, latissimus dorsi and teres major.

6

For shoulder joint lateral rotation – infraspinatus, teres minor and the posterior fibres of the deltoid.

For shoulder joint extension – posterior fibres of the deltoid, latissimus dorsi assisted by teres major.

For maintaining spine stability – the combined action of the pelvic floor, anterior abdominal wall muscles and erector spinae.

For thoracic spine rotation to the right – the left external oblique abdominals and left erector spinae acting together with the right internal oblique abdominals.

For return to neutral from rotation – the left external oblique abdominals and left erector spinae together with the right internal oblique abdominals acting eccentrically

Body position

Sitting erect with the spine elongated and the legs hip distance apart. The feet are on the floor or raised on blocks to achieve approximately 90 degrees of hip/knee flexion. The glenohumeral joints are neutral in rotation so that the arms hang from the shoulders to align beside the body with the thumbs facing directly forwards. Raise the arms diagonally forwards and flex the elbows approximately 90 degrees to allow the fingertips to lightly touch in front of the sternum. The palms face the floor (Fig. 6.9A).

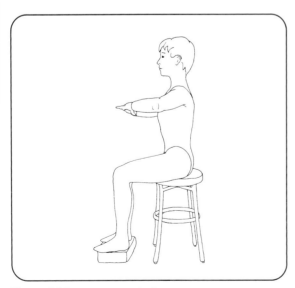

Figure 6.9A   Spine twist – body position.

Action

Breathing in – to prepare.

Breathing out – gently activate the pelvic floor muscles and lengthen the spine from the sacrum through to the crown of the head.

Breathing in – maintaining breadth across the front and back of the chest, stabilize the pectoral girdle and rotate the upper torso to the left. The hands remain aligned with the sternum and the head moves with the spine, the eyes continuing to look directly forwards (Fig. 6.9B).

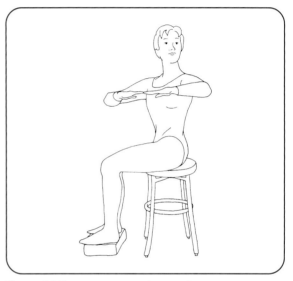

Figure 6.9B   Spine twist – end range of motion.

Breathing out – increase pelvic floor muscle engagement, spine elongation and scapular stabilization to further rotate the spine to its end range of motion as the left elbow flexes more to draw the hands to align with the left side of the ribcage. The head turns gently as the upper torso rotates so that by the end of the motion the eyes look over the left shoulder towards the left elbow.

Breathing in – maintaining spine length and pectoral girdle stabilization with breadth across the front and back of the chest, return through the starting position to commence rotation to the right side.

Breathing out – complete rotation to the right side as before (Fig. 6.9C).

Breathing in – to repeat to the left side.

Repeat three to five times to each side.

Modification

Perform with the arms wrapped around a small theraball in front of the body. Rotate the torso and ball as a unit.

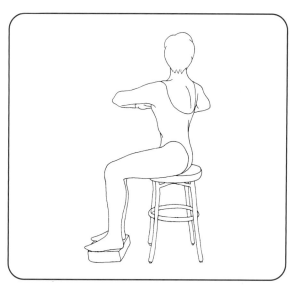

Figure 6.9C Spine twist to right side.

Progression

Body position

Perform the basic exercise until the spine has reached its apparent end range of rotation motion and the head is turned to look over the left shoulder.

Action

Breathing normally – keeping the head still, move the eyes as quickly as possible from right to left for 15–30 seconds, then again look over the left shoulder.

Breathing in – improve pelvic floor muscle engagement and spine length.

Breathing out – maintain spine elongation and scapular stability to further rotate the spine and draw the left elbow more behind the body. Stabilize the scapulae more strongly and allow the action of the left elbow reaching behind the body to assist and improve spine rotation.

Breathing in – return to the starting position as before. Repeat once or twice to each side.

Common problems

- Arms move before spine rotation begins: Cue to keep the hands in front of the sternum and visualize the motion initiating from within the vertebral column.
- Lumbar spine rotation: Ensure that the starting position is correct (see sitting posture) and spine elongation is maintained throughout; cue for improved pelvic floor muscle control and to rotate the torso from above the waist; consider assisting pelvic stability by sitting the subject astride a chair/box.

- Lumbar spine extension as the thoracic spine rotates: Cue for stronger pelvic floor muscle engagement, spine elongation and to maintain the balance of the upper torso over the pelvis; consider performing with the spine supported against a wall or foam roller to assist body awareness; cue to release the throat muscles and encourage a relaxed approach.

See Table 6.8 for Teaching points.

⚠ Precautions

- Neck, shoulder and spine pathology – monitor for pain-free activity, seek medical advice if unsure.

➕ Contraindications

- Painful neck, shoulder or spine pathology – for onward referral.

Tactile cue suggestions

1. To correct spine alignment and promote spine elongation – lightly run the fingers from above the sacrum up along the spine towards the skull to rest with the thumb and forefinger supporting the base of the skull gently directing the spine upwards. Lightly touch the crown of the head to direct it upwards.
2. To correct the relationship between the upper and lower torso – use the hands to improve spine elongation and alignment. Correct the relationship between the upper torso and the pelvis by directing the lower ribs in and down towards the pelvis.
3. To release unwanted shoulder and neck tension – sweep the hands lightly down the sides of the neck to the tips of the shoulders as if 'dusting' the neck and shoulders.
4. To assist scapular depression and improve scapular stability – place the hands over the shoulders, fingers forwards and thumbs on the spines of the scapulae, then use the fingers to draw the collarbones away from each other as the thumbs depress the scapular spines. Follow this by moving the hands down so that they wrap around the inferior angles of the scapulae and sides of the ribcage, thumbs behind, fingers forwards. Continue to direct the scapulae down and across the back.

6

Tactile cue suggestions—cont'd

5. To cue thoracic spine mobilization – anticipate the motion, lightly touching the vertebrae involved.
6. To cue shoulder extension – lightly touch the elbow to direct it slightly downwards and backwards.

Exercise UBE9 – Side bending (lateral spine flexion)

Note: Spine twist and side bending should be repeated sequentially to improve mobility in both rotation and lateral flexion.

Aim
To enhance postural awareness.
To promote spine elongation.
To improve pelvic stability during spine mobilization.
To increase spine mobility in lateral flexion.
To improve pectoral girdle alignment and stability.

Equipment
Firm bed or table.

Target muscles
For scapular stability – all three parts of trapezius acting together to pull each scapula towards the midline, assisted by the rhomboids, latissimus dorsi and teres major.

For shoulder joint flexion – the anterior fibres of the deltoid, pectoralis major and coracobrachialis assisted by biceps brachii and subscapularis.

For maintaining spine stability – the combined action of the pelvic floor and anterior abdominal wall muscles together with erector spinae.

For spine flexion to the right – rectus abdominis, right quadratus lumborum, right internal and external obliques and right erector spinae (intertransversarii and multifidus) acting concentrically to pull the right side of the ribcage down sideways, so curving the spine to the right.

Note: Once approximately 10 degrees of lateral flexion has been produced the motion is controlled by the eccentric contraction of the muscles on the opposite side. During lateral flexion to the right there is associated contralateral rotation of the thoracic vertebrae to the left so that the spinous processes of the thoracic vertebrae point to the concavity of the curve (to the right).

For vertebral rotation – multifidus and rotators (transversospinalis) produce thoracic spine rotation, moving each vertebra individually as well as in vertebral segments.

Body position
Sitting erect with the spine elongated and the legs hip distance apart. The feet are on the floor or raised on

Table 6.8	Teaching points – Spine twist
Focus on	**Examples of verbal/visual cues**
A neutral and stable lumbar spine throughout to allow independent thoracic spine movement	Tighten the pelvic floor muscles and draw the lower abdominal muscles gently towards the spine Lengthen from the sitting bones through to the crown of the head and turn the ribcage from above the waist
Shoulder alignment and girdle stability	Imagine the shoulder blades sliding diagonally down and across the back
Limiting neck tension	Relax the tongue in the throat and allow the head to balance on the top of the spine Imagine wearing long, dangling earrings
Initiating the movement from the spine	To begin turning the body to the side, imagine the upper body pivoting on the spine from above the waist
Maximum spine rotation	As you turn to the right, imagine the left lower ribs gliding around the body to float above the right hip bone
Stronger pectoral girdle activation when fully rotated to one side	Open the upper outer corner of the shoulder to reach the elbow behind you and draw the shoulder blade down and across the back

blocks to achieve approximately 90 degrees of hip/knee flexion. The glenohumeral joints are neutral in rotation so that the arms hang from the shoulders to align beside the body with the thumbs facing directly forwards. Flex the left glenohumeral joint approximately 160 degrees to raise the left arm in front of the body (Fig. 6.10A).

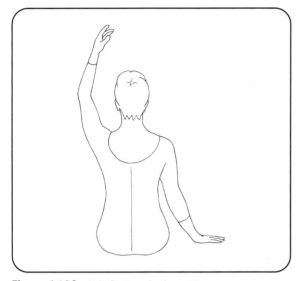

Figure 6.10A Side flexion – body position.

Flex the left elbow joint, rounding the left arm to frame the face. Rest the right palm on the bed (Fig. 6.10B).

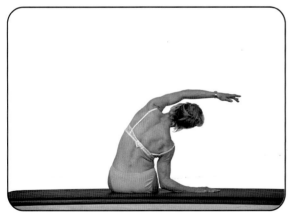

Figure 6.10B

Action

Breathing in – gently activate the pelvic floor and lower abdominal muscles and simultaneously stabilize the pectoral girdle.

Breathing out – reach through the crown of the head, further lengthening the spine and begin flexing the body to the right, drawing the lower right ribs in to curve the body sideways as if over a ball.

Breathing in – maintaining breadth across the front and back of the chest, further engage the abdominal and pectoral girdle stabilizing muscles to begin returning from flexion, stacking the vertebrae sequentially from the base of the spine upwards and lengthening the spine to return to the starting position.

Breathing out – reach the left arm to the side and return it to the starting position.

Repeat to the left side, first flexing the right glenohumeral joint approximately 160 degrees to raise the right arm and placing the left palm on the bed.

Perform three to four times to each side.

Progression 1

Perform two to three times to one side, aiming to increase the range of side flexion motion with each repetition.

Progression 2

Body position

Flex the right glenohumeral joint approximately 160 degrees to raise the right arm in front of the body. Flex the right elbow joint, rounding the right arm to frame the face. Place the left hand over the left lower ribs. Perform as in the basic exercise but use light pressure through the left hand to direct the ribs in towards the centre of the body to increase side flexion. Allow the upper torso to curl over the hand as the spine flexes sideways.

Action

Breathing in – remain in side flexion, maintaining abdominal muscle and pectoral girdle muscle engagement.

Breathing out – improve abdominal muscle control and draw the lower left ribs in further towards the centre of the body. Allow the body to drape over the hand, increasing side flexion.

Breathing in – use pelvic floor and abdominal muscle control to gradually return from flexion, stacking the vertebrae sequentially from the base of the spine upwards and lengthening the spine to return to the starting position.

6

Repeat once or twice to perform side bending to the right followed by a side twist to the left (previous exercise). Repeat the whole sequence to opposite sides.

Common problems

■ Arm moves ahead of the torso: Cue to maintain the hand slightly in front of and above the sternum.

■ Pelvic instability: Monitor the sitting position and ensure the thighs are fully supported; consider sitting astride a chair or box; cue for stronger preparatory pelvic floor and lower abdominal muscle control and spine lengthening.

■ Lumbar spine extension: Ensure the starting position is correct with the pelvis balanced above the ischial tuberosities, the upper torso balanced directly over the pelvis, the spinal curves lengthened and the superficial neck muscles appearing comparatively relaxed; cue to release the throat muscles and allow the motion to occur rather than 'trying too hard'; consider performing with the back support against a wall.

See Table 6.9 for Teaching points.

Precautions

■ Neck, shoulder and spine pathology – monitor for pain-free activity, seek medical advice if unsure.

Contraindications

■ Painful neck, shoulder or spine pathology – for onward referral.

Tactile cue suggestions

1. To correct spine alignment and promote spine elongation – lightly run the fingers from above the sacrum up along the spine towards the skull to rest with the thumb and forefinger supporting the base of the skull gently directing the spine upwards. Lightly touch the crown of the head to direct it upwards.

2. To correct the relationship between the upper and lower torso – use the hands to direct the ribs in and down towards the pelvis. Consider performing the exercise with the back supported against a wall.

3. To assist scapular depression and improve scapular stability – place the hands over the shoulders, fingers forwards and thumbs on the spines of the scapulae, then use the fingers to draw the collarbones away from each other as the thumbs depress the scapular spines. Follow this by moving the hands down so that they wrap around the inferior angles of the scapulae and sides of the ribcage, thumbs behind, fingers forwards. Continue to direct the scapulae down and across the back.

4. To cue spine mobilization – anticipate vertebral mobilization by lightly touching the vertebrae to be involved.

5. To cue side flexion to the right – standing behind, place the right hand on the right lower ribs to gently assist moving them inwards. Allow the torso to drape over the hand. Lightly tap the spaces between the left ribs to assist mobilization.

Exercise UBE10 – Spine curls (spine flexion)

Aim
To enhance postural awareness.
To promote spine elongation.
To improve pelvic stability during spine mobilization.
To increase spine mobility in flexion.
To improve upper back muscle flexibility.

Equipment
Stool or chair, back support or wall as required, bolster or chi ball for between the thighs, support for feet as required.

Target muscles
For scapular stability – all three parts of trapezius acting together to pull each scapula towards the midline, assisted by the rhomboids, latissimus dorsi and teres major.
For maintaining spine stability – the combined action of the pelvic floor and anterior abdominal wall muscles together with erector spinae.
For spine flexion – flexion is initiated by rectus abdominis and the oblique abdominals and then the effect of gravity is counteracted by cervical and thoracic erector spinae contracting eccentrically.
For return from spine flexion – erector spinae.

Body position
Sitting erect with the spine elongated and the legs hip distance apart. The feet are on the floor or raised on blocks to achieve approximately 90 degrees of hip/ knee flexion. The glenohumeral joints are neutral in rotation so that the arms hang from the shoulders

Table 6.9 Teaching points – Side flexion

Focus on	Examples of verbal/visual cues
Maintaining a lengthened, correctly aligned spine	Lengthen from the crown of the head to the sitting bones
Efficient abdominal control and core stability throughout	Tighten the pelvic floor and lower abdominal muscles
Shoulder alignment and girdle stability	Imagine the shoulder blades sliding down across the back
A softly rounded arm	Imagine draping the arm over a rainbow
Avoiding lumbar extension	Imagine the body is curling sideways between two panes of glass
Achieving maximum lateral flexion to the right	Think of the right lower ribs moving inwards
Maintaining the correct relationship between the head and the cervical spine	Keep the eyes looking straight ahead and move the head with the spine
Initiating the movement from the spine and creating a long, C-shaped spine from above the sacrum to the top of the cervical spine	Imagine the spine is made of chocolate and the vertebrae warm and melt one by one as the spine curls as if over a ball

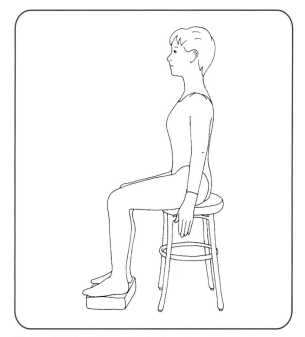

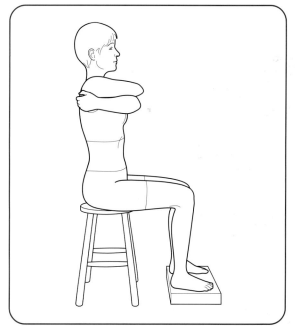

Figure 6.11A Spine curls – body position.

Figure 6.11B Spine curls – wrapping arms around the body.

6

to align beside the body with the thumbs facing directly forwards. Wrap the arms around the body to clasp the opposite scapula (Figs 6.11A&B).

Action
Breathing in – gently activate the pelvic floor and lower abdominal muscles, stabilize the pectoral girdle and lengthen the spine.

Breathing out – nod the head and allow the upper spine to flex, drawing the scapulae down the back as the elbows draw downwards and inwards.
Breathing in – maintain pelvic floor and lower abdominal control. Direct the breath more into the posterior ribcage and simultaneously draw the scapulae further down the back.

Table 6.10 Teaching points – Spine curls

Focus on	Examples of verbal/visual cues
Correctly lengthening and mobilizing the spine	Lengthen from the crown of the head to the sitting bones To curl the body, imagine the spine is made of chocolate and the vertebrae warm and melt one by one To return to the sitting position, imagine the vertebrae as building bricks smoothly stacking one above the other
Efficient abdominal control and core stability throughout	Tighten the pelvic floor and lower abdominal muscles
Correct shoulder alignment and stability	Imagine the shoulder blades sliding down across the back
Limiting unwanted tension	Relax the tongue in the throat and allow the body to softly round Imagine draping the upper body over a ball
Flexing the spine from above the waist	Think of the lower ribs moving inwards to curl the upper body as if over a ball

Breathing out – maintain the pelvis neutral and stable and allow the upper back to release and curve as the scapulae slide further down the back.

Breathing in – return to the starting position using pelvic floor and abdominal muscle control to stack the vertebrae sequentially as the spine lengthens.

Breathing out – to repeat spine flexion.

Repeat three to five times.

Common problems

- Lumbar spine flexion: Ensure the starting position is correct with the pelvis balanced above the ischial tuberosities and the upper torso balanced directly over the pelvis; cue for stronger pelvic floor and lower abdominal muscle control to keep the lower back lengthened and lifted; consider performing with the back against a wall or other support.
- Restricted spine mobility: Cue to allow the upper back to release as the body curls as if over a ball; use tactile cues to assist vertebral mobilization.

See Table 6.10 for Teaching points.

① Precautions
- Neck, shoulder and spine pathology – monitor for pain-free activity, seek medical advice if unsure.

✚ Contraindications
- Painful neck, shoulder or spine pathology – for onward referral.

Tactile cue suggestions

1. To correct spine alignment and promote spine elongation – lightly run the fingers from above the sacrum up along the spine towards the skull to rest with the thumb and forefinger supporting the base of the skull gently directing the spine upwards. Lightly touch the crown of the head to direct it upwards.
2. To correct the relationship between the upper and lower torso – use the hands to direct the ribs in and down towards the pelvis. Consider performing the exercise with the back supported against a wall.
3. To cue spine mobilization – direct the sternum inwards and downwards and direct the scapulae downwards to initiate thoracic spine flexion. Anticipate vertebral mobilization by lightly touching the vertebrae to be involved.

PRONE PECTORAL GIRDLE MOBILIZATION AND STABILIZATION (EXERCISES UBE11–12)

Exercise UBE11 – Batman (scapular adduction, abduction and stabilization)

Aim

To improve rhomboid, middle and lower trapezius performance.

To improve shoulder joint mobility, scapular alignment and stability.

To improve abdominal muscle control over spine stability during independent pectoral girdle mobilization.

Equipment

Mat or firm bed, a small support for the forehead or supports in the axillae as required for comfort, a foam roller.

Target muscles

For maintaining spine stability – the combined action of the pelvic floor and anterior abdominal wall muscles together with erector spinae.

For scapular stability – all three parts of trapezius acting together to pull each scapula towards the midline, assisted by the rhomboids, latissimus dorsi and teres major.

For scapular adduction – the trapezius and the rhomboids.

For spine extension and return from spine extension – erector spinae acting concentrically during spine extension and eccentrically on the return from extension.

Body position

Prone with the arms reaching over the head, the wrists resting on a foam roller. The shoulders are relaxed, the elbows softly extended with the palms of the hands facing the floor. The forehead may rest on a small support to correct cervical spine alignment. The chin is slightly dropped towards the sternum so that the back of the neck is lengthened. The crown of the head reaches away from the top of the spine (Fig. 6.12A).

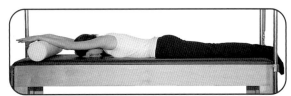

Figure 6.12A

Action

Breathing in – to prepare.

Breathing out – broaden across the front of the chest. Begin drawing the scapulae down and across the back as if placing them in back hip pockets and simultaneously activate the pelvic floor and lower abdominal muscles to lengthen and stabilize the lumbar spine. Slide the shoulder blades further down the back, flexing the elbows and using the weight of the arms on the foam roller to roll it towards the head. Allow the glenohumeral joints to be comparatively relaxed so that the elbows drop towards the floor (Fig. 6.12B).

Breathing in – as the roller almost touches the head, adduct the scapulae to lift the elbows towards the ceiling (Fig. 6.12C).

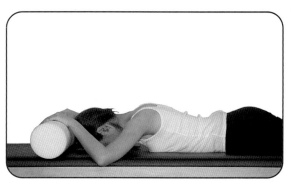

Figure 6.12B

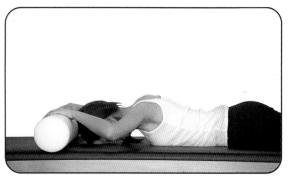

Figure 6.12C

Breathing out – increase abdominal muscle activation to maintain lumbar spine stability and allow upper trapezius to be comparatively relaxed so that the neck remains long with the shoulders dropping away from the ears.

Breathing normally – maintain this position for a few seconds.

Breathing in – keeping the elbows lifted, gradually release scapular adduction.

Breathing out – extend the elbows, reaching the roller away and simultaneously depress the scapulae as the arms return to their starting position (Fig. 6.12D).

Repeat three to five times.

6

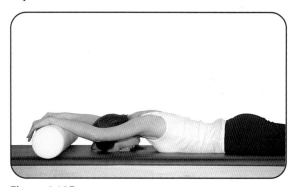

Figure 6.12D

Modification

Limit the range of shoulder flexion and/or scapular adduction.

Progression 1

Perform without the foam roller for support. Begin in the same starting position. Lift the arms away from the floor as if supported on a roller, flex the elbows to take the hands behind the head for scapular adduction and then continue as in the basic exercise.

Progression 2

Perform Progression 1 and once the scapulae have been adducted, further engage the pelvic floor and lower abdominal muscles before moving into thoracic spine extension. Return from spine extension and then continue as in the basic exercise.

Note: As the spine moves into extension the pelvis and lumbar spine are stabilized through pelvic floor and abdominal muscle control. If required, the lower fibres of gluteus maximus may be activated to assist lumbar spine stability. The back of the neck is lengthened and the chin is softly dropped towards the sternum (craniovertebral flexion). The gaze is to the floor and the head moves with the spine as the sternum moves forwards and up.

Repeat the sequence three to five times in each direction.

Common problems

- Upper body/neck tension: Provide sufficient head/neck support for correct alignment and comfort and instruct the student to keep the gaze to the floor.
- Shoulders lift towards the ears during flexion: Cue to maintain breadth across the collarbones and space between the tips of the shoulders and the ears.
- Insufficient abdominal muscle control over lumbar spine stability: Cue for improved pelvic floor and lower abdominal muscle control to lengthen the lumbar spine; consider activating the lower fibres of gluteus maximus to assist lumbar spine stability.

See Table 6.11 for Teaching points.

Precautions
- Back, neck or shoulder pathology – monitor for pain-free activity, provide sufficient support for comfort.
- Monitor the shoulder girdle position and range of motion.
- Ensure sufficient abdominal muscle control over the lumbar spine throughout – seek medical advice if unsure.

Contraindications
- Painful neck, arm, shoulder or back pathology – for onward referral.

Table 6.11   Teaching points – Batman

Focus on	Examples of verbal/visual cues
Maintaining a lengthened, correctly aligned spine	Reach the crown of the head away from the sitting bones
Efficient abdominal control and core stability throughout	Tighten the pelvic floor and lower abdominal muscles
Limiting neck tension	Keep the gaze towards the floor Imagine holding a soft peach between the chin and the breastbone
Placing emphasis on trapezius muscle activation	Imagine strings drawing the outer tips of the elbows towards the ceiling as the shoulder blades move together Imagine the shoulder blades sliding towards the heels as the arms reach over the head
Correct thoracic spine extension	Move the spine inwards between the shoulder blades as the chest lifts away from the floor Move the spine inwards just under the bra strap
Lumbar spine stability during thoracic spine extension	Maintain abdominal muscle control and imagine the lower front ribs are loosely stitched to the hipbones as the spine moves into extension

6

Tactile cue suggestions

1. To correct the relationship between the upper and lower torso – use the hands to assist the ribs to funnel down towards the pelvis.
2. To assist spine elongation – lightly touch the crown of the head to direct it forwards.
3. To assist scapular depression and stability – place the hands over the shoulders, fingers forwards and thumbs on the spines of the scapulae. Use the fingers to draw the collarbones away from each other as the thumbs depress the scapular spines. Follow this by moving the hands down so that they wrap around the inferior angles of the scapulae and sides of the ribcage, thumbs behind, fingers forwards. Continue to direct the scapulae down and across the back.
4. To improve scapular mobility – use the hands to guide the scapulae through adduction and abduction.
5. To direct thoracic spine extension whilst maintaining the correct relationship between the head and the cervical spine – gently place the thumb and third finger of the left hand just below the occipital tuberosities whilst extending the right forearm across and lightly supporting the collarbones.

Exercise UBE12 – Sphinx (pectoral girdle stabilization for upper limb body weight bearing)

Aim
To collectively strengthen the pectoral girdle muscles.
To improve scapular alignment and stability for efficient weight bearing with the upper limbs.

Equipment
Mat or bed.

Target muscles
For maintaining spine stability – the combined action of the pelvic floor and anterior abdominal wall muscles together with erector spinae.
For scapular stability – all three parts of trapezius acting together to pull each scapula towards the midline, assisted by the rhomboids, latissimus dorsi and teres major.
For weight bearing with the upper limbs – serratus anterior and the middle fibres of trapezius.

Note: During 'push-ups' the serratus anterior and middle fibres of trapezius act together to stabilize the scapula and keep it flat against the ribcage.

Body position
Four-point kneeling with the hips flexed 90 degrees, the knees no more than hip distance apart and the soles of the feet facing the ceiling. Move the hands forwards approximately 30 cm and keep the fingers pointing forwards. The little fingers press lightly into the floor to assist engagement of the pectoral girdle muscles. The back of the neck is lengthened with the cervical curve intact and the superficial neck muscles comparatively relaxed. The gaze is directly down (Fig. 6.13A).

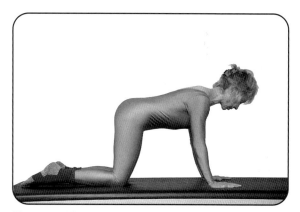

Figure 6.13A

Action
Breathing in – to prepare.
Breathing out – broaden across the front of the chest, stabilize the pectoral girdle and activate the pelvic floor and lower abdominal muscles.
Breathing normally – maintaining the neutral spine, flex both elbows to place the forearms on the floor parallel and in line with the shoulders.
Breathing in – reach the left leg backwards then the right and dorsiflex the toes (the toes curl under) so the weight is placed over the balls of the feet (Fig. 6.13B).
Breathing out – increase abdominal muscle control and pectoral girdle stabilization before fully extending both knees so that the body is supported away from the floor with the weight evenly distributed between the shoulders and the feet.
Breathing normally – maintain this plank position for up to five breathing cycles.
Bend one leg and then the other to release and return the legs to the starting position.

6

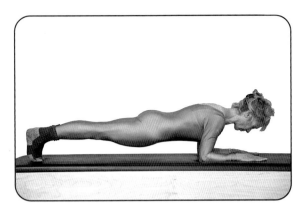

Figure 6.13B

Modification 1

Perform standing with the forearms resting on a desk or table with the hips flexed and the spine in neutral.

Modification 2

Perform with hips and knees flexed approximately 90 degrees (Figs 6.13C&D).

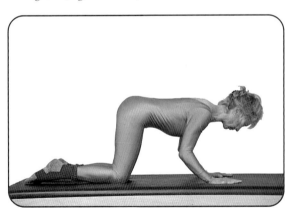

Figure 6.13C

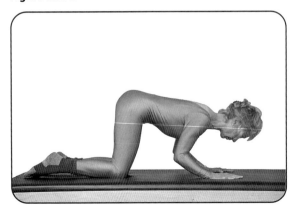

Figure 6.13D

Progression 1

Perform with the elbows extended so that the arms support the body weight as in a press-up. The spine is stabilized in a neutral position (Fig. 6.14).

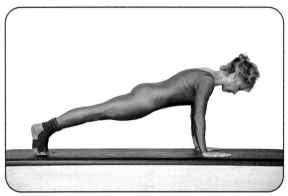

Figure 6.14

Progression 2

Perform with the lower limbs supported on a gym ball and the arms supporting the body weight as in a press-up. Flex and extend the elbows (traditional 'push-ups') three to five times, maintaining spine and pectoral girdle stability throughout.

Common problems

- Spine sag between the shoulder blades: Cue to draw the breastbone up towards the spine and for stronger scapular stabilization; emphasize length through the spine from the crown of the head to the tailbone.
- Shoulders tense and lift towards the ears: Cue for stronger scapular stabilization and to maintain space between the ears and tips of the shoulders.
- Lumbar spine instability: Cue for improved pelvic floor and abdominal muscle activation and consider adding lower gluteus maximus activation; emphasize length through the spine from the crown of the head to the tailbone.

See Table 6.12 for Teaching points.

> **! Precautions**
> - Lower limb, hip, back, neck, shoulder or upper limb pathology – ensure the student has sufficient strength for safe exercise performance; monitor alignment and technique throughout; seek medical advice if unsure.

6

Table 6.12   Teaching points – Sphinx

Focus on	Examples of verbal/visual cues
Maintaining a lengthened, correctly aligned spine	Lengthen from the crown of the head to the sitting bones
Efficient abdominal control and core stability throughout	Tighten the pelvic floor and lower abdominal muscles
The correct relationship between the upper and lower torso as the spine extends	On breathing out, funnel the ribs down towards the pelvis Draw the breastbone up between the shoulder blades
Limiting neck tension	Imagine a soft peach being held between the chin and the collarbones Maintain space between the tips of the ears and the shoulders Keep the gaze towards the floor
Shoulder alignment and girdle stability	Imagine the shoulder blades sliding down across the back
Keeping the scapulae flat on the ribcage	Imagine you are pushing the floor away and press through the little fingers as you slide the shoulder blades down the back Draw the breastbone up towards the spine and maintain space between the shoulder blades

 Contraindications

■ Painful limb/spine pathology – for onward referral.

Tactile cue suggestions

1. To correct the spine sagging between the ribs – lightly touch the sternum to direct it up towards the spine.
2. To correct the relationship between the upper and lower torso – use the hands to direct the ribs in and down towards the pelvis.
3. To assist spine elongation – lightly touch the crown of the head to direct it forwards.
4. To assist scapular depression and improve stability – place the hands over the shoulders, fingers forwards and thumbs on the spines of the scapulae. Use the fingers to draw the collarbones away from each other as the thumbs depress the scapular spines. Follow this by moving the hands down so that they wrap around the inferior angles of the scapulae and sides of the ribcage, thumbs behind, fingers forwards. Continue to direct the scapulae down and across the back.
5. To maintain breadth across the collarbones – lightly sweep the fingers from the sternum to the distal ends of the collarbones.

SIDE LYING PECTORAL GIRDLE STABILIZATION AND STRENGTHENING (EXERCISE UBE13)

Exercise UBE13 – Side lifts (unilateral pectoral girdle stabilization for upper limb)

Aim
To collectively strengthen the pectoral girdle stabilizing muscles.
To improve scapular alignment and stability for efficient body weight bearing with the upper limbs.

Equipment
Mat or firm bed.

Target muscles
For maintaining spine stability – the combined action of the pelvic floor and anterior abdominal wall muscles, together with erector spinae.
For scapular stability – all three parts of trapezius acting together to pull each scapula towards the midline, assisted by the rhomboids, latissimus dorsi and teres major.
For resisted glenohumeral adduction – pectoralis major, teres major, latissimus dorsi and coracobrachialis.
For resisted lower limb abduction – gluteus medius, gluteus minimus and tensor fasciae latae.

Body position
Lying on the right side with the upper body supported away from the floor with the right arm. The right elbow is flexed approximately 90 degrees and the

6

right shoulder aligns above the right elbow. The right shoulder joint is in medial rotation so that the forearm points directly forwards. The upper arm lies along the body with the palm of the hand resting on the thigh. The body is lengthened with the normal spinal curves intact and the legs align with the body (Fig. 6.15A).

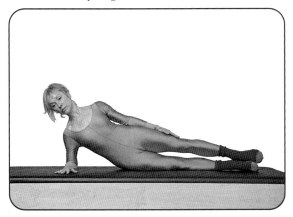

Figure 6.15A

Action

Breathing in – to prepare.

Breathing out – activate the pelvic floor and lower abdominal muscles and lengthen the spine.

Breathing in – increase abdominal muscle control, stabilize the pectoral girdle and reach the legs away from the body to float the pelvis from the floor to align with the body as in standing (Fig. 6.15B).

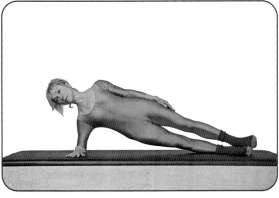

Figure 6.15B

As the pelvis lifts, laterally rotate the left arm to reach it over overhead with the elbow slightly flexed to frame the face.

Breathing out – maintaining abdominal and pectoral girdle muscle control, hold the position, lengthening the spine and reaching the legs away from the body.

Breathing in – still lengthening through the spine, control a gradual return to the starting position.

Common problems

- Insufficient abdominal muscle control over lumbar spine stability: Cue for improved pelvic floor and lower abdominal muscle control to lengthen the lumbar spine; consider activating the lower fibres of gluteus maximus to assist lumbar spine stability; emphasize lengthening from the crown of the head through to the heels.
- Pectoral girdle protraction as the pelvis lifts: Cue for breadth across the front of the chest and stronger pectoral girdle stability.
- Spine sag as the pelvis returns to the floor: Cue to maintain spine elongation and to slowly release 'resisted glenohumeral adduction'.

See Table 6.13 for Teaching points.

⚠ Precautions
- Lower limb, hip, back, neck, shoulder or upper limb pathology – ensure the student has sufficient strength for safe exercise performance; monitor alignment and technique throughout; seek medical advice if unsure.

✚ Contraindications
- Painful limb/spine pathology – for onward referral.

Tactile cue suggestions

1. To correct spine alignment and promote spine elongation – lightly run the fingers from above the sacrum up along the spine towards the skull to rest with the thumb and forefinger supporting the base of the skull gently directing the spine out of the pelvis. Lightly touch the crown of the head to direct the spine to lengthen away from the heels.

2. To correct the relationship between the upper and lower torso – use the hands to direct the ribs in and down towards the pelvis.

3. To release unwanted shoulder and neck tension – sweep the hands lightly from the occiput down the sides of the neck to the tips of the shoulders as if 'dusting' the neck and shoulders.

Table 6.13 Teaching points – Side lifts

Focus on	Examples of verbal/visual cues
Achieving a correctly aligned and supported spine throughout	Lengthen from the crown of the head to the sitting bones Reach the head away from the heels as the pelvis floats up
Efficient abdominal control	Tighten the pelvic floor muscles and lower abdominal muscles
Achieving the correct relationship between the upper and lower torso throughout	On breathing out, funnel the ribs down towards the pelvis Imagine floating the pelvis up between two panes of glass
Limiting neck tension	Imagine a soft peach being held between the chin and the collarbones Maintain space between the tips of the ears and the shoulders Keep the gaze directly forwards
Shoulder alignment and girdle stability	Draw the shoulder blades gently down and across the back
Keeping the scapulae flat on the ribcage	To float the pelvis up, imagine pulling the elbow towards the body and press the fingers into the floor Imagine the shoulder blades hugging the ribs as they slide down the back
Maintaining lower limb stability	Imagine a wall at the base of the feet that the heels are to reach towards for support

STRETCHING, JOINT MOBILIZATION AND EXERCISES TO IMPROVE FOOT ALIGNMENT, MOBILITY AND STRENGTH

Stretching assists joint mobility, contributes to postural fault correction and chronic pain management, and may help to improve overall musculoskeletal function.

The section describes:

1. guidelines for safe and effective stretching and joint mobilization
2. foot mobilization routines
3. easy and developmental stretches to address specific postural faults.

Safe effective stretching requires a thorough understanding of the following:

- *Controlled breathing* – this facilitates relaxation. Use slow, rhythmical and controlled cycles, 'breathing out' assisting muscle relaxation and mental focus. If breathing is inhibited or stressed during sustained stretching, ease the tension off a little until the body can relax and resume more natural breathing patterns.
- *Timing stretching* – this helps the development of self-knowledge. Until an individual knows how their muscles react to stretching it is helpful to time the duration of every stretch. This is done by the clock or through counting a slow heartbeat rate of about 60 beats per minute. Eventually people learn to feel and interpret the way their muscles react to stretching and then adjust the length of each stretch accordingly.
- *The stretch reflex* – this protects muscles and helps to prevent injuries. When muscle fibres are overstretched a nerve reflex responds by signalling the muscle to contract and prevent further stretching. This response occurs during extreme stretching – beyond what is comfortable or manageable – and when bouncing up and down in a stretch.
- *Extreme stretching and bouncing stretching* – these may cause microscopic trauma to muscle fibres leading to permanent damage and scarring in muscle tissue. Holding a stretch as far as it can go and bouncing up and down strains the muscles and activates the stretch reflex. Both practices can be painful and lead to tight, sore muscles that lose rather than gain flexibility.
- *The easy stretch* – this stretch gently releases muscle tightness in preparation for developmental stretching. Stretch to the point where mild tension is felt, then relax and hold the position for 10–30 seconds. The feeling of tension should subside as the position is held. If tension does not subside, the stretch should be eased off a little to find a more comfortable position. Continue in this more comfortable position for the required length of time.

6

■ *The developmental stretch* – this stretch fine-tunes the muscles and increases muscle flexibility. Perform the easy stretch, and once the feeling of tension has subsided, gently stretch a little further to once again feel mild tension. As with the easy stretch, the feeling of tension should subside as the position is held; if this does not happen, ease off a little. Hold the position for 20–30 seconds.

Therefore, in summary:

■ Ensure body and limb alignment are correct throughout.
■ Incorporate breathing to assist muscle relaxation.
■ Encourage relaxed sustained stretching and discourage bouncing up and down in a stretch.
■ Promote mental concentration on specific target areas during sustained stretches.
■ Advise levels of stretching that can be experienced but are not stressful or painful.
■ Promote non-competitive and enjoyable stretching, using care and common sense to appreciate how flexibility and pain thresholds vary.
■ For exercise preparation (warm-up), gently move joints through their functional ranges of motion without bouncing or force.
■ During exercising perform easy stretching as required for improved mobility and more flowing movement.
■ After exercising (warm-down), perform easy and developmental stretching to help prevent muscle soreness and promote overall body flexibility and a feeling of well-being.
■ Encourage students to take responsibility for their level of stretching and to release tight muscles as required.
■ Encourage stretching as a part of the daily routine.

(For details of specific bones, joints and muscles, see the anatomical charts on pp. xii–xiii.)

IMPROVING FOOT ALIGNMENT, MOBILITY AND STRENGTH (EXERCISES FM1–3)

Exercise FM1.1 – Exercising the forefoot (clasping with fingers and toes)

Aim/Target muscles
To exercise the intrinsic foot muscles.
To improve foot mobility.
To strengthen the foot's supporting arches.
To improve lower limb alignment.

Equipment
Chair, a raised support for sitting on the floor (e.g. a yoga block).

Body position
Sitting on a chair in a relaxed position with the backs of the thighs being supported by the chair. Bend the left leg to rest it on the right thigh supporting it with the left hand.

Action 1
Open the fingers of the left hand and place the fingers between the toes of the right foot, gently separating them. Lightly squeeze the toes together against the fingers and hold for 10 seconds. Release and repeat up to three times with each foot (Fig. 6.16A).

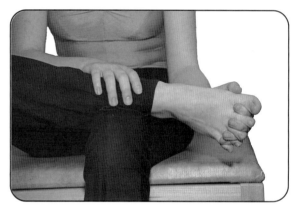

Figure 6.16A   Squeezing fingers between the toes.

Action 2
Place the left fingers over all the toes (heel of the hand underneath the toes) and apply sufficient pressure to plantarflex the right forefoot. Hold for 10 seconds (Fig. 6.16B).

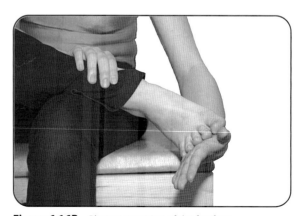

Figure 6.16B   Plantar extension of the forefoot.

Lift the fingers of the left hand away from the toes and use pressure through the heel of the left hand to plantarextend the forefoot. Hold for 10 seconds. Repeat three times in both directions with each foot.

Action 3

Use the left hand to gently mobilize each toe of the right foot through flexion, extension, abduction and adduction. Repeat on the other side.

For increased mobility through resisted stretching, apply opposing pressure with the fingers or through the use of rubber bands as the toes actively flex or extend. Hold the resistance for 10–15 seconds. Release and use the hand to passively mobilize the joints involved.

Exercise FM1.2 – Exercising the forefoot (instep lifts)

Aim/Target muscles

To exercise the intrinsic foot muscles.
To improve foot mobility.
To strengthen the foot's supporting arches.
To improve lower limb alignment.

Equipment

Chair or low bed.

Body position

Sitting on a chair with the backs of the thighs supported and both feet flat on the floor (Fig. 6.17A).

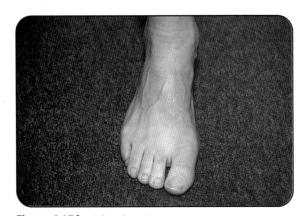

Figure 6.17A   Relaxed position.

Action

Keeping the heel and toes in contact with the floor, lift the instep. Aim to keep the toes lengthened and comparatively relaxed as the lumbrical muscles engage. Their muscular action is felt under the foot and above between the metatarsal bones, and can be observed as the spaces between them narrow.

Perform slowly, checking to see that the instep lifts evenly and correct alignment is maintained (Figs 6.17B&C).

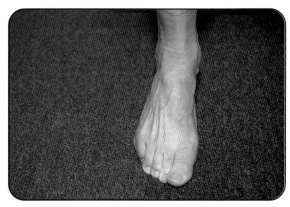

Figure 6.17B   Engaging the lumbrical muscles.

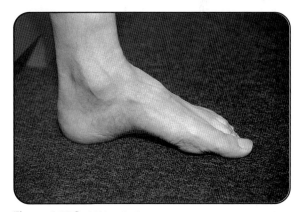

Figure 6.17C   Lifting the instep.

Exercise FM1.3 – Exercising the forefoot (instep lifts with toe action)

Aim/Target muscles

To exercise the intrinsic foot muscles.
To improve foot mobility.
To strengthen the foot's supporting arches.
To improve lower limb alignment.

Equipment

Chair or low bed, a tissue or light cloth.

Body position 1

Sitting on a chair with the backs of the thighs supported and both feet flat on the floor.

Body position 2

Lying supine with the hips and knees flexed approximately 60–90 degrees and the feet resting on a wall.

6

Action

Place the tissue or cloth on the floor under the ball of one foot. Plantarflex the foot and pick the tissue off the floor with the toes. Extend the toes and place the tissue back on the floor to repeat the motion (Fig. 6.18).

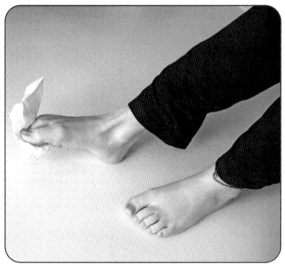

Figure 6.18

Note: Perform slowly and smoothly, observing for correct foot alignment throughout and that the instep lifts evenly during plantarflexion. Repeat 5–10 times with each foot.

⊘ Precautions
- Osteoporosis; back problems (ensure correct sitting posture); lower limb or foot pathology – monitor for pain-free activity, seek medical advice.

✚ *Contraindications*
- Provided the patient's health professional has prescribed foot mobilization, there are no specific contraindications.

Exercise FM2 – Ankle mobilization

Aim/Target muscles

To improve mobility of the muscles of the ankle joint.

Equipment

Chair or low support for sitting on the floor (e.g. a yoga block).

Body position

Sitting on a chair in a relaxed position with the backs of the thighs being supported by the chair. Bend the left leg to rest it on the right thigh, supporting it with the left hand. Hold the left foot with the right hand (Fig. 6.19A).

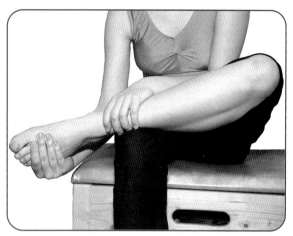

Figure 6.19A

Action 1

Applying slight resistance with the right hand, rotate the left ankle in both clockwise and anticlockwise directions, gradually increasing the range of motion with each repetition. Repeat 10–15 times in each direction on both sides (Figs 6.19B&C).

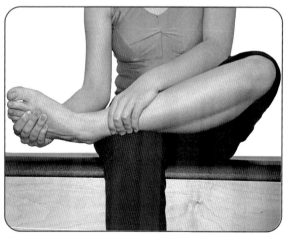

Figure 6.19B

Action 2

Perform the circling motions with the left foot without the support and resistance of the right hand, aiming to increase the range of motion with each

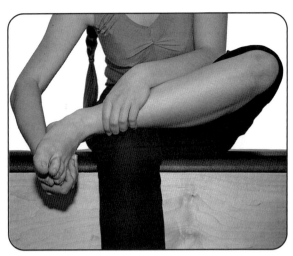

Figure 6.19C

repetition. Repeat 10–15 times in each direction on both sides.

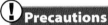**Precautions**

■ Osteoporosis; back problems (ensure correct sitting posture); lower limb or foot pathology – monitor for pain-free activity, seek medical advice.

➕ *Contraindications*

■ Provided the patient's health professional has prescribed ankle mobilization, there are no specific contraindications.

Exercise FM3.1 – Exercising the lower limb and foot (heel lifts)

Aim/Target muscles
To exercise gastrocnemius and soleus together.
To improve foot mobility and strength.
To improve lower limb alignment and strength.
To improve balance and proprioception.

Equipment
Sturdy chair or similar support, soft support for between the ankles to help maintain foot alignment.

Body position
Standing upright with the feet approximately one foot width apart and the knees extended, the hands supported on the back of a chair and the eyes looking directly ahead.

Action 1
Plantarflex the ankle and lift the heels as high as possible to balance over the toes. Lower the heels to the floor, maintaining correct upright posture throughout. Repeat smoothly and slowly for up to 12–14 repetitions

Action 2
Repeat as quickly as possible through the complete range of movement 8–10 times.
Note: To help maintain correct spine alignment and balance, keep the gaze directly ahead and cue to keep the body weight balanced between the feet throughout; to assist foot and ankle alignment during ankle plantarflexion, cue to balance the weight over the second metatarsal head and to imagine a line following the path of tibialis anterior down the front of the leg to between the great and second toes.

Action 3
Repeat Actions 1 and 2 without support.

Action 4
Repeat Actions 1 and 2 with the eyes closed.

Action 5
Repeat all the above standing on one leg.

Exercise FM3.2 – Exercising the lower limb and foot (heel lifts with flexed knees)

Aim/Target muscles
To exercise soleus with reduced gastrocnemius involvement.
To improve foot mobility and strength.
To improve lower limb alignment and strength.
To improve balance and proprioception.

Equipment
Sturdy chair or similar support, soft support for between the ankles to help maintain foot alignment.

Body position
Standing upright, feet approximately one foot width apart and turned to face very slightly outwards – 'toeing outwards'. The knees are flexed to approximately 45 degrees with the hands supported on the back of a chair and the eyes looking directly ahead.

Action 1
Maintaining knee flexion throughout, plantarflex the ankles and lift the heels as high as possible

6

to balance over the toes. Lower the heels to the floor. Repeat smoothly and slowly for up to 12 repetitions

Note: To help maintain correct spine alignment and balance, keep the gaze directly ahead and cue to keep the body weight balanced between the feet throughout; to help prevent foot/lower limb instability during hip/knee flexion, cue to direct the knees over the second and third toes during knee flexion; to assist foot and ankle alignment during ankle plantarflexion, cue to balance the weight over the second metatarsal head; to avoid tibialis anterior being overactive (it presents as a tight band at the front of the ankle during knee flexion), cue to spread the feet and think of lifting the little toes just slightly as the knees sink into flexion.

Action 2

Prepare as in Action 1. Maintaining knee flexion, plantarflex the ankles and lift the heels as high as possible to balance over the toes. Maintain ankle plantarflexion and fully extend the knees. Lower the heels and repeat rhythmically and smoothly 8–10 times.

Action 3

Reverse Action 2.

Action 4

Repeat Actions 1 and 2 without support.

Action 5

Repeat Actions 1 and 2 with support and the eyes closed.

Action 6

Repeat all the above standing with light support on one leg.

Exercise FM3.3 – Exercising the lower limb and foot (heel drops over step)

Aim/Target muscles

To improve the performance of soleus during deceleration.
To improve foot mobility and strength.
To improve lower limb alignment and strength.
To improve balance and proprioception.

Equipment

Step or similar standing support, hand support.

Body position

Standing upright with the balls of the feet on the step and the heels aligned as if standing on the floor. The hands are supported on a stair rail or similar support and the spine is correctly aligned so that the eyes look directly ahead. Transfer the weight to stand balanced on the left leg and flex the right hip and knee to lift the right foot from the step (Fig. 6.20A).

Action 1

Plantarflex the left ankle and lift the left heel as high as possible to balance over the toes.
Maintaining ankle plantarflexion, flex the left knee approximately 45 degrees, sending the knee forwards over the second and third toes (Fig. 6.20B).
Maintaining knee flexion, lower limb and ankle alignment, reach the left heel below the level of the step to stretch the calf muscles and the back of the ankle (Fig. 6.20C).
Maintaining the heel position, extend the knee and hip, then lift the heel to align once more as if standing on the floor (Fig. 6.20D).
Repeat smoothly and with control for up to 10 repetitions.

Action 2

Reverse Action 1. Begin with lowering the heel below the level of the step and continue by flexing the knee with the heel below the step before moving into plantarflexion with the knee still flexed and then finally into knee extension whilst in ankle plantarflexion.

Note: To help maintain correct spine alignment and balance, keep the gaze directly ahead and cue to keep the body weight balanced more over the balls of the feet throughout; to help prevent foot/lower limb instability during hip/knee flexion, cue to direct the knees over the second and third toes during knee flexion; to assist foot and ankle alignment during ankle plantarflexion, cue to balance the weight over the second metatarsal head.

STRETCHING THE POSTERIOR HIP AND LOWER LIMB (EXERCISES ST1–18)*

Exercise ST1 – Calf muscle stretch

Aim/Target muscles

To improve gastrocnemius and soleus muscle flexibility.

---

*For a comprehensive overview of muscle stretching, see Anderson R 2000 Stretching. Shelter Publications, Bolinas, CA

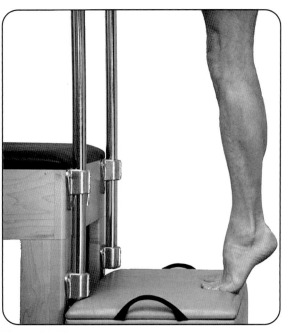

Figure 6.20A   Ankle plantar flexion.

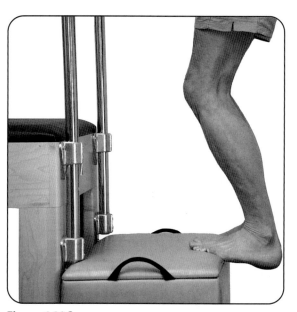

Figure 6.20C

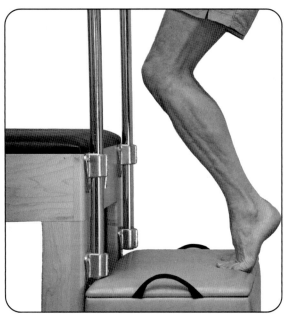

Figure 6.20B

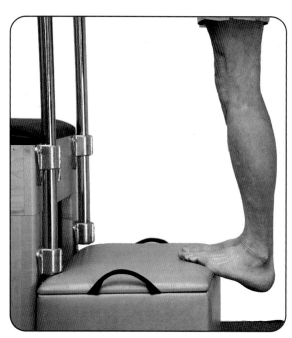

Figure 6.20D

6

Equipment
Sturdy chair, wall for body support.

Body position
Standing facing the wall (or chair), approximately 3 feet away from the wall with the hips neutral in rotation, the legs aligned with the axes of the hips and the feet pointing directly forwards. Maintaining the same leg alignment, step the right foot forwards and place the hands on the wall in front of the chest. The body weight is still more over the left leg and the right knee is slightly flexed (Fig. 6.21).

Action 1
Keeping the heels on the floor and the spine/pelvis in neutral, flex the elbows to the body forwards in one piece and transfer the body weight to be more over the right foot, allowing the right knee to flex more.
Hold the stretch for 20 seconds, increasing the stretch if required through moving the pelvis (still in a neutral position) further forwards.
Repeat on the other side.

Action 2
Develop the stretch by holding it longer but for no more than 40 seconds.

Action 3
To target the lower calf and Achilles tendon, perform Action 1 and hold the stretch for 10–15 seconds, then bend the left knee until a gentle stretch is felt in the Achilles tendon and lower calf. Hold for no more than 25 seconds.
Note: To help maintain correct spine alignment and balance, keep the gaze directly ahead and cue to keep the body weight balanced between the feet throughout; to maintain correct foot/leg alignment, cue for the knees to face directly ahead and align over the second and third toes of the feet, and to maintain the heels in contact with the floor with each foot distributing weight evenly between the heel and the forefoot.

Hamstring muscle stretching

- Individuals with very tight hamstrings may feel them stretching when performing the calf stretch series above.
- Individuals with osteoporosis should avoid spinal flexion when performing standing and sitting routines – keep the spine neutral and stable, and hinge forwards from the hips.

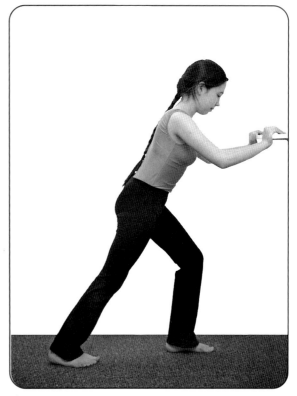

Figure 6.21   Calf muscle stretch (right leg).

Precautions
- Pregnancy; shoulder, hip, lower limb or foot pathology; injury rehabilitation, particularly during the early stages – seek medical advice.

Contraindications
- Painful hip, lower limb or foot pathology – for onward referral.

Exercise ST2.1 – Hamstring muscle stretch in standing

Aim/Target muscles
To improve semitendinosus, semimembranosus and biceps femoris muscle flexibility.

Equipment
Sturdy chair or low table.

Body position
Standing facing a chair approximately 3 feet away. With the hips neutral in rotation, stand on the

left leg and lift the right leg to rest on the chair (Fig. 6.22A).

Align both legs with the axes of the hips. Allow the right knee to flex slightly. Maintain leg alignment and, keeping the pelvis stable, flex the body forwards and place the hands lightly on the leg.

Note: Ensure the supporting surface is low enough to maintain a stable position.

Action

Breathing in – lengthen through the crown of the head, elongating the spine.

Breathing out – maintaining spinal length, draw in the lower abdominal muscles and curl the body forwards as if over a large ball to begin walking the fingers down the right leg (Fig. 6.22B).

Note: When the hamstrings begin to stretch, hold the position and rest. Focus on releasing unwanted muscle tension, particularly in the face, throat and

toes whilst breathing quietly for two or three breaths. Continue when the feeling of stretching in the hamstrings has reduced.

Breathing in – further elongate the spine, drawing the body out of the pelvis to move it slightly up away from the leg as it reaches forwards.

Breathing out – draw in the lower abdominal muscles and walk the fingers further down the right leg again, allowing the body to drop and curl as if over a large ball.

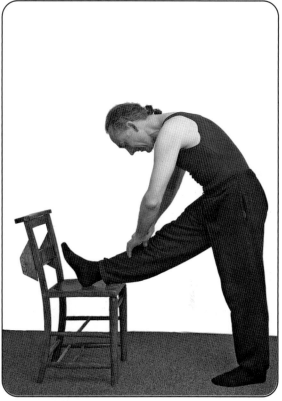

Figure 6.22B Hamstring stretch – position 2.

Note: Cue to imagine the hamstrings stretching from the back of the knee to the sitting bones and the calf muscles from the back of the knee to the heel.

Breathing normally – rest again, allowing hamstring tension to release. The hips remain neutral in rotation and the foot and ankle of the raised leg are relaxed. Develop the stretch for 20–30 seconds, allowing the breathing to assist muscle relaxation, spine elongation, mobilization and stabilization.

Repeat two to three times. Repeat on the left side.

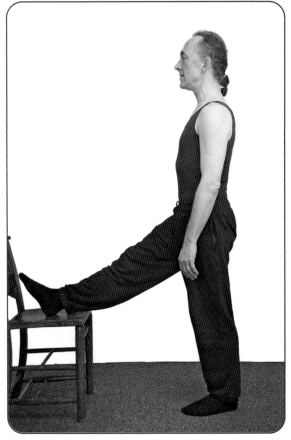

Figure 6.22A Hamstring stretch – position 1.

Precautions

■ Pregnancy; osteoporosis (perform with spine in neutral and hinged forward from the hips); shoulder, back, lower limb or foot pathology; injury rehabilitation, particularly during the early stages – seek medical advice.

Contraindications

■ Painful back, hip or lower limb pathology – for onward referral.

Exercise ST2.2 – Hamstring muscle stretch in sitting

Aim/Target muscles
To improve semitendinosus, semimembranosus and biceps femoris muscle flexibility.

Equipment
Bench or firm bed.

Body position
Sitting on a bench or firm bed with the left foot on the floor, the right leg extended on the bench and the body facing the leg (Fig. 6.23A).

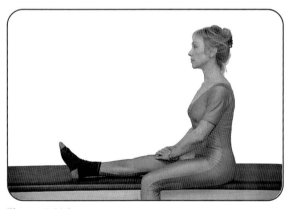

Figure 6.23A   Action 1.

A small rolled towel can be placed under the knee to flex it slightly. As flexibility improves, remove the towel and encourage lengthening through the back of the knee to progress the exercise.

Action
Place the hands lightly on the right thigh or beside the leg on the bed.

Breathing in – lengthen through the crown of the head, elongating the spine.

Breathing out – maintaining spinal length, draw in the lower abdominal muscles and curl the body forwards as if over a large ball to begin walking the fingers down the right leg or bed (Fig. 6.23B).

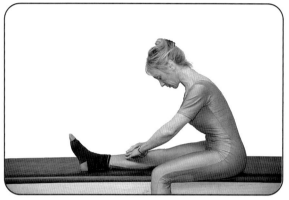

Figure 6.23B   Action 2.

Note: When the hamstrings begin to stretch, hold the position and rest. Focus on releasing unwanted muscle tension, particularly in the face, throat and toes, whilst breathing quietly for two or three breaths. Continue when the feeling of stretching in the hamstrings has reduced.

Breathing in – further elongate the spine, drawing the body out of the pelvis to move it slightly up away from the leg as it reaches forwards (Fig. 6.23C).

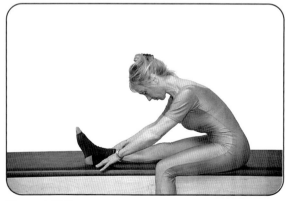

Figure 6.23C   Action 3.

Breathing out – draw the lower abdominal muscles in and walk the fingers further down the right leg/bed, curling the body as if over a large ball (Fig. 6.23D).

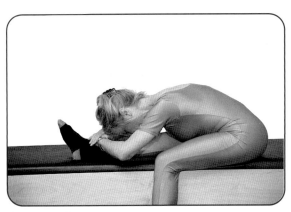

Figure 6.23D   Action 4.

Note: Cue to imagine the hamstrings stretching from the back of the knee to the sitting bones and the calf muscles from the back of the knee to the heel.

Breathing normally – rest again, allowing hamstring tension to release. The right knee stays facing the ceiling and the right toe, foot and calf muscles are relaxed.

Develop the stretch for 20–30 seconds, allowing the breathing to assist muscle relaxation, spine elongation, mobilization and stabilization.

Repeat two to three times. Repeat on the left side.

Note: When 90 degrees of hip flexion can be achieved in supine with the pelvis neutral and stable, perform Exercise ST2.3.

> (!) **Precautions**
> ■ Pregnancy; osteoporosis (individuals with osteoporosis should avoid spinal flexion when performing standing and sitting routines – keep the spine neutral and stable, and hinge forwards from the hips); shoulder, back, lower limb or foot pathology; injury rehabilitation, particularly during the early stages – seek medical advice.

> (+) **Contraindications**
> ■ Advanced stages of pregnancy; osteoporosis; painful back, hip or lower limb pathology – for onward referral.

Exercise ST2.3 – Hamstring muscle stretch in supine

Aim/Target muscles
To individually and collectively improve semitendinosus, semimembranosus and biceps femoris muscle flexibility.

Equipment
Exercise mat or firm bed, a yoga belt or similar non-elastic strap, head supports to correct head/neck alignment and prevent neck tension.

Body position
Supine position with both legs flexed 90 degrees at hip/knee or with one knee flexed and the other leg extended along the mat. Hold the strap between the hands and bend the right knee and place the right foot in the strap. Keeping the pelvis neutral and stable and the hip neutral in rotation, extend the right knee to align the right leg with the axis of the right hip (Fig. 6.24A).

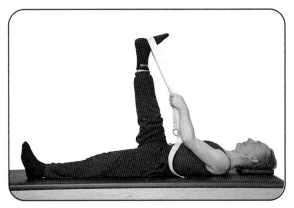

Figure 6.24A

Adjust the hands on the strap so that the arms extend until the elbows are still slightly flexed and the scapulae are able to draw down the back and stabilize on the ribcage. Allow the weight of the right leg to drop the femoral head down into the hip socket.

Action 1
Note: This stretches the hamstring muscles collectively.

Breathing in – lengthen through the crown of the head, elongating the spine.

Breathing out – maintaining spinal length, activate the lower abdominal muscles and begin drawing the leg towards the body in line with the axis of its hip.

Note: When the hamstrings begin to gently stretch, rest in that position, breathing normally for two or three breaths. Focus on maintaining a feeling of

6

space between the thigh and the pelvis (check with the thumb as in the illustration) and allowing the face, throat, back legs and toes to relax whilst breathing easily. Keep the hip neutral in rotation throughout.

Breathing in – lengthen through the crown of the head, elongating the spine.

Breathing out – continue, allowing the stretch to increase with each breathing cycle.

Develop the stretch for 25–30 seconds.

Repeat two to three times to each side.

Action 2

This stretches the medial aspect of the hamstring muscles. Prepare as in Action 1 and extend the right leg in line with the axis of the hip. Take the belt in the right hand and place the left hand on the left hip to assist pelvic stability (Fig. 6.24B).

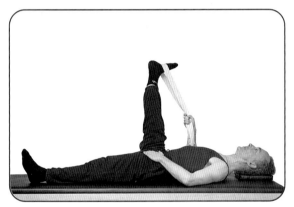

Figure 6.24B

Laterally rotate the right hip and perform the breathing and stretching sequence, drawing the right leg towards the right shoulder. A stretch will be felt more down the medial aspect of the hamstrings and the back of the knee.

Repeat two to three times to each side.

Action 3

This stretches the lateral aspect of the hamstring muscles. Prepare as in Action 1 and extend the left leg in line with the axis of the hip. Take the belt in the right hand and place the left thumb in the left groin area to assist pelvic stability and hip placement (Fig. 6.24C).

Medially rotate the left hip and perform the breathing and stretching sequencing, drawing the left leg towards the right shoulder. A stretch will be felt more down the lateral aspect of the hamstrings and the back of the knee.

Repeat two to three times to each side.

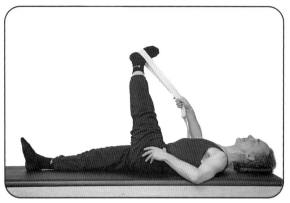

Figure 6.24C

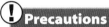

Precautions

■ Pregnancy; osteoporosis; shoulder, back, lower limb or foot pathology; injury rehabilitation, particularly during the early stages – seek medical advice.

Contraindications

■ Painful back, hip or lower limb pathology – for onward referral.

Exercise ST3.1 – Tensor fasciae latae stretch in standing

Aim/Target muscles

To improve flexibility in the upper, outer hip muscles.

Equipment

Sturdy chair or a wall.

Body position

Standing facing the wall (or chair), approximately 3 feet away from the wall with the hips neutral in rotation, the legs aligned with the axes of the hips and the feet pointing directly forwards. Maintaining the same leg alignment, step the right foot forwards and place the hands on the wall in front of the chest. The body weight is still more over the left leg and the right knee is slightly flexed (Fig. 6.25A).

Action 1

Keeping the heels on the floor and the spine/pelvis in neutral, flex the elbows to move the body forwards in one piece and transfer the body weight to be more over the right foot, allowing the right knee to flex more. Maintain this forward position and gently rotate the left hip forwards and the right hip backwards (Fig. 6.25B).

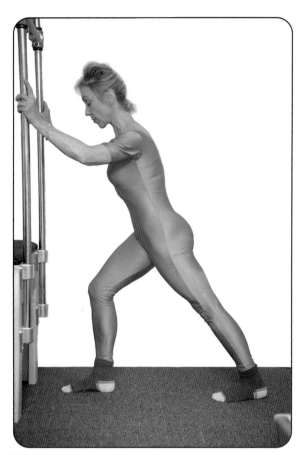

Figure 6.25A   Tensor fasciae latae stretching.

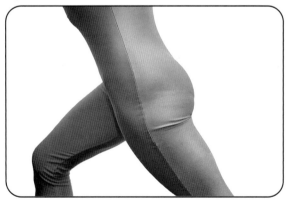

Figure 6.25B

Then still keeping the medial aspect of the left foot in contact with the floor, allow the body weight to shift more forwards, diagonally to the left, stretching the outer aspect of the left hip (Fig. 6.25C).

Hold the stretch for 20–25 seconds, possibly moving the pelvis further forwards to the right to increase the stretch.

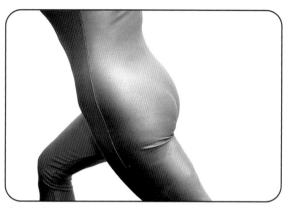

Figure 6.25C

Repeat two to three times to each side.

Note: Progress to Action 2 when 90 degrees of hip flexion can be achieved whilst maintaining a neutral and stable pelvis lying in the supine position.

> **⚠ Precautions**
> ■ Pregnancy; osteoporosis; shoulder, back, knee or foot pathology; injury rehabilitation, particularly during the early stages – seek medical advice.

> **➕ Contraindications**
> ■ Painful back, hip or knee pathology – for onward referral.

Exercise ST3.2 – Tensor fasciae latae stretch in supine

Aim/Target muscles
To improve tensor fasciae latae muscle flexibility.

Equipment
Mat or firm bed, a yoga belt or similar non-elastic strap, head supports to correct head/neck alignment and prevent neck tension.

Body position
Supine position with the knees bent and lumbar spine in neutral. Holding the strap between the hands, bend the left knee and place the left foot in the strap (Fig. 6.26A).

Keeping the pelvis neutral and stable and the hip neutral in rotation, extend the left knee to align the left leg with the axis of its hip.

6

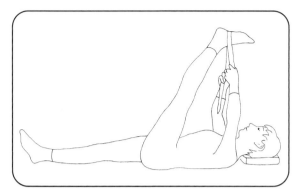

Figure 6.26A Supine tensor fasciae latae stretch.

Adjust the hands on the strap so that the arms extend until the elbows are still slightly flexed and the scapulae are able to draw down the back and stabilize on the ribcage.

Allow the weight of the left leg to drop the femoral head down into the hip joint.

Take the belt in the right hand and place the left thumb in the left groin area to assist pelvic stability and hip placement (Fig. 6.26B).

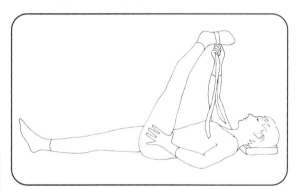

Figure 6.26B

Action

Breathing in – lengthen through the crown of the head, elongating the spine.

Breathing out – maintaining spinal length, activate the lower abdominal muscles and begin drawing the leg towards the body in line with the axis of its hip.

Breathing normally – maintaining spinal length and abdominal muscle control, slightly medially rotate the left hip to face the left knee more towards the right. Allow the left foot to slightly pronate and turn in the strap so that the sole faces more towards the right.

Breathing in.

Breathing out – maintaining spine length and abdominal muscle control, draw the leg gently

across the body to stretch the outer, upper aspect of the right hip.

Breathing normally – sustain the stretch for 25–30 seconds if possible, but no longer than is reasonably comfortable. Focus on maintaining a feeling of space between the thigh and the pelvis (check with the thumb as in the illustration) and use the breathing to assist relaxation of the target muscles as well as the face, throat, back, legs and toes.

Note: The pelvis remains neutral and stable throughout.

Repeat two to three times to each side.

Exercise ST4.1 – Gluteal and hamstring stretch (hip and thigh stretch with strap)

Aim/Target muscles
To improve gluteal and hamstring muscle flexibility.

Equipment
Mat or firm bed, a yoga belt or similar non-elastic strap, head supports to correct head/neck alignment and prevent neck tension.

Body position
Supine with the knees bent and lumbar spine in neutral. Hold the strap between the hands and bend the right knee and place the right foot in the strap (Fig. 6.27A).

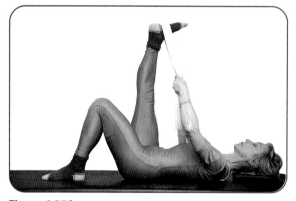

Figure 6.27A

Action
Take the strap in the left hand, flex the right knee and laterally rotate the right hip, pulling the foot in the strap towards the chest (Fig. 6.27B).

Keeping the pelvis neutral and stable, gently draw the leg more towards the centre of the body. If a stretch is felt in the buttocks and the upper back of the thigh, hold this position for 15–20 seconds then repeat on the other side (Fig. 6.27C).

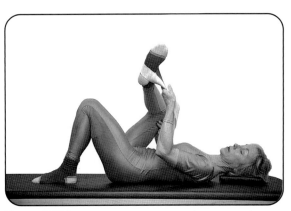

Figure 6.27B

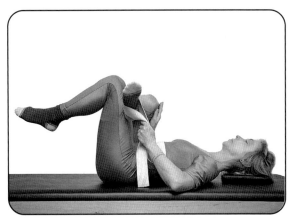

Figure 6.27C

For a deeper stretch, further flex the left hip, lifting the left foot off the floor and use the left leg to draw the right foot nearer to the body as you gently press the right hand on the right inner thigh to assist laterally rotating and stretching the right hip. Use the breath to increase the stretch.

Breathing in.

Breathing out – relax the face, throat, upper back and toes and gently draw the right foot more towards and across the body.

Breathing normally – hold for 15–20 seconds.

Repeat two to three times to each side.

Note: The lower back will flatten as the leg moves towards the chest to establish the stretch position. Aim to keep the lumbar spine and pelvis stable to develop the stretch.

Exercise ST4.2 – Gluteal and hamstring stretch (knee hugs with crossed thighs)

Aim/Target muscles

To improve gluteal and hamstring muscle flexibility.

Equipment

Mat or firm bed, head supports to correct head/neck alignment and prevent neck tension.

Body position

Supine with the knees bent and the lumbar spine in neutral. Flex the right hip and move the thigh in an arc until it is perpendicular to the floor in approximately 90 degrees of hip/knee flexion. Flex the left hip, bringing the left thigh to align with the right (Fig. 6.28A).

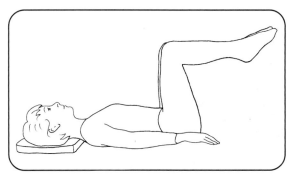

Figure 6.28A Knee hugs with crossed thighs – action 1.

Cross the thighs and hold the left foot in the right hand and the right foot in the left hand (Fig. 6.28B).

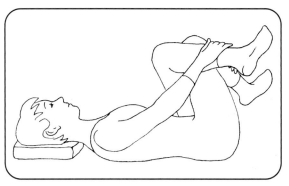

Figure 6.28B Knee hugs with crossed thighs – action 2.

Note: Keep the lumbar spine and pelvis in neutral and the groins soft and deep as the hips flex.

Breathing in – lengthen through the crown of the head and breathe deeply into the sides of the chest.

Breathing out – relax the face, throat, back and toes and gently cross the legs further, drawing them towards the chest to stretch the gluteal and upper hamstring muscles (Fig. 6.28C).

Breathing normally – hold for 15–20 seconds.

Repeat on both sides two to three times.

6

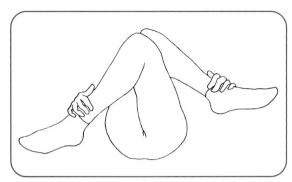

Figure 6.28C

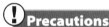**Precautions**
- Pregnancy; osteoporosis; shoulder, back, knee or foot pathology; injury rehabilitation, particularly during the early stages – seek medical advice.

➕ *Contraindications*
- Painful back, hip or knee pathology – for onward referral.

Exercise ST4.3 – Sacroiliac release

Aim/Target area
To improve flexibility in the lower back.

Equipment
Mat or firm bed, head supports to correct head/neck alignment and prevent neck tension.

Body position
Supine with the knees bent and the lumbar spine in neutral. Flex the right hip and move the thigh in an arc until it is perpendicular to the floor, approximately 90 degrees of hip/knee flexion. Clasp the hands behind the back of the thigh.

Action
Keeping the lumbar spine flattened and stable, try to gently extend the right thigh away from the torso whilst resisting the movement with the hands (this will create a sensation of tightening around the right sacroiliac region). Maintain this position and effort for approximately 15 seconds.
Breathing in – expand the sides and back of the chest and lengthen the spine from the crown of the head through to the ischial tuberosities.
Breathing out – keeping the pelvis in a neutral position, draw the right thigh in towards the chest to gently stretch the right sacroiliac region.
Repeat three to five times.
Repeat the whole sequence on the left side.

❗**Precautions**
- Pregnancy; osteoporosis; shoulder, spine/lower back, hip and knee pathology; back injury rehabilitation, particularly in the early stages – seek medical advice.

➕ *Contraindications*
- Advanced stages of pregnancy; painful spine, lower back or hip pathology – for onward referral.

Exercise ST5.1 – Iliopsoas stretch in supine

Aim
To improve iliopsoas muscle flexibility.

Equipment
Bench or firm raised bed, head supports to correct head/neck alignment and prevent neck tension.

Target muscles
Iliopsoas.

Body position
Supine with the lower back supported on the bed and the knees hugged to the chest. The ischial tuberosities are aligned with the edge of the bed (Fig. 6.29).

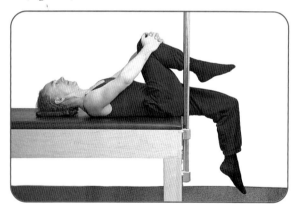

Figure 6.29

Action
Keeping the lumbar spine flattened and stable, keep holding the right leg and gently lower the left leg so that it hangs over the edge of the bed.
Breathing normally – relax the face, back, legs and toes and allow the weight of the leg to gently stretch the groin area. Maintain for 30–60 seconds.
Repeat once or twice to each side.
Note: Ideally there will be 90 degrees of hip and knee flexion in this position (see postural assessment, Chapter 1).

Exercise ST5.2 – Iliopsoas stretch in standing

Aim
To improve iliopsoas muscle flexibility.

Equipment
Mat or firm bed.

Target muscles
Iliopsoas.

Body position
Standing with the hips neutral in rotation and each leg in line with the axis of its hip. Bend the right knee and reach the left leg back into a lunge. Allow the body to bend to rest the hands on the floor. Keep the left leg extended and its knee off the floor. Adjust the position so that the right knee is directly over the right lower leg and ankle and the left leg is in line with the axis of the left hip (Fig. 6.30A).

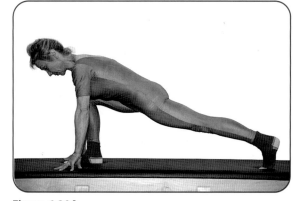

Figure 6.30A

Action
Breathing in – reach from the crown of the head through to the ischial tuberosities and lift the body away from the left knee to achieve a neutral spine. Level the pelvis so that both hips face the floor. Aiming to maintain the neutral spine, deepen the right knee bend and reach the left leg further back to rest its knee on the floor (Fig. 6.30B).

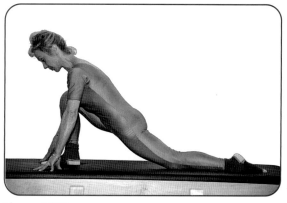

Figure 6.30B

Breathing out – Engage the lower abdominal muscles to assist pelvic stability and move the pelvis slightly forwards, increasing the stretch in the groin.
Breathing normally – hold for 20–30 seconds.
Repeat on both sides two to three times.

Exercise ST6 – Quadriceps stretch

Aim
To improve quadriceps muscle flexibility.

Equipment
Mat or firm bed, rolled towel if needed for head or thigh support, a yoga belt if needed to create space at the back of the knee.

Target muscles
Quadriceps group.

Body position
Lying face down, preferably on a mat or a raised bed that enables the ankles to relax as the feet drop over the edge. The arms are bent with the elbows pointing to the side, and the hands resting one on top of the other to make a support for the forehead. Leave the right hand supporting the head and reach the left hand back to grasp the left foot (Fig. 6.31A).

6

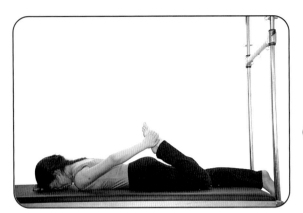

Figure 6.31A

Action 1

Breathing in – to prepare.

Breathing out – tighten the lower abdominal muscles, lengthening and stabilizing the lumbar spine to press both groins into the mat whilst keeping the gluteal muscles comparatively relaxed.

Draw the left foot towards the left ischial tuberosity, stretching the centre front of the left thigh.

Breathing normally – hold for 10–12 seconds, allowing the front thigh muscles to release.

Repeat on the right side. Perform on each leg two to three times.

Note: To develop the stretch, repeat the motion using the exhalation to draw the foot nearer to the body. Hold for up to 30 seconds, breathing normally whilst maintaining spine stability and relaxing into the stretch.

Action 2

Perform Action 1, drawing the foot to the lateral aspect of the pelvis to stretch the medial front thigh muscles (Fig. 6.31B).

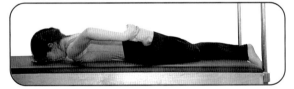

Figure 6.31B

Perform once or twice as required to achieve more balanced thigh muscle flexibility.

Action 3

Perform Action 1, drawing the foot to the medial aspect of the thigh to stretch the lateral front thigh muscles. Perform once or twice as required to achieve more balanced thigh muscle flexibility.

Note: When rehabilitating knee problems, place a slim support such as a yoga belt or thin rolled towel at the back of the knee to maintain space during knee flexion. This helps to prevent knee joint discomfort and/or strain. A rolled towel may also be placed to support the thigh and extend the hip a little to increase stretch of rectus femoris and psoas muscles. Ensure the pelvis remains neutral and stable.

! Precautions

■ Pregnancy; lower back, hip or knee/ankle pathology. For rehabilitation of knee injuries, seek medical advice as to the stage of recovery.

+ Contraindications

■ Advanced stages of pregnancy; painful hip or knee pathology – for onward referral.

Exercise ST7 – Adductor stretch

Aim

To improve adductor muscle flexibility.

Equipment

Mat, wall.

Target muscles

Adductor group.

Body position

Supine with the lumbar spine relaxed. The body lies approximately 10–12 cm from a wall with the legs up and resting together on the wall. The hips are neutral in rotation so the knees face directly forwards. The arms are laterally rotated and bent with the fingers of the hands interlacing behind and supporting the head, or resting down beside the body, the palms rotated to the ceiling or the floor (Fig. 6.32).

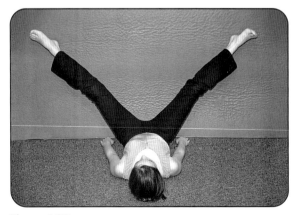

Figure 6.32

Breathing in – to prepare.

Breathing out – allow the whole body to relax as if imprinting itself into the mat.

Breathing normally – remain in this position, relaxing both mind and body for 30–60 seconds.

Breathing in – lengthen from the crown of the head through to the ischial tuberosities.

Breathing out – gently engage the lower abdominal muscles to stabilize the lumbar spine and begin opening the legs, allowing gravity to then draw them towards the floor. Keep the hips neutral in rotation.

Note: When a gentle stretch begins, focus on relaxing the toes, feet, back and throat.

Breathing normally – relax into the stretch and hold for up to 30 seconds.

Breathing in.

Breathing out – allow the legs to rotate laterally and relax more into the stretch.

Breathing normally – notice specific areas of tightness and adjust the legs to stretch those areas. Hold for up to 15 seconds.

To return to the starting position, flex the knees and use the hands to assist moving the legs back up the wall. To return to sitting, bend the knees towards the chest and roll over to one side to rest for a few moments before gently getting up. Gradual recovery from the 'feet higher than head' position helps to prevent dizziness or loss of balance when moving to sitting and standing.

⊘ Precautions
- Pregnancy; spine, lower back, hip and lower limb pathology – seek medical advice.

➕ Contraindications
- Advanced stages of pregnancy; painful hip or lower back pathology – for onward referral.

Exercise ST8 – Supine back stretch

Aim
To improve flexibility in the lower back muscles.

Equipment
Mat or firm bed, head supports to correct head/neck alignment and prevent neck tension.

Target muscles
Lower back.

Body position
Supine with the knees bent and lumbar spine in neutral. Flex the right hip and move the thigh in an arc until it is perpendicular to the floor in approximately 90 degrees of hip/knee flexion. Flex the left hip, bringing the left thigh to align with the right.

Action
Keeping the lumbar spine flattened and stable, place the hands lightly on the knees (Fig. 6.33A).

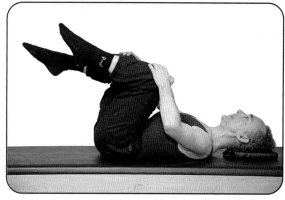

Figure 6.33A

Breathing in – expand the sides and back of the chest and lengthen the spine from the crown of the head through to the ischial tuberosities.

Breathing out – keeping the left leg still and the pelvis stable, gently draw the right knee towards the chest (Fig. 6.33B).

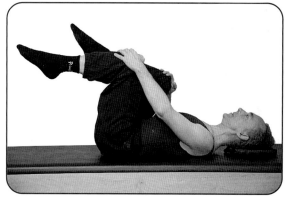

Figure 6.33B

Breathing in – return the right leg to align with the left.

Breathing out – draw the left knee to the chest.

Breathing in – return the left leg to align with the right.

Breathing out – draw both legs towards the chest, lengthening from the crown of the head to the ischial tuberosities and maintaining the lumbar spine neutral and stable (Fig. 6.33C).

6

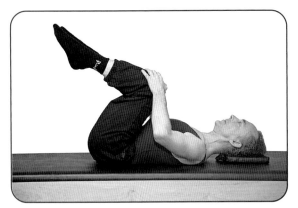

Figure 6.33C

On *breathing out*, relax the face, back, legs and toes and use just sufficient abdominal muscle control to assist lumbar spine stability.

Repeat the whole sequence three to five times.

Precautions
- Pregnancy; osteoporosis; shoulder, spine/lower back, hip and knee pathology; back injury rehabilitation, particularly in the early stages – seek medical advice.

Contraindications
- Advanced stages of pregnancy; painful spine, lower back or hip pathology – for onward referral.

Exercise ST9 – Spine stretch

Aim
To improve flexibility in the spine and lower back muscles.

Equipment
Mat or firm bed, head supports to correct head/neck alignment and prevent neck tension.

Target muscles
Spinal and back.

Body position
Supine with the knees bent and lumbar spine in neutral. Flex the right hip and move the thigh in an arc until it is perpendicular to the floor in approximately 90 degrees of hip flexion with the lower legs and feet relaxed. Flex the left hip, bringing the left thigh to align with the right and place the hands below the knees (Fig. 6.34A).

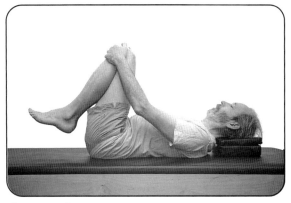

Figure 6.34A

Action
Breathing in – to prepare.
Breathing out – drawing the abdominal muscles gently towards the spine, drop the chin towards the chest and curl the upper torso away from the bed, drawing the knees towards the chest. Hug the knees with the arms and allow the lumbar spine to flex with the leg action, stretching the lower back (Fig. 6.34B).

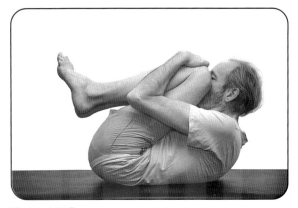

Figure 6.34B

Breathing in – draw the abdominal muscles to the spine to control the return to starting position.
Breathing out – rest the head back on its support and totally relax the back.
Breathing in – to prepare.
Breathing out – repeat the hugging action.
Repeat 5–10 times.
Note: To increase the stretch, maintain the hugging position, breathing normally for 10–25 seconds before returning to the starting position. Allow the gaze to follow the movement of the head, and the throat and upper back muscles to relax throughout.

Precautions
- Pregnancy; shoulder, spine/lower back, hip and knee pathology; back injury rehabilitation, particularly in the early stages – seek medical advice.

Contraindications
- Advanced stages of pregnancy; osteoporosis (spinal flexion to be avoided); painful spine, lower back or hip pathology – for onward referral.

Exercise ST10 – Neck stretch

Aim
To improve flexibility in the neck and upper back muscles.

Equipment
Chair or firm bed.

Target muscles
Neck and upper back.

Body position
Sitting with normal cervical curve intact and the eyes looking directly ahead. The hips are flexed approximately 90 degrees and the backs of the thighs are fully supported by the chair. Gently activate the pectoral girdle stabilizing muscles if needed to maintain their alignment.

Action 1
Cervical spine flexion and extension. Keeping the upright sitting position, allow the weight of the head to drop the chin, flexing the cervical spine and gently stretching the back of the neck.
Hold and relax into the stretch if this feels comfortable before reversing the motion and stretching the chin up towards the ceiling. Return to the starting position.
Note: Maintain length through the back of the neck and move the gaze with the head motion.

Action 2
Atlantoaxial rotation. Keeping the left shoulder still, gently reach the crown of the head away from the top of the spine and rotate the head to the right. A stretch will be felt down the left side of the neck, perhaps even to the lateral aspect of the left collarbone. If desired, hold and relax into the stretch before repeating to the left.

Note: For greater neck mobility the stretch reflex may be inhibited by the following: hold the rotated position with the eyes looking to the right, then move them rapidly from left to right for 20–30 seconds. Cease the eye motion and rotate the head even further to the right, looking over the right shoulder. Return to the starting position and repeat on the other side.

Action 3
Lateral flexion, from the same starting position with the eyes looking directly forwards. Allow the weight of the head to drop it towards the right side until a stretch is felt down the left side of the neck and possibly down the front and back of the chest. Hold and relax into the stretch if this feels comfortable before performing to the right.
Note: As the head drops to one side the nose and eyes face directly forwards to prevent unwanted cervical spine flexion or rotation.

Action 4
Head circles. Maintaining the upright sitting position, allow the weight of the head to flex the cervical spine then continue to move it slowly through right side flexion, extension, left side flexion and back to flexion. Repeat to the left.
Repeat again to each side, stopping to stretch tight areas as required, providing this is comfortable.

Precautions:
- Osteoporosis (avoid spinal flexion) cervical spine and shoulder pathology, neck muscle strain/injury in the early stages of rehabilitation: seek medical advice.

Contraindications:
- Painful neck or shoulder pathology; seek medical advice

6

Exercise ST11 – Neck, shoulder and upper back stretch

Aim
To improve flexibility in the neck and upper back muscles.

Equipment
Chair or firm bed, a long theraband of medium elasticity.

Target muscles
Neck and upper back.

Body position

Sitting with normal cervical curve intact and the eyes looking directly ahead. The hips are flexed approximately 90 degrees and the backs of the thighs are fully supported by the chair. Gently activate the pectoral girdle stabilizing muscles if needed to maintain their alignment (Fig. 6.35A).

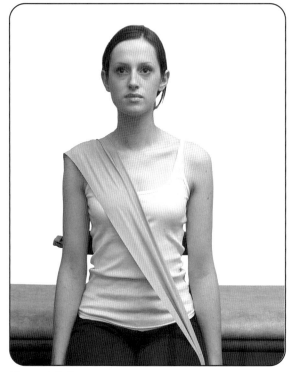

Figure 6.35A

Before action

Before setting the body position, tie the ends of the theraband to form an elastic circle. Fix the theraband under the front left and back right chair legs and sit on the chair with the theraband resting over the right shoulder. It should feel firmly in place so as not to slip during the motion. Maintaining the upright position, elevate and depress the right pectoral girdle.

Action 1

Slow controlled motions (1–2 seconds/slow counts up; 2–3 seconds/slow counts down). Allow the shoulder and neck muscles to release fully at the end of the motion (Fig. 6.35B).

Perform six to eight times to each side.

Note: Use the gentle resistance of the theraband during shoulder elevation and work against its assistance during shoulder release to achieve

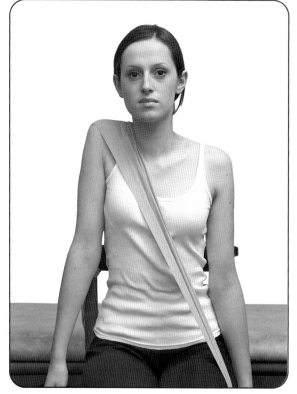

Figure 6.35B

controlled muscle action. The controlled, resisted eccentric muscle action during shoulder release assists muscle flexibility and performance.

Action 2

Perform circular motions with the pectoral girdle, first taking the shoulder back, up, forwards and down six to eight times before reversing the motion. Perform six to eight times.

Perform Actions 1 and 2 on the left side.

If one side of the neck/shoulder feels tighter than the other, adjust the number of repetitions accordingly.

Precautions

■ Shoulder pathology; neck muscle strain/injury in the early stages of rehabilitation – seek medical advice.

Contraindications

■ Painful neck or shoulder pathology – for onward referral.

Exercise ST12 – Sitting back stretch

Aim

To improve hamstring, gluteal and back muscle flexibility.

Equipment

Mat or firm bed, a yoga block or small box, rolled towel, foam roller, triangle.

Target muscles

Spinal, back and hamstring group.

Body position

Sitting with the hips abducted approximately 45–60 degrees. Individuals with tight back muscles, short hamstring and/or tight gluteal muscles may sit on a yoga block or small box and rest their hands on a foam roller or triangle (Fig. 6.36A).

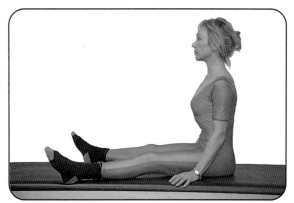

Figure 6.36A

Action 1

Breathing in – lengthen from the sitting bones through to the crown of the head and reach the body forwards as if over a large ball. Allow the fingers to slide or move their support forwards (the foam roller can turn away from the body) (Fig. 6.36B).

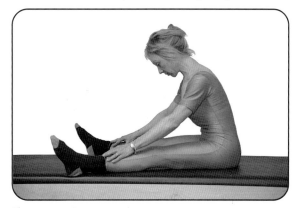

Figure 6.36B

Breathing out – keeping the spine lengthened and the pelvis stable, keep curling the body as if over a ball and allow its weight to gently move it towards the floor (Fig. 6.36C).

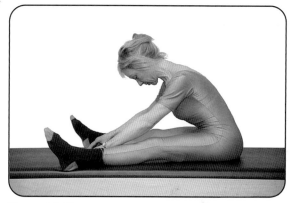

Figure 6.36C

Breathing normally for three or four breaths – maintain this position, relaxing the face, back, legs and toes, and allow the weight of the body to gently stretch the back.

Breathing in – maintaining pelvic stability, lift the body slightly away from the legs, aiming for a stretch from the sitting bones through to the crown of the head.

Note: Imagine the hamstrings stretching from the back of the knees to the sitting bones and the calf muscles from the back of the knees to the heels.

Breathing out – keeping the spine lengthened and the pelvis stable, further curl the body up and over an imaginary ball and allow its weight to gently move it towards the floor.

Note: The roller or triangle moves forwards with the body. The cervical spine curves remain intact with the gaze being soft and following the movement of the head.

Breathing normally – maintain this position, relaxing the face, back, legs and toes, and allow the weight of the body to gently stretch the back.

Hold for 30 seconds and develop the stretch further if required. Repeat once or twice.

Action 2

Perform with spine rotation. To prepare, maintain the pelvis neutral and stable, rotate the upper torso from above the waist to the right and continue as in Action 1. Repeat to the left (Figs 6.37A&B).

Action 3

Perform Actions 1 and 2 with increased hip abduction to further stretch the adductors and allow increased spine/hip flexion.

6

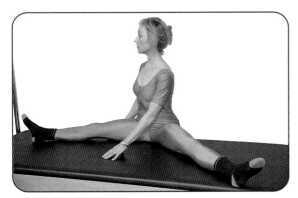

Figure 6.37A

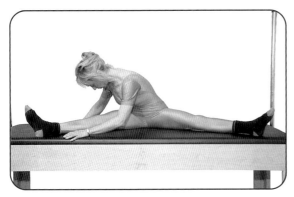

Figure 6.37B

Note: Aim to keep the pelvis stable with the hips neutral in rotation and the knees facing the ceiling as the body curls up and over towards the floor.

6

> ⊘ **Precautions**
> - Pregnancy; hip, spine/lower back pathology – seek medical advice.

> ⊕ **Contraindications**
> - Advanced stages of pregnancy; osteoporosis (spinal flexion to be avoided); painful spine, lower back or hip pathology – for onward referral.

Exercise ST13 – Prone back stretch (child pose)

Aim
To improve spine and back muscle flexibility.

Equipment
Mat or firm bed; a yoga block if needed for shoulder, head or pelvic support; rolled towel if needed for

head, pelvic or ankle support; a yoga belt if needed to create space at the back of the knee.

Target muscles
Spinal, pectoral girdle, torso and gluteal.

Body position
Four-point kneeling with the hips flexed 90 degrees, the knees no more than hip distance apart and the feet facing away from the body. The hands are placed approximately in line with or just in front of the glenohumeral joint (if the arms are comparatively long) and the arms are slightly rotated laterally. The little fingers press lightly into the floor to assist engagement of the pectoral girdle stabilizing muscles. The back of the neck is lengthened with the cervical curve intact and the superficial neck muscles comparatively relaxed. The gaze is between the thumbs.

Keep the hands still and move the hips back to rest the pelvis on the heels.

Lengthen the spine and feel the weight of the pelvis as it drops to the heels. Stretch the back from the coccyx through to the crown of the head (Fig. 6.38A).

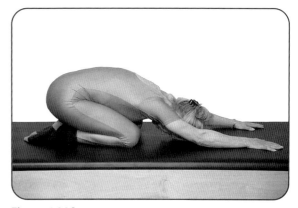

Figure 6.38A

Action 1
Breathing in – inhale into the back and sides of the ribcage.

Breathing out – relax the back, press lightly down with the hands (particularly press through the little fingers) and reach the crown of the head forwards and down and the ischial tuberosities to the heels.

Breathing normally – relax the whole body for 10–20 seconds, allowing the back muscles to release and the spine to lengthen.

Repeat the breathing cycle, allowing the muscles to further release.

Note: If the position is uncomfortable for the shoulders and arms, flex the elbows and move the hands more towards the head or relax the arms beside the body (medially rotated with the palms to the ceiling and with the head resting on a support for comfort). Alternatively, allow the pelvis to be supported above the heels with a yoga block or rolled towel. As overall flexibility improves, alter the position to stretch the arms and shoulders more.

Action 2
Progress from Action 1, stretching one arm and then the other further forwards along the floor.

Action 3
Assisted back stretch. Place the hands as illustrated in the diagram and, during *breathing out*, firmly but gently apply pressure through the heels of the hands to create a diagonal stretch across the back. Perform on both sides (Figs 6.38B & 6.39A).

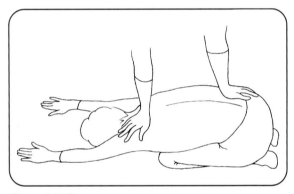

Figure 6.38B

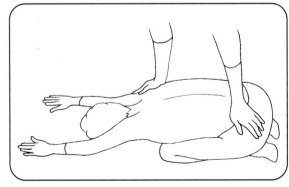

Figure 6.39A

Stretch the spine by placing the hands above the sacrum and thoracic spine and, during *breathing out*, firmly but gently apply pressure through the heels of the hands. Direct the heels of the hands away from each other to create the stretch (Figs 6.39B&C).
Note: Perform this stretch with care, making sure pressure is not applied downwards towards the spine.

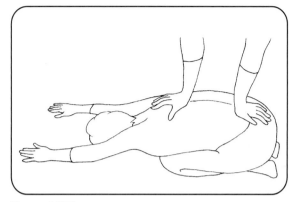

Figure 6.39B

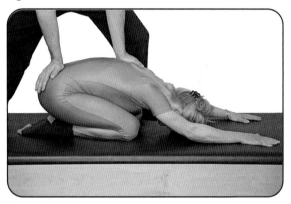

Figure 6.39C

Action 4
Prepare as in Action 1. Keep the right arm stretching forwards, flex the left elbow and turn the left palm towards the ceiling and slide it under the right arm as the upper torso rotates towards the right (Fig. 6.39D).

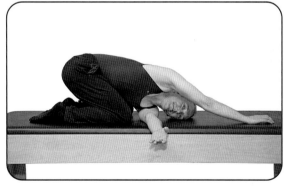

Figure 6.39D

Breathing in – inhale into the back and sides of the ribcage.
Breathing out – draw in the abdominal muscles, lengthen the spine and rotate the upper torso to the left, sliding the right hand under the left arm.

6

Note: Relax and lengthen the back as the spine rotates.

Breathing normally – hold the position for 15 seconds, allowing the back muscles to release to further lengthen and rotate the spine.

Breathing in – rotate the spine back to its starting position.

Breathing out – repeat the motion.

Perform two to three times to each side.

> ⊘ **Precautions**
> - Pregnancy; hip, spine/lower back, knee and ankle pathology – seek medical advice.

> ⊕ *Contraindications*
> - Advanced stages of pregnancy; osteoporosis (spinal flexion to be avoided); painful spine, lower back or hip pathology – for onward referral.

Exercise ST14 – Standing back stretch

Aim
To improve back muscle flexibility.

Equipment
Mat or firm bed, sturdy chair, half barrel or small box, a yoga belt if performing the stretch with a partner.

Target muscles
Back.

Body position
Standing facing the wall (or chair), place the hands on the wall or rest them on a bed with a half barrel or small box placed for support at a suitable height. Step back so that the hips flex approximately 60–90 degrees with the legs in an upright standing position, the spine in neutral and the arms reaching overhead to rest on the wall/box or to hold a sturdy chair.

Action 1
Breathing in – to prepare.

Breathing out – tighten the lower abdominal muscles, lengthening and stabilizing the lumbar spine to reach the crown of the head and ischial tuberosities in opposite directions.

Breathing normally – hold for 20–30 seconds, using the breath to assist back muscle release and spine elongation.

Repeat two to three times.

Bend the knees a little and walk towards the wall to come out of the position.

Action 2
Partner stretching. Place the yoga belt around the pelvis at approximately the level of the ASIS. A partner stands behind holding the belt.

During *breathing out* the partner gently applies traction to assist spine elongation.

Repeat two to three times.

Bend the knees a little and walk towards the wall to come out of the position.

> ⊘ **Precautions**
> - Shoulder, lower back/hip pathology – seek medical advice.

> ⊕ *Contraindications*
> - Painful shoulder, back or hip pathology – for onward referral.

Exercise ST15 – Spine roll down and up (free standing or with back against a wall)

Aim/Target muscles
To improve spine and back and posterior hip muscle flexibility.

Body position
Standing with the feet hip distance apart and the knees slightly flexed. The normal spinal curves are intact with the eyes looking directly ahead. The arms hang beside the body with the thumbs facing forwards (Fig. 6.40A).

Action
Breathing in – tighten the lower abdominal muscles and lower the chin towards the chest (Fig. 6.40B).

Breathing out – continue sequential cervical, thoracic and lumbar spine flexion, curling it to the floor to its end range of spine/hip flexion (Fig. 6.40C).

Note: The spine articulates vertebra by vertebra from the cervical spine to the lumbar spine and the body curls as if up and over a large ball. The gaze moves with the head. The knees remain slightly flexed during the motion.

Breathing in – fill the back and sides of the ribcage with air.

Breathing out – increase abdominal muscle engagement and allow the back muscles to release so that the weight of the head and trunk produces traction for the spine, lower back and posterior hip muscles.

6

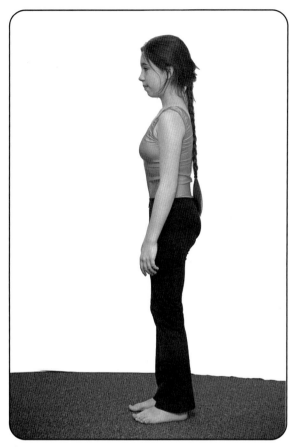

Figure 6.40A

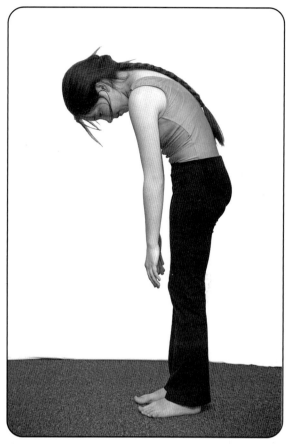

Figure 6.40B

Note: The head hangs from the top of the spine and the arms hang from the shoulders.

Breathing in – fill the back and sides of the ribcage with air.

Breathing out – increase abdominal muscle engagement and allow the posterior pelvis to slide down a little to initiate the motion (if using a wall, the posterior pelvis slides down the wall). Then continue return from flexion with simultaneous spine and hip extension to re-establish the starting position.

Note: The spine articulates vertebra by vertebra from the lumbar spine upwards to the cervical spine, the gaze moves with the head and the knees remain slightly flexed during the motion.

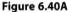

Precautions
- Spine, lower back, hip and knee pathology – seek medical advice.

Contraindications
- Advanced stages of pregnancy; osteoporosis; painful shoulder, spine or hip pathology – for onward referral.

6

Exercise ST16 – Spine curl

Aim
To improve spine and upper back muscle flexibility.

Equipment
Chair.

Target muscles
Spinal, gluteal and hamstrings.

Body position
Sitting with normal cervical curve intact and the eyes looking directly ahead. The hips are flexed approximately 90 degrees and the backs of the

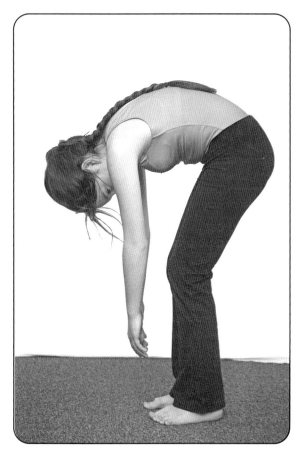

Figure 6.40C

thighs are fully supported by the chair. The arms rest beside the body.

Action

To prepare – maintaining the upright position, gently activate the pectoral girdle stabilizing muscles and cross the arms to wrap around the body.

Breathing in – tighten the lower abdominal muscles, lengthen through the crown of the head and allow the chin to drop towards the sternum.

Breathing out – lengthen the spine more to flex and curl it as if up and over a ball.

Note: The spine articulates vertebra by vertebra from the cervical spine to the thoracic spine. The lumbar spine is not involved and remains stable. The gaze moves with the head.

Breathing in – fill the back and sides of the ribcage with air.

Breathing out – hug the body, curling the spine more as the elbows draw in towards the waist and the shoulder blades slide further down the back.

Breathing normally – hold for 5–10 seconds, allowing the spine and upper back muscles to release.

Breathing in – maintaining good abdominal muscle control, return from flexion, lengthening the spine as it articulates back to its starting position.

Breathing out – repeat forward flexion etc. Perform three times.

> **⊘ Precautions**
> ■ Spine, lower back, hip and knee pathology – seek medical advice.

> **✚ Contraindications**
> ■ Advanced stages of pregnancy; osteoporosis; painful shoulder, spine or hip pathology – for onward referral.

Exercise ST17 – Hip rolls with stretch

Aim

To improve chest, side torso, lower back, spine and posterior hip muscle flexibility.

Equipment

Mat, firm bed, half barrel, small box.

Target muscles

Torso and anterior hip.

Body position

Supine with the pelvis in neutral and the legs a little wider than the hips with the knees/hips flexed approximately 90 degrees. The arms are laterally rotated and bent with the fingers of the hands interlacing behind and supporting the head, or the arms laterally rotate and bend to frame the head so that the hands can hold the uprights of a trapeze bed or other support (Fig. 6.41A).

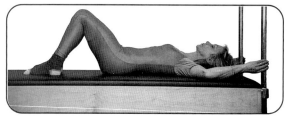

Figure 6.41A

Note: The feet may be slightly raised on a half barrel or small box to assist abdominal muscle control over the lumbar spine and pelvis during the motion.

Action

Breathing in – to prepare.

Breathing out – tighten the pelvic floor and lower abdominal muscles, allow the upper back to relax to the bed and roll the pelvis from below the waist to the right (Fig. 6.41B).

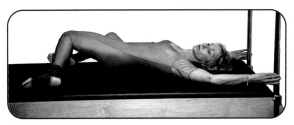

Figure 6.41B

Breathing normally – remain in the position briefly to accommodate the stretch across the front of the hips and chest.

Note: Aim to keep the normal lumbar curve intact and avoid lumbar extension.

Lift the right foot and rest it on the left thigh above the knee (Fig. 6.41C).

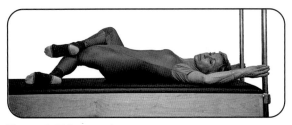

Figure 6.41C

Breathing in.

Breathing out – ensure good lower abdominal muscle control and allow the weight of the right leg to draw the left side of the pelvis more towards the right, increasing the stretch down the left side of the body.

Note: The right knee reaches away from the body rather than down to the floor. Allow the head to turn gently away from the motion and drop the lower back ribs towards the bed as the pelvis moves to the right.

Breathing normally – with the chest facing the ceiling and the back ribs in contact with the bed, lengthen the front and back of the torso and slide the left back hip towards the heels. Maintaining a stable pelvis, allow the back muscles to relax, reach the left knee away from the left hip and lengthen through the left groin. Relax into the stretch for up to 30 seconds.

Note: A stretch may be felt along the left side or back of the torso, in the lumbar spine and/or in the front thigh, hip and chest. The stretch should feel beneficial as opposed to causing muscle cramping or pain. If the stretch is not comfortable, consider reducing the range of motion or assisting core control by raising the feet or allowing the right knee to rest on a support.

Breathing in.

Breathing out – increase abdominal muscle control over the lumbar spine and return the pelvis and legs to the starting position.

Repeat to the left.

Repeat three times to each side.

! Precautions

- Shoulder, spine, lower back and hip/knee pathology – this stretch can relieve sciatic pain, symptoms associated with sacroiliac strain and other lower back problems; seek medical advice as to when it may be helpful.

✚ Contraindications

- Painful lower back problems, hip or knee pathology – for onward referral.

Exercise ST18.1 – Front of chest stretch (using wall or trapeze bed)

Aim
To improve pectoral muscle flexibility.

Equipment
Wall or trapeze bed.

Target muscles
Anterior crest and torso.

Body position
Standing near a wall so one arm can be extended in lateral rotation with the palm on the wall. The hand is approximately in line with the centre of the glenohumeral joint and the body is turned a little away from the arm (Fig. 6.42A).

Action
Breathing in – to prepare.

Breathing out – tighten the lower abdominal muscles and slide the hand a little way down the wall, pressing with the little finger to engage the pectoral girdle stabilizing muscles.

6

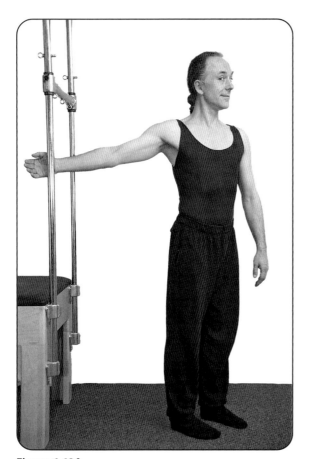

Figure 6.42A

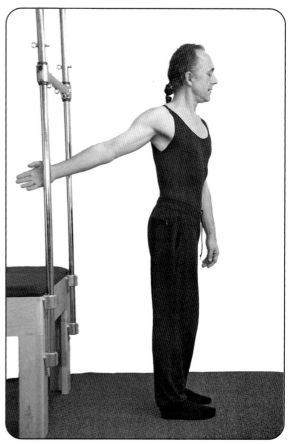

Figure 6.42B

Breathing normally – remaining in this position, press the hand into the wall to begin gently stretching the front of the glenohumeral joint.

Note: Press with about 60% of possible effort for 15 seconds.

Breathing in – maintaining spine and shoulder stability, cease the pressing action.

Breathing out – maintaining spine and shoulder stability, turn the feet and body more away from the hand to increase the front chest stretch (Fig. 6.42B).

Breathing normally – relaxing the fingers, front chest, throat and face muscles, hold the stretch for 15 seconds. Repeat to the other side.

Repeat three times to each side.

> **⊘ Precautions**
> ■ Pregnancy; wrist, shoulder and neck problems – seek medical advice.

> **✚ Contraindications**
> ■ Painful wrist, shoulder or neck pathology – seek medical advice before stretching.

Exercise ST18.2 – Front of chest stretch (with a towel or stick)

Aim
To improve pectoral muscle flexibility and shoulder mobility.

Equipment
Towel or stick.

Target muscles
Pectoral girdle.

Body position
Standing upright with the towel or stick between the hands held above the head. The arms are wider than the shoulders but only as far apart as is comfortable (Fig. 6.43A).

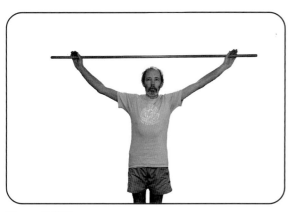

Figure 6.43A

Action

Breathing in – to prepare.

Breathing out – tighten the lower abdominal muscles and bring the stick forwards to approximately mid-chest level. Reach the hands along the stick whilst sliding the shoulder blades down the back. Aim to broaden across the front of the chest and gently stretch the front chest and shoulder muscles (Fig. 6.43B).

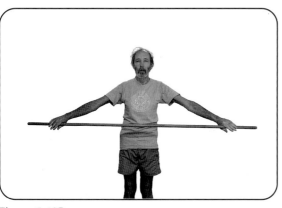

Figure 6.43B

Breathing in – return the arms to their starting position.

Breathing out – tighten the lower abdominal muscles and bring the stick overhead behind the body, adjusting the hands along the stick for wrist and shoulder comfort during the motion. Only go as far as necessary to feel gentle stretching in the glenohumeral joints before returning the arms to their starting position (Fig. 6.43C).

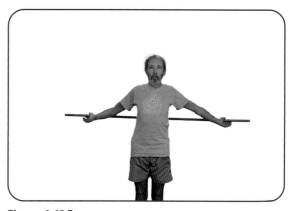

Figure 6.43C

Repeat the forwards and backwards motions smoothly, incorporating the breath to assist spine stability and muscle relaxation, and gradually increase the range of glenohumeral joint motion.

Note: Throughout the exercise keep the front of the chest open with correct shoulder alignment to allow optimum glenohumeral joint mobilization.

Precautions
- Pregnancy; wrist, shoulder and neck problems – seek medical advice.

Contraindications
- Painful wrist, shoulder or neck pathology – for onward referral.

6

Chapter 7

The teaching process

Teaching Pilates is a bit like teaching somebody to play the violin. You can observe Nigel Kennedy in concert but this will not teach the skills required to play the violin. You could also come up with a list of the characteristics of a good violin player, such as in time, in tune, right notes, expresses emotion and so on, but this will not enable anybody to play the violin. A more technical list about how to hold the violin, how to hold the bow, how to tune the violin, which fingers to use for which notes and so on might be more useful. But watching a master at work, and giving information about what a good violin player does are not enough to teach somebody how to play the violin. The problem is the same in teaching Pilates.

If imparting information and watching a master are not enough, how can Pilates be taught? Many teachers of Pilates may know what to do instinctively, but looking at it in a more theoretical way may be helpful for those who are just beginning or for more experienced teachers to reflect on what they do.

I shall start with a basic model of skills training:

- Describe how to do the exercise/demonstrate how to do the exercise
- Watch the learner do the exercise
- Give the learner feedback/instruction
- Ask the learner to do it again.

This is a well-accepted model of skills teaching for adults. Skills are taught by breaking them down into their components and by the learner practising and working on each component incrementally. Of course you do not have to go through just one cycle. After the learner has done the exercise again you may want to provide further feedback/instruction. And you may want to start in the middle, by watching the learner. Overall, the goal of this model of practice and feedback is that the learner gets a bit better every time.

This teaching cycle can be further analysed under the following headings.

- While the learner is doing the exercise:
  - Assess the standard
  - Identify the problems
  - Select one (or a limited number) of elements to comment on
- Instruction:
  - Explain the element you are going to comment on
  - Describe how to do it better, and/or
  - Demonstrate how to do it better, and/or
  - Guide the learner to do it better using tactile cues
  - Ask the learner to do it again.

The rest of this section will break down and elaborate on these ideas.

WHILE THE LEARNER IS DOING THE EXERCISE

In a mat class or a studio class you will have only a short time to watch the learner's performance. During that time you will have to analyse the way the learner is doing exercises and decide what should be worked on. The quality of your teaching will depend on how well you assess what is happening and prepare to comment on it.

ASSESS THE STANDARD

Your teaching must be appropriate to the standard of the learner. Each learner will have a unique mix of understanding, experience, skill and ability. Some learners may, for instance, have a very good theoretical understanding of Pilates but not be able to reflect this in their own bodies. Others may have a lot of experience but have been taught in a very different way elsewhere. You need to make a judgement about the learner's standard so that your teaching can be directed to this.

Identify the problems

Identify where and why the learner is having difficulties and how the learner might improve. You will need to go beyond thinking about *what* the learner is doing wrong and start to think about *why* the learner is doing it wrong. In this way you should be able to identify specific problems which can be worked on and which cause the difficulties.

For example, the learner may be having difficulty with mobilizing specific vertebral joints during spine flexion and extension. You will need to go beyond this to thinking about the underlying causes. These might, for example, be postural faults and/or faulty abdominal muscle length, strength and recruitment. Thus, by recognizing and then addressing the underlying problems, spinal mobility may be improved.

SELECT ONE ELEMENT (OR A LIMITED NUMBER OF ELEMENTS) TO COMMENT ON

There is no point in telling the learner everything at once. If too much information is given, learners will be unable to take it in. In addition, there is a danger of making the learner feel inadequate. How should you go about choosing what to comment on?

Fundamental

Try to choose something which is fundamental and may underlie other problems. Choosing a small detail which is really only a manifestation of more fundamental problems will be of much less help to the learner.

Suppose, for instance, that the learner is having problems with neck tension and strain during exercises performed in the supine position. Then the fundamental issue that might need addressing is that of poor resting head, neck and upper spine alignment. The answer may be found in taking time to prepare for exercises and in doing so paying attention to details such as correcting the head/neck position with appropriate supports, checking body alignment, etc. Attention to these fundamental issues may help to avoid many different problems during exercising.

Recurrent

Think also about whether the topic you have chosen is a recurrent problem for this learner. Obviously you will be better able to do this if you have worked with the learner on a number of occasions. Clearly working on recurrent problems which may manifest themselves in different ways in different exercises will be much more beneficial for the learner.

What would help the learner improve most

A further guide in deciding what to comment on is to think about what is holding the learner back most. What single element would help the learner to improve most? If you are uncertain of the answer to the question you may find it helpful to think back to the underlying Pilates exercise principles. They will very often provide an answer.

Appropriate to a learner of that level

Make sure that you are dealing with something that a learner of that standard should be able to understand and apply. For a learner at a basic level it might be appropriate to concentrate on issues such as enhanced body awareness, good body alignment, correct breathing patterns, pelvic floor and abdominal muscle control, etc. so as to improve core stability, spine mobility and overall musculoskeletal function. For an experienced learner with good body awareness and movement integration skills you might want to concentrate on challenging mental focus, breathing patterns and dynamic control of posture, alignment, spine mobility and stability.

7

Can be dealt with in the time

Choose something that can be dealt with in the available time. Some points take longer to explain and demonstrate than others.

Variety

If the learner is someone you work with regularly you will also need to provide some variety and challenge in your instruction, ensuring that you cover a range of topics over a period of time. If you comment on the same issue over a number of sessions, try to add something new or to do so in a different way. One way to provide variety is through the imaginative use of equipment – for example, pelvic tilts and femur arcs might be performed lying on a roller, and the double leg stretch or the hundreds might be performed lying on a slope.

Something others can learn from

If you are providing instruction in a class setting where other learners may be listening, you might also take into account that the other learners will be watching and learning from your instruction of any individual. Sometimes a learner will need instruction in relation to a particular problem that is unique to them such as a medical condition. However, you should be aware that if you choose an element to comment on that is also relevant to other learners, you will be providing instruction that has a more general benefit.

Make sure that you are clear about how the learner did the exercise, not just how it should be done, so that you can explain this to the learner later.

Selection of an appropriate element to work on is one of the most important steps in the teaching process. Indeed, a teacher's ability to perform the 'observing and analysing' stage of the teaching cycle is of vital importance to the quality of their teaching and is one of the factors distinguishing really exceptional teachers.

7 INSTRUCTION

EXPLAIN THE ELEMENT YOU ARE GOING TO COMMENT ON AND WHAT THE LEARNER DID

So that your instruction can be specific and precise, it may be useful to start by explaining what you are going to comment on and maybe also what the learner did.

DESCRIBE HOW TO DO IT BETTER AND/OR SHOW HOW TO DO IT BETTER AND/OR GUIDE THE LEARNER TO DO IT BETTER USING TACTILE CUES

Different people have different ways of learning. Some people learn and remember best through what they see, some through what they hear, and so on. Often you can tell how people learn and remember by listening to what they say. If somebody talks a lot about how things looked, then that person will probably learn and remember best through visual images. Others may learn and remember best from how their body feels and will respond better to being told how their body should feel or being guided into a better position. You should take this into account in deciding the best way(s) to help the learner. Over time you will need to develop an effective and imaginative range of ways to describe, demonstrate and guide learners to perform exercises better and learn to be sensitive to which ways are working and which are not. Also remember to work with what the learner did, not how you would do it. As the purpose is to assist learners at their level, start from what they are doing and how it can be improved.

Describe how to do it better

'Talking through'

Describing how exercises should look and feel and how component parts relate to create flowing movements is challenging. You will need a precise knowledge of how exercises are structured to be able to find the language to guide the learner accurately through movement sequences. 'Talking through' the sequential order of exercises several times may help new learners to understand inherent patterns within the exercise.

Verbal cues

It may also be helpful to give verbal cues as a learner is performing an exercise. These can be given just before the movement and then, once it occurs, further anticipatory cues can be used to guide a learner through a series of movements. Paraphrases and words that highlight specific technical points can be added pertinently as 'aides-mémoire' as expertise progresses.

Visual imagery

Visual imagery is vital to your descriptions. The use of visual imagery is a powerful tool for teaching physical skills and may be enormously useful to improve performance and quality of movement. Descriptive words that evoke ideas of space, length, light, support or smooth movement are powerful in their ability to stimulate the brain to influence correct musculoskeletal function (see Verbal cues) and can also enhance perception and knowledge.

However, even tried and tested visual imagery cues may not work for everyone. Ideally you should develop a range of different ways of describing how to overcome and improve basic problems since what may help one learner may mean nothing to another. Then, if your initial approach fails, you have something to fall back on. Or you can use different descriptions on different occasions for the same learner. You need to experiment with images with other teachers and with learners. Experimentation and time and practice will help you develop this area of your teaching until it becomes really imaginative and effective.

Discussion

When teaching an individual, particularly a person recovering from illness or injury, discussion and verbal feedback throughout the lesson may be essential for safe, effective teaching. When teaching a group, however, lengthy discussion will be untimely. If important issues arise it may be helpful to suggest that they are discussed after the class.

Demonstrate how to do it better

Demonstrate at the learner's level. Your demonstration should be aimed at showing the learner how they can improve, not at showing how well you can do the exercise, or what the next stage in the exercise is. If the learner is not at the same level, demonstrating at your level may not be of much help and may make them feel irritated with your showing off. However, for many learners, demonstration will be an important part of the learning process so you must be ready to demonstrate. You may find it useful to demonstrate at the same time as, or before, explaining an exercise.

Guide the learner to do it better using tactile cues

Sometimes a 'hands on' approach may be the best one. It provides information for the teacher and assists the learner to experience correct musculoskeletal function. For example, the teacher's touch can encourage spine lengthening, stabilization and mobilization, and correct muscle action and anatomical placement.

You will need to use your hands to give clear direction and to apply confidently just sufficient pressure to direct a message. Individuals will respond differently as some people are more sensitive to tactile stimuli and you should take this into account. The following should assist more effective 'hands on' teaching.

- Before you do anything, discuss 'hands on' teaching with the learner and understand their comfort zone boundaries.
- Know what is to be achieved through physical contact and select appropriate cues.
- Consider the anatomical orientation of the learner and how to use cues without invading their personal space.
- Ensure that correct anatomical landmarks are identified on initial contact through prior visualization of the underlying bony and muscular structures.
- Alert the learner and place your hands gently but firmly (be aware that some people may react adversely despite prior agreement).
- Direct the cues correctly – for example, to facilitate or improve latissimus dorsi activity the hands would travel in the direction of its muscular contraction; to improve spinal elongation in sitting the hands would trace upwards from the base of the vertebral column.
- Use the hands confidently but gently and always be aware that individuals will respond differently – some people may be ticklish, have low pain thresholds, etc.
- Once the cue has been given, remove the hands carefully but surely.
- Evaluate the effect of cueing before reapplying.

Throughout this text are suggestions for tactile cues that are advocated by leaders in the field.

Timing of the cues is also important. For instance, in latissimus dorsi activity in shoulder adduction and extension the hands are placed as the muscle action is about to occur and then used to guide as the movement occurs. Allow the learner to find a comfortable rhythm and pace.

FURTHER WAYS TO IMPROVE YOUR TEACHING

7

CONSIDER THE LEARNER'S FEELINGS

Confidence

Learners' views of themselves, their confidence about exercise and their bodies will vary enormously. Take this into account. Some learners will feel embarrassed about their bodies and awkward about being in the studio.

Painful learning memories involving exercise or sport, particularly during childhood and adolescence, may result in poor self-image and an overall lack of confidence when exercising.

As a teacher you may have to recognize and tackle these issues and this can be challenging. The teacher's approach can be crucial in facilitating change and persuading learners that exercise can be enjoyable and enriching. A non-judgemental, encouraging and positive approach that subtly hands responsibility for learning to the learner will assist self-assurance and self-esteem.

Learners who do not like being touched

This is clearly a difficult issue and one which may be a real barrier to learning. Obviously you should adjust your teaching to favour demonstrations together with verbal and visual imagery cueing. You may be able to discuss and agree an acceptable level of physical contact with your learner. If learning does not progress by trying these other approaches and the learner still insists that being touched is unacceptable, you should consider onward referral, perhaps to a health professional. Or it may be that the learner has a particular issue with you so the right person may be another Pilates teacher.

Sufficient personal space

You should ensure that all learners have sufficient personal space to feel comfortable. Learners may not tell you if they are uncomfortable but you should be able to see from their body language. If learners are crowding each other this may mean moving them to different positions in the class. Or you may need to ensure that throughout the lesson you favour verbal and visual cues over tactile ones and do not 'stand over' or 'crowd' the learner. Additionally, whenever using tactile cues, make sure that there is a distance between your body and the learner's body.

The relationship with the teacher

How close a relationship should you have with learners? You must assess and control this, which means measuring out personal boundaries that feel comfortable while reflecting each learner's needs. Learners requiring support and mentoring may respond to a more personalized approach while others may dislike or even resent it. The initial assessment and early sessions should indicate the best approach to take but it is important to be observant and intuitive and be prepared to change as required.

AVOID AND OVERCOME BARRIERS TO COMMUNICATION

Language

Keep language direct, clear and simple. Avoid jargon and ambiguity. Be aware of the speed with which you speak. Be aware also of the quality, tone, volume and cadence of your voice. For instance, appropriate use of phrasing and pace can assist communication whereas a dull, atonal voice can make learners 'switch off'. Use silence and pauses to help learners reflect on and absorb what you have said.

Cultural differences

Misunderstandings may occur particularly when teaching learners from other cultures or learners whose first language differs from your own. Where there are language differences you may want to rely less on describing how exercises are done and more on other methods of instruction. It will also help with effective communication and avoid misunderstandings if you have an awareness of your learners' cultural backgrounds and value systems.

Hearing impairments

Be aware also that some of your learners may have hearing impairments. Hearing impairments are common, particularly as people age. Again you will need to be sensitive to the situation and take steps to ensure that effective learning is not prevented. All that may be required may be to move the position of the learner in the class, or you may need to rely more on non-verbal methods of instruction.

Other distractions

Distractions may take the form of external noise such as traffic or noise from the streets outside, particularly when windows are open in warm weather. If problems are ongoing and really serious, it may be necessary to find another venue. Other distractions may be learners arriving late, talking within the class, squeaky floorboards as the teacher moves around the room, noisy heating systems, etc. Loud or poor quality music production or the use of music can be distracting. Do what you can to minimize distractions.

BE POSITIVE BUT DON'T OVERDO IT

This means concentrating not on what went wrong but on how it can be improved. Where learners have made progress be sure to say so. However, don't overdo it and say everything is excellent when it isn't, otherwise you may sound disingenuous and learners will not be able to distinguish real praise from general platitudes.

MODEL WHAT YOU ARE TEACHING

Remember that you are the model. Everything you do will be watched by the learners. Much of their learning will come from watching you when both you and they may be unaware of it. Therefore, everything you do must be consistent with what you are teaching. This means not only when you are demonstrating but also for instance when you are standing or walking round the studio.

7

Chapter **8**

Health and safety

SAFE, EFFECTIVE PRACTICE

This encompasses a wide range of issues including the safety of the working environment, the teacher's fitness for work, the appropriate application of exercise, protocols for ongoing referrals and the legal implications of good and ethical practice.

Official guidance is available from a variety of sources, with which all teachers and trainers should be familiar.

The Health and Safety Executive provides a Code of Practice as required by the Health and Safety Commission, under the auspices of the Secretary of State for Health.

Although failure to comply with any of the provision of this Code is not in itself an offence, such failure to comply may be taken by a court in criminal proceedings as proof that a person has contravened a regulation or sections of the 1974 Act to which a provision relates. In such a case, however, it will be open to that person to satisfy the court that the regulation has been complied with in some other way.

For up-to-date information on approved codes of practice it is advisable to refer to the most recent publication of Workplace Health, Safety and Welfare Regulations. There is an array of such publications issued by the Health and Safety Commission (HSC) and published and sold by The Stationery Office (TSO).

Important issues Pilates teachers must consider are highlighted below.

THE WORKING SPACE

This could range from a space in your own home, a village hall or a health club to a customized Pilates studio. Although it is not always possible to have total control over the physical parameters of a space, the following are guidelines to provide a safe working area.

Ideally this space should:

- be well lit with as much natural light as practicable and have emergency lighting facilities
- be well ventilated and a comfortable temperature for the wearing of light exercise clothing
- provide appropriate, maintained and accessible fire prevention equipment and emergency exits
- provide sufficient floor area and unoccupied space for the teacher to move around safely without obstruction
- provide a flat floor surface that is clean but not slippery
- have adequate changing space and washroom facilities etc.
- provide safe electrical arrangements for the use of sound systems and other electrical appliances

- provide adequate security and have well-lit public entrance and exit routes
- have a no smoking policy.

Other important considerations include:

- valid certification of teaching staff, including first aid certification with an organization such as the British Red Cross or St John's Ambulance services
- professional insurance
- public liability insurance
- building and contents insurance
- personal injury prevention
- prevention of injury to others within the environment, including members of staff, students and clients.

8

Appendix 1

SAMPLE CLIENT RECORD FORM			
Name		Date of birth	
Address			
Home Tel No:		Work Tel No:	
Medical referral	Y/N	Referral letter	Y/N
Occupation			
Contact in case of injury			
Basic Medical History			
Do you have or have you suffered from:			
High blood pressure	Epilepsy	Diabetes	Asthma
Heart problems	Arthritis	Stomach problems	
Do you/have you suffered from:			
Neck problems	Back problems	Joint problems	
Past injuries/surgery:			
Any medication:			
General Health			
Height (m)	Weight (kg)		
Do you smoke	Y/N	Alcohol units per week	
Current exercise sessions and number of times per week			
Marketing			
Where did you hear about us?			
I accept that I exercise at my own risk			
Signed:		**Date:**	

Appendix 2

SAMPLE POSTURAL ASSESSMENT FORM

Name		Date of 1st exam	
Occupation		Date of 2nd exam	
Handedness	Age	Sex	

Plumb Alignment

Side view	Left		Right	
Back view	Deviated left		Deviated right	

Static Observations

Feet	Pronation	Supination	Pigeon toed		Toeing out	
Ankles	Shortened Achilles	Thickened Achilles	Medial malleoli level			
Calves	Overdeveloped	Underdeveloped				
Knees	Hyperextended	Bow legged	Rolling in		Popliteal crease level	
Buttock	Overdeveloped	Underdeveloped	Gluteal crease level			
Pelvis	Lateral leg rotation	Medial leg rotation	Tilt		Twist operation	
Low back	Lordosis	Flat	Kyphosis		Operation	
Up. back	Kyphosis	Flat	Scapula adduct/abduct		Scapula elevated	
Spine align.	Head – C.spine	C.spine – T.spine	Thorax – pelvis		Pelvis – legs	
Muscle dev.	Trapezius	Rhomboid	Latissimus dorsi		Erector spinae	
Thorax	Depressed chest	Elevated chest	Rotation		Level	
Shoulder	Low	High	Forward		Med.rotated	
Arms	Pronated	Supinated	High L/R		Low L/R	
Neck	Hyperextended	Shortened	Muscle under developed		Muscle over developed	
Head	Forward	Retracted	Tilt		Rotation	

Tests for Flexibility and Muscle Length

Forward bending	Range		Obs	
Arms overhead	Left		Right	
Hip flexors	Left		Right	
Tensor fasciae latae	Left		Right	
Hamstrings	Left		Right	
Trunk lateral flexion	To left		To right	
Where do you feel your weight is?	Balls of feet		Heels	

Postural Observations

Notes

Recommended programme

Suggested shorthand for postural assessment form:
X = postural defect present; L = left; R = right; B = both; E = even;
Ant = anterior; Post = posterior; + = overdeveloped; – = underdeveloped

Appendix 3

SUGGESTED FURTHER READING ON ANATOMY

Anatomy is a thrilling subject; the way in which a human body is put together has been the subject of scholars from the ancient Greeks through to Leonardo Da Vinci. There are now many different ways of representing this knowledge, examples include: anatomical charts and posters, textbooks and study guides, dissections and autopsies.

Now in the 21st century there are many CDs, DVDs and other interactive media to help students who need to learn more on human anatomy. Before we go on to suggest these sources of information it is worth remembering what is perhaps the most valuable resource – your own body. When it when it comes to anatomy, never forget that you carry your own syllabus around with you, and the careful student can learn a great deal from studying their own bodies and those of their fellow students.

Finally, having taught anatomy for over a decade and being frequently asked about which the best book for anatomy is, my answer is this: if it is a book which you find easy to read and to learn from then it is the best book for you.

Stuart Porter, Salford 2008

Suggested useful sources of further information on human anatomy:

1. Palastanga, Field and Soames: Anatomy and human movement, 5E Elsevier 2006
   This book is an extremely well illustrated and detailed yet user-friendly guide for upper, lower limb and spinal anatomy. It is also useful for its detailed presentation of biomechanics and functional anatomy.

2. Porter: The anatomy colouring and workbook, 2E Elsevier 2008
   This beginner's level book is a more light-hearted guide to human anatomy which is designed to jog one's memory by the use of rhymes and other memory aids and gives the reader interactive study and colouring tasks to assist in their understanding of human anatomy.

3. Drake, Vogl & Mitchell: Gray's anatomy for students: with Student Consult Access, Elsevier 2004
   This book has a companion website which includes an Image Bank, Interactive Surface Anatomy tool, as well as a bank of hundreds of anatomy questions. The book presents the essentials of clinical anatomy in a way that furthers complete understanding and firmly relates the study of anatomy to clinical practice. This textbook is organized by body region, and each chapter, an overview that describes the function of structures within that region. Particularly useful for those learning Pilates, each chapter also contains a section on Surface Anatomy with outstanding photographs overlaid with anatomic diagrams

4. Thomas Myers: Anatomy Trains: Myofascial meridians for manual and movement therapists, 2E, Elsevier 2008
   Understanding the role of fascia in healthy movement and postural distortion is of vital importance to body workers and movement therapists. *Anatomy Trains: Myofascial Meridians for Manual and Movement Therapists* presents a unique 'whole systems' view of myofascial/locomotor anatomy in which the body wide connections among the muscles within the fascial net are described in detail for the first time. Using the metaphor of railway or train lines, Myers explains how patterns of strain communicate through the myofascial 'webbing', contributing to postural compensation and movement stability. Written in a style that makes it easy to understand and apply, *Anatomy Trains* provides an accessible and comprehensive explanation of the anatomy and function of the myofascial system in the body.

INDEX

Note: Page numbers in **bold** refer to figures.